Clinical Virology

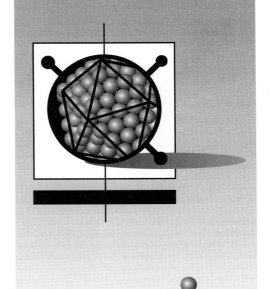

DIANE S. LELAND, Ph.D.
Department of Pathology and Laboratory Medicine
Indiana University School of Medicine
Indianapolis, Indiana

W.B. SAUNDERS COMPANY
A Division of Harcourt Brace & Company
Philadelphia London Toronto Montreal Sydney Tokyo

W.B. SAUNDERS COMPANY
A Division of Harcourt Brace & Company

The Curtis Center
Independence Square West
Philadelphia, Pennsylvania 19106

Library of Congress Cataloging-in-Publication Data

Leland, Diane Schultze
   Clinical virology / Diane S. Leland — 1st ed.

    p.   cm.

   ISBN 0–7216–4958–0

   1. Diagnostic virology.   I. Title.
   [DNLM: 1. Viruses—isolation & purification—laboratory manuals.
2. Virus Diseases—diagnosis—laboratory manuals.   QW 25 L537c 1996]

  QR387.L45 1996   616′.0194—dc20

  DNLM/DLC   95–30881

Clinical Virology   ISBN 0–7216–4958–0

Printed in the United States of America

Last digit is the print number: 9   8   7   6   5   4   3   2   1

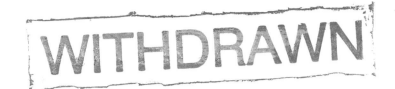
Clinical
Virology

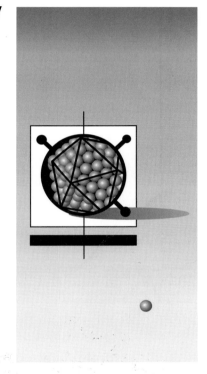

The purpose of this book is to provide the information needed by clinical laboratory scientists who wish to contribute effectively in the diagnosis of viral infections. Viral diagnostic techniques and procedures are presented, each one with an explanation of the scientific basis and concept involved. Only those methods that are useful in the clinical diagnostic virology laboratory are presented. Techniques that are highly specialized and primarily used in research are not included. Viruses and viral infections that can be diagnosed through routine virology laboratory techniques are emphasized. Viruses that are rare and viral infections that cannot be diagnosed through routine virology laboratory methods may not be included.

This book is intended for use by both students and practitioners of clinical laboratory virology. It does not provide complete information on basic virology, immunologic mechanisms, or viral disease pathogenesis.

A topic outline and educational objectives are provided at the beginning of each chapter. These define the scope of the material included and indicate the information emphasized. At the end of each chapter, review questions are provided. All answers are given at the end of the last chapter.

Test procedures, written in accordance with the National Committee for Clinical Laboratory Standards' (NCCLS) guidelines, are provided in the *Appendix* of this text. For some of the procedures, a commercial source of reagents is indicated. This mention of the commercial source is not intended to serve as an endorsement of the particular product but rather to ensure that each procedure is used only with the reagents intended. Other manufacturers may produce products that are equally suitable. Products may vary, however, and modifications in procedure may be necessary if reagents from other suppliers are substituted. In any procedure in which commercially prepared reagents are utilized, the directions of the particular manufacturer should be followed carefully.

DIANE S. LELAND, PHD

ACKNOWLEDGMENTS

To my family for their support and for their never-ending patience.

With special thanks to Theresa Mason for her technical advice, editing, and encouragement throughout the writing process; Elizabeth Cunningham for her technical advice; Dr. Nat U. Hill and Eric Powell for their help with photography; Nancy Coppaway for her help in preparing this manuscript; and the staff of the Virology and Serology Laboratories at the Indiana University School of Medicine who, through their day-to-day performance of laboratory assays, provided the ideas, information, and data that are the bases of this text.

CONTENTS

Viruses and the Clinical Diagnostic Laboratory

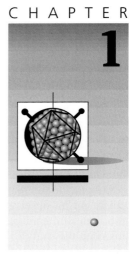

O B J E C T I V E S

At the completion of this unit of study, the student will be able to do the following:

1. Compare the sizes of viruses and other common microscopic entities and indicate which type of microscope should be used to observe each virus or entity.

2. Diagram and describe the arrangements and components of viral structure.

3. Provide family names and identify the type of nucleic acid found in common human viral pathogens, including herpes simplex virus, cytomegalovirus, the enteroviruses, hepatitis B virus, respiratory syncytial virus, and human immunodeficiency virus.

4. List and describe the steps in viral replication.

5. Identify routes of transmission and mechanisms of pathogenesis for various types of viruses.

6. Describe interferon, discuss the viral response to interferon, and explain why antimicrobial agents are not effective against viruses.

7. List and describe four approaches for viral disease diagnosis that are important in the clinical virology laboratory for definitively identifying viruses.

8. Give at least three reasons why a definitive diagnosis of viral disease is important.

INTRODUCTION

The science of microbiology was initiated centuries ago when Anton van Leeuwenhoek devised the first microscope and observed tiny "animalcules" swimming in water. Since that time, progress in the various areas of microbiology, including bacteriology, mycology, and mycobacteriology, has been constant and enormous. This progress was largely due to the discovery that microorganisms could be cultivated through growth on nonliving media such as broths and agar; in this way, various bacteria and fungi could be isolated and characterized. With the use of improved light microscopes, these organisms were carefully observed, and improved diagnostic tests were developed for use by physicians and in laboratories to aid in infectious disease diagnosis.

Progress in one of the areas of microbiology—virology—lagged behind that of the other areas. The word **virus,** meaning "poison," was used early on to denote invisible agents that produced disease. Although physicians worked with viruses and viral infections, as demonstrated by Jenner's development of smallpox vaccine in 1796 and Pasteur's rabies vaccine in 1885, the nature of viruses was unknown, and no specific viruses were identified. The nature of viruses was initially characterized by Ivanowski in Russia in 1892, when he showed that sap from tobacco plants with tobacco mosaic disease maintained its infectivity for other healthy plants after it was passed through a filter. The name **filterable** viruses was then applied. Filterable animal viruses were demonstrated in 1898 for foot-and-mouth disease of cattle and in 1900 for yellow fever in humans.

Despite the fact that the existence of viral agents was suspected or confirmed, the actual agents could not be observed with existing light microscopes. Because these agents also failed to proliferate on nonliving media, they could not be isolated in the laboratory. Both of these facts impeded the study of viruses and stymied the progress of scientists who attempted to provide laboratory protocols for use in diagnosing viral infection.

Viral biology and physiology advanced rapidly during the 1930s with the development of electron microscopes that allowed actual viral particles to be observed. Likewise, the discovery by Scherer in 1953 that viruses replicated in single layers of cells grown in test tubes allowed viral replication to be examined and provided for the isolation and identification of many viruses.

VIRAL SIZE, COMPOSITION, AND CLASSIFICATION

Size of Viruses

Because viruses are very small (i.e., filterable, indicating that they can pass through a filter with pore sizes of 0.45 to 0.22 μm or smaller), they cannot be seen with a light microscope. Some of the smaller viruses, the picornaviruses, are 25 to 30 nm in diameter, and the largest viruses, the poxviruses, measure 250×400 nm. How do viruses compare with other microbes in terms of size? In Figure 1–1, viruses and other microscopic entities are compared in regard to size, and the ranges of resolution of the light and electron microscopes are indicated. The largest viruses are just slightly smaller than the smallest bacteria. These viruses are just below the resolution limit of the light microscope, whereas the smallest viruses are much smaller than bacteria and are slightly larger than certain macromolecules. The viruses, in general, can be observed only with the electron microscope.

Viral Composition and Arrangement

Through the use of the electron microscope and various molecular biology techniques, viral composition and arrangement have been characterized. Viruses are the least complex type of organism that scientists have studied, consisting of a **nucleic acid core** surrounded by a coat of protein called a **capsid**. The nucleic acid core may be either **RNA** or **DNA** but **never both**. The nucleic acid may be single stranded or double stranded, and most viral nucleic acid is linear, although papovavirus has circular nucleic acid. The nucleic acid constitutes the viral genome that encodes all viral structural proteins and enzymes. Viral nucleic acid has been described as "the software program for making a copy of the virus" [1].

The **capsid,** which is made of protein, is rigid and determines the shape of the virus. It functions in protecting the nucleic acid. The capsid is composed of repeating protein subunits called **capsomeres.** There are two general capsid configurations: **icosahedral (20 sided),** also described as "cubic" (Fig. 1–2), and **helical (rod shaped)** (Fig. 1–3). Icosahedral capsids resemble crystals, with each capsid showing 20 facets, each of which is an equilateral triangle. Helical capsids are

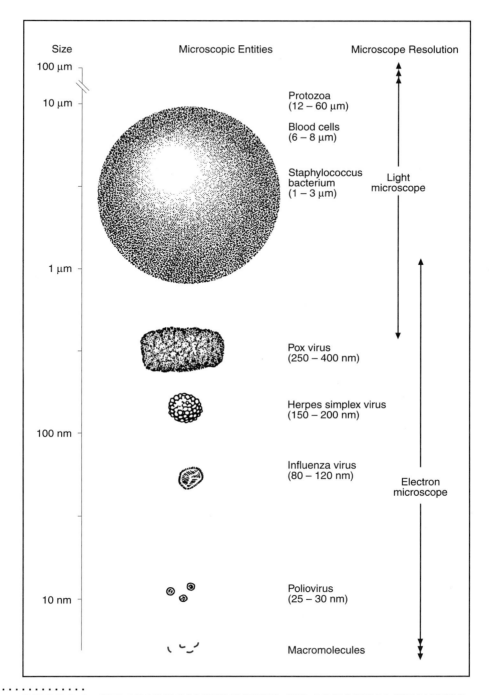

FIGURE 1–1 SIZE OF MICROSCOPIC ENTITIES AND MICROSCOPE RESOLUTION.
Viruses are smaller than the smallest bacteria and larger than macromolecules. They can be seen with the electron microscope. (Illustration demonstrates relative sizes and is not drawn to scale.)

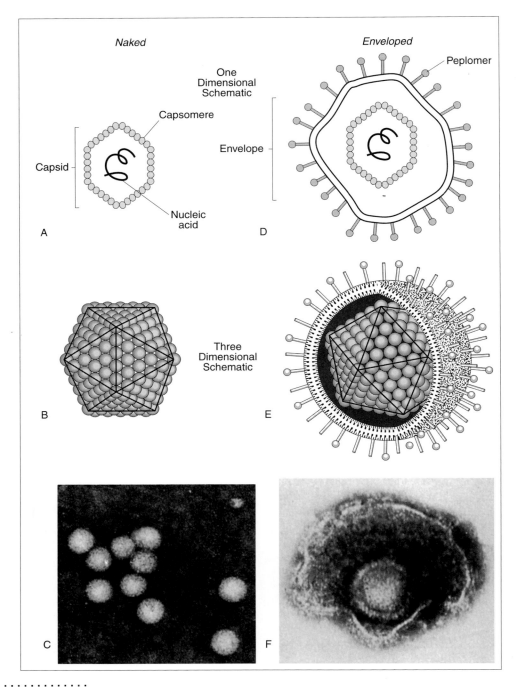

FIGURE 1–2 ICOSAHEDRAL CAPSID CONFIGURATION IN NAKED AND ENVELOPED VIRUSES. Naked icosahedral viruses appear cubic or crystalline (A, B, and C). Enveloped icosahedral viruses appear nearly spherical (D, E, and F). (Fig. 1–2C from Ryan KJ (ed), Sherris Medical Microbiology: An Introduction to Infectious Diseases, 3rd ed. Norwalk, CT: Appleton & Lange, 1994. Fig. 1–2F from Murray PR, Kobayashi GS, Pfaller MA, Rosenthal KS. Medical Microbiology, 2nd ed. St. Louis: Mosby-Year Book, 1994, p 573.)

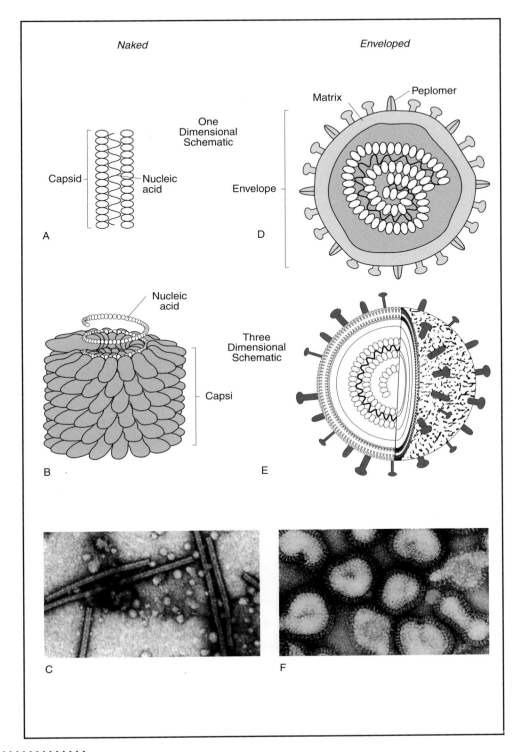

FIGURE 1–3   HELICAL CAPSID CONFIGURATION IN NAKED AND ENVELOPED VIRUSES.
Naked helical viruses are cylindrical or rod shaped (A, B, and C). Enveloped helical viruses appear nearly spherical because the nucleocapsid (capsid and nucleic acid) may curl inside the envelope (D, E, and F). (Fig. 1–3C from Tortora et al. Microbiology, 4th ed. Redwood City, CA: Benjamin Cummings 1992, p 336. Fig. 1–3F from Ryan KJ (ed), Sherris Medical Microbiology: An Introduction to Infectious Diseases, 3rd ed. Norwalk, CT: Appleton & Lange, 1994.

cylindrical. A few viruses have capsids that are neither icosahedral nor helical; these capsid configurations are termed **complex** and may appear spiral or brick shaped or may have other nonstandard appearances.

The capsid and the nucleic acid core together form the **nucleocapsid.** Some viral nucleocapsids are surrounded by a loose membranous **envelope.** Both icosahedral viruses and helical viruses may have envelopes (see Figs. 1–2 and 1–3). Enveloped viruses are nearly spherical but highly pleomorphic because the envelope is not rigid. Also, the rod-shaped nucleocapsid of helical virions may bend or coil inside the envelope. Viruses that do not have envelopes are called **naked** viruses.

The envelope is acquired by the virus during replication as the newly formed nucleocapsids bud through the host cell membrane. Envelopes are lipid bilayers that contain proteins, both glycoproteins and matrix proteins. The glycoproteins may span the membrane, protruding outside the envelope to appear as projections (spikes) called **peplomers** (see Figs. 1–2 and 1–3). They function in mediating attachment of the virus to host cell receptors. **Matrix proteins,** found only in certain viruses, are not glycosylated and form a layer on the inner surface of the envelope, apparently connecting the envelope and the capsid. Proteins in the envelope are specified by viral genes, whereas the lipids and carbohydrates are specified by the host cell genes [2]. Chemical agents and other adverse conditions that affect the envelope can inactivate the virus. These include drying, high temperatures, freezing and thawing, pH below 6 or above 8, lipid solvents, and chemicals containing chlorine, hydrogen peroxide, or phenol [3]. Enveloped viruses are maintained *in vivo* in aqueous environments and are often transmitted in body fluids. In contrast, naked viruses, which are more stable than enveloped viruses and can withstand drying, acid, and detergents, are often transmitted via the fecal-oral route.

The term **virion** is applied to describe the mature animal virus particle that is capable of infecting vertebrate cells and is free of its host [4]. For nonenveloped viruses, the nucleocapsid alone is correctly identified as the virion. For enveloped viruses, the nucleocapsid and the envelope make up the virion. Important terms to know concerning viral structure are listed in Table 1–1.

Viral Classification

Several systems for classification of viruses have been used in the past. Most of these have been based on viral disease symptoms or on the agent's mode of transmission. In 1966, the

. . . .
TABLE 1–1   TERMS TO KNOW CONCERNING VIRAL STRUCTURE

TERM	DEFINITION
Capsid	A rigid protective protein coat that surrounds the nucleic acid
Capsomere	Identical proteins that make up the capsid
Complex	Nonstandard viral capsid configuration that is neither helical nor icosahedral and may appear spiral or brick shaped or may have other nonstandard characteristics
Envelope	A nonrigid additional coat that surrounds the capsid in some of the more complex viruses; the envelope consists of protein and lipid
Helical	Capsid arrangement in the form of a long tube surrounding the nucleic acid
Icosahedral	Viral capsid arrangement that has the shape of a 20-sided polygon (icosahedral), each face being an equilateral triangle; also called "cubic"
Matrix proteins	Nonglycosylated proteins that form a layer on the inner surface of the viral envelope and connect the envelope and the capsid
Naked virus	A virus without an envelope
Nucleic acid	Either DNA or RNA; not both in the same virus
Nucleocapsid	Nucleic acid and capsid together
Peplomers	Glycoproteins that protrude outside the envelope and appear as projections or spikes; they function in attachment of the virus to host cell receptors
Virion	The mature animal virus particle that is capable of infecting other cells; for nonenveloped viruses, the nucleocapsid alone is the virion; for enveloped viruses, the nucleocapsid and the envelope make up the virion

International Committee on the Nomenclature of Viruses was formed. This committee devised the following criteria for use in classifying viruses:

1. Nucleic acid type, composition, and molecular weight
2. Virus morphology
3. Serological cross-reactivity of group antigens

The DNA-containing viruses important in human infection are listed in Table 1–2, and the RNA-containing viruses are listed in Table 1–3. The family names and the more common viruses included in each family are listed, along with the capsid configuration, the size, and the nucleic acid configuration. The names assigned to viral families often indicate the structure or disease association of the viruses in the family or may indicate where the viruses were discovered or by whom. Explanations of family naming as well as disease associations for the specific viruses are also given in Tables 1–2 and 1–3.

VIRAL REPLICATION

Viruses are simple particles that lack the constituents required for growth and multiplication. They have no ribosomes, enzyme systems required for synthesis of nucleic acid and proteins, or systems for generating adenosine triphosphate. Therefore, viruses are not capable of growth on artificial media or of reproducing by binary fission, budding, or other methods common to other microorganisms. Viruses are **obligate intracellular parasites** and can replicate only within living cells. Richard Preston characterized the virus-host relationship and viral replication in his book *The Hot Zone* [1].

> ome biologists classify viruses as "life forms," because they are not strictly known to be alive . . . . A virus is a parasite. It can't live on its own . . . . Viruses that are outside cells merely sit there; nothing happens. They are dead . . . . Once the virus enters the cell, it becomes a Trojan horse. It switches on and begins to replicate. [Viruses] can only make copies of [themselves] inside a cell using the cell's materials and machinery to get the job done. A virus makes copies of itself inside a cell until eventually the cell gets pigged with virus and pops, and the viruses spill out of the broken cell. Or viruses can bud through a cell wall, like drips coming out of a faucet—drip, drip, drip, drip, copy, copy, copy, copy. The faucet runs and runs until the cell is exhausted, consumed, and destroyed.

Viral replication consists of synthesis of the separate viral components. In subsequent steps, the newly synthesized components are assembled into new virions. The six steps in viral replication—attachment, penetration, eclipse (uncoating), replication, maturation (assembly), and release—are described next and illustrated in Figure 1–4.

Attachment
Attachment is mediated by specific binding of proteins on the viral capsid or envelope to complementary receptors on the cell surface. This is a specific receptor-mediated reaction that determines which viruses can infect which types of cells. For example, wart viruses can attach to skin cells, whereas rhinoviruses attach to respiratory mucosal cells. Some viruses may attach to many different types of cells. Attachment sometimes leads to irreversible changes in the structure of the virion [5].

Penetration
Penetration rapidly follows attachment and may occur by engulfment or endocytosis (called **viropexis**) in which the cell membrane folds in to surround the virion and then closes to create a cytoplasmic vacuole. For enveloped viruses, penetration may involve fusion of the viral envelope with the host cell membrane, which allows only the nucleocapsid to enter the cell [6]. Some small, nonenveloped viruses may pass directly through the cell membrane [4].

TABLE 1–2 DNA VIRUSES IMPORTANT IN HUMAN INFECTION

FAMILY NAME COMMON VIRUSES	NAMING INFORMATION AND DISEASE ASSOCIATION	SIZE (nm)	NUCLEIC ACID	CAPSID	ENV
Adenoviridae	Named for the tissue (adenoids) from which the virus was first isolated	70–90	DS	Icos	0
Adenovirus	Upper and lower respiratory tract infections, keratitis, cystitis, gastroenteritis				
Hepadnaviridae	"Hep" = liver (associated with liver disease), "dna" = DNA virus	40–42	DS	Complex*	+*
Hepatitis B	Agent of "serum" hepatitis				
Herpesviridae	From "herpes" (to creep), describing herpes fluid-filled vesicles, which coalesce ("creep") to form lesions such as cold sores	150–200	DS	Icos	+
Herpes simplex types 1 and 2	Recurrent oral and genital lesions, congenital infections				
Varicella-zoster	Chickenpox and shingles				
Cytomegalo-virus	Mononucleosis-like infection and congenital anomalies; virus causes cells ("cyto") to enlarge ("megalo")				
Epstein-Barr virus	Described by Epstein, Barr, and Achong; causes infectious mononucleosis				
Papovaviridae	"Pa" = papilloma, "po" = polyoma, "va" = vacuolating	45–55	DS	Icos	0
Polyomavirus	Polyoma is an agent of many tumors; tumor-producing viruses (in animals)				
Papillomavirus	Papilloma is a benign wart; these viruses produce warts				
Parvoviridae	"Parvus" = small; the smallest DNA viruses	18–26	SS	Icos	0
Human parvovirus B19	Implicated in fifth disease, fetal hydrops, and aplastic crisis				
Poxviridae (poxviruses)	Produce vesicular lesions called pocks	25 × 400	DS	Complex†	+
Variola (smallpox)	Severe, often fatal systemic illness with large pocks covering the body; smallpox now believed to be eradicated worldwide				

*Three structures: an enveloped double-shelled Dane particle, a nonenveloped spherical form, and a nonenveloped filamentous form.
†Nonstandard brick-shaped capsid.
DS = double stranded; Env = envelope; Icos = icosahedral capsid; SS = single stranded; + = envelope present, 0 = nonenveloped (naked).

....
TABLE 1–3 RNA VIRUSES IMPORTANT IN HUMAN INFECTION

FAMILY NAME COMMON VIRUSES	NAMING INFORMATION AND DISEASE ASSOCIATION	SIZE (nm)	NUCLEIC ACID	CAPSID	ENV
Arenaviridae	"Arena" = sand; named for the unique electron microscopic appearance of the virions; cause aseptic meningitis, hemorrhagic fever	50–300	SS	He	+
Bunyaviridae	Named for Bunyamera, Uganda, where the original virus was isolated	100	SS	He	+
California encephalitis virus*	Initially isolated in the San Joaquin Valley, CA; causes encephalitis				
Caliciviridae	Named for cuplike depressions (chalices or calices) in viral particles observed by electron microscopy	35–40	SS	Icos	0
Norwalk agent	Named for Norwalk, OH, where the virus was first observed by electron microscopy in stools of patients with acute gastroenteritis; causes epidemic gastroenteritis				
Coronaviridae	"Corona" = crown; viral capsid resembles a crown of thorns or solar corona; cause upper respiratory infection and colds	100	SS	He	+
Filoviridae	Long, filamentous viruses, often with hook shapes	80 × 800	SS	He†	+
Marburg and Ebola	Severe hemorrhagic fevers; found in Africa				
Orthomyxoviridae	"Ortho" = normal, correct; "myxo" = mucus	80–120	SS	He	+
Influenza A and B	"Influentia" = influence; reflects importance of epidemic and pandemic influenza				
Paramyxoviridae Measles	Structure resembles orthomyxoviruses Causes "measles," a 7- to 10-day systemic febrile illness usually with cough, conjunctivitis, and rash	150–300	SS	He	+
Mumps	Causes "mumps," a systemic febrile illness usually accompanied by swelling of the parotid glands				
Parainfluenza	Respiratory illness resembling influenza				
Respiratory syncytial virus	Produces syncytia in cell cultures; causes mild to severe respiratory disease, especially in children				
Picornaviridae	"Pico" = small; "rna" = RNA virus	25–30	SS	Icos	0
Poliovirus‡	Orignally poliomyelitis: "polios" = gray, "myelitis" = inflammation of the matter of anterior horn of spinal cord; virus attacks CNS to cause paralysis				

Table continued on following page

. . . .

TABLE 1–3 RNA VIRUSES IMPORTANT IN HUMAN INFECTION *Continued*

FAMILY NAME COMMON VIRUSES	NAMING INFORMATION AND DISEASE ASSOCIATION	SIZE (nm)	NUCLEIC ACID	CAPSID	ENV
Coxsackie virus A, B‡	Originally isolated in Coxsackie, NY; cause a variety of enteric and CNS symptoms				
Echovirus‡	"E" = enteric, "c" = cytopathogenic, "h" = human, "o" = orphan; viruses grow from human feces to cause cytopathogenic effect in cell cultures; relationship to human disease not clear (i.e., orphan)—some infections similar to coxsackievirus, others totally asymptomatic				
Hepatitis A‡	Agent of "infectious" hepatitis				
Rhinovirus	"Rhino" = nose; major cause of the common cold				
Reoviridae	"R" = respiratory, "e" = enteric, "o" = orphan	60–80	DS	Icos	0
Rotavirus	Viral capsid resembles a wheel ("rota" = wheel); severe diarrhea in infants and in malnourished or debilitated adults				
Retroviridae	"Retro" = backward; viruses have reverse transcriptase that allows them to make DNA from RNA—in reverse order of usual nucleic acid synthesis	100	SS	Icos	+
HIV types 1 and 2	Agents of acquired immunodeficiency syndrome				
Rhabdoviridae	"Rhabdos" = rod; viruses have rod- or bullet-shaped capsids	75 × 180	SS	He	+
Rabies	"Rabidus" = rabid or mad; virus named for symptoms demonstrated by infected individuals				
Togaviridae	"Toga" = coat (i.e., envelope)	40–70	SS	Icos	+
Rubella	German measles; mild (3-day) illness, usually with rash and mild fever; can damage fetus of infected pregnant women				
Eastern and western equine encephalitis*	Encephalitis-producing viruses transmitted through mosquito bites				
Unclassified	Non-A, non-B hepatitis agents remain unclassified; some of these have been named hepatitis C virus				

*Common name = arboviruses ("ar" = arthropod, "bo" = borne); viruses transmitted by arthropod vector.
†Bacilliform.
‡Common name = enteroviruses (produce enteric illness).
CNS = central nervous system; DS = double stranded; SS = single stranded; HE = helical capsid; Env = envelope;
+ = envelope present; 0 = nonenveloped (naked); HIV = human immunodeficiency virus.

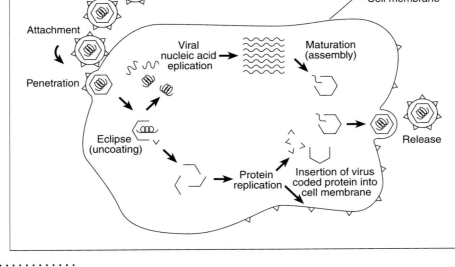

. . . .
FIGURE 1–4   VIRAL REPLICATION. The virus first attaches to the cell surface and then penetrates and uncoats. The nucleic acid and the viral proteins are then replicated in different areas within the cell. The newly formed nucleic acids and viral proteins are assembled to make new viral nucleocapsids, which are then released from the cell.

Eclipse
In the **eclipse phase (uncoating),** after penetration, the capsid structure undergoes a configurational change that results in uncoating, which frees the nucleic acid. During this period, the intact virion cannot be detected within the cell.

Replication
In the **replication phase,** after uncoating, the viral nucleic acid inhibits synthesis of host cell nucleic acid and directs the host cell to produce viral nucleic acid and viral proteins, beginning with the synthesis of viral enzymes for viral genome production. Transcription, translation, and replication of viral proteins and nucleic acids follow. For DNA viruses, most replication takes place in the nucleus, whereas for RNA viruses, replication is centered in the cytoplasm. Newly synthesized viral glycoproteins may be inserted into the cell membrane of the host cell during this time.

Maturation
In the **maturation phase (assembly),** new virions are assembled from the newly synthesized viral nucleic acid, viral structural proteins, and viral enzymes. Assembly may occur in the cytoplasm or in the nucleus.

Release
Release of newly formed nucleocapsids may result in total lysis of the cell or may occur by "budding" with relatively little distortion of cellular morphology. Cell lysis, which kills the host cell, is the mechanism through which most nonenveloped viruses are released. The nucleocapsids of viruses that will be enveloped are released by budding through the cell membrane in areas where virus-encoded glycoproteins have been inserted [6]; the membrane surrounds the nucleocapsid to form the envelope. This budding may or may not kill the cell. Released virions may infect adjacent cells or may be carried by fluids to distant cells.

ROUTES OF TRANSMISSION AND VIRAL PATHOGENESIS

In an otherwise healthy individual who has a functioning immune system and intact natural barriers to infection (e.g., healthy, intact skin and mucous membranes; saliva; gastric acids) and who has been immunized according to the currently recommended schedule, many viral illnesses can be avoided. However, because of failure of immunization programs, breaches in natural barriers, and encounters with viruses that can bypass natural barriers and are not excluded by currently available immunizations, viruses remain a major factor in disease in the United States. Because virus-infected cells fail to produce the proteins needed for cell maintenance and function, the infected cells cannot carry out their usual biological processes, and the host soon experiences signs and symptoms that signal infection and illness. A vast array of clinical syndromes are associated with virus-induced illness. The type and severity of disease symptoms depend on many factors. The location and type of the cells infected and the type and quantity of the infecting virus determine the sort of infection that will follow. However, the body's immune response to the infection and accompanying tissue damage are important factors in determining the severity of the disease.

A common route of viral infection is through the respiratory tract (Fig. 1–5). Viruses are transmitted by inhalation of virus-infected aerosols or by hand-to-hand contact. Viruses such as the **rhinoviruses** and **coronaviruses** reach the upper respiratory mucosa, where they attach to and infect epithelial cells. These cells cease to function normally and release bradykinin and histamine, which are chemical modulators associated with anaphylactic responses. The activity of these chemicals produces inflamed mucosal cells that initially release a watery discharge and later a mucopurulent discharge containing many neutrophils. These infections last only a few days and resolve without treatment.

Other respiratory viruses, such as the **influenzas** and **parainfluenzas,** attach to ciliated columnar epithelial cells by means of viral structures called hemagglutinins, which project from the viral envelope. The ciliated epithelial cells are also the target of **respiratory syncytial virus** and certain **adenoviruses.** The virus-infected cells lyse, releasing enzymes and activating complement, resulting in a local mononuclear cell inflammatory response. Normal airway clearance mechanisms fail because the infected ciliated epithelial cells cease to function normally and may slough off. Cell debris from dead and dying cells may plug the airways [7]. The host becomes very susceptible to bacterial superinfection. The immune response to influenza infection may be responsible for systemic symptoms such as fever and muscle aches. **Influenza** and, less frequently, **parainfluenza, respiratory syncytial virus,** and **adenovirus** may progress to lower respiratory involvement and pneumonia. After replication in respiratory epithelial cells, **adenovirus** travels via the blood to the lymphoid tissues in all areas of the body. During acute infection, these distant sites show inflammation.

Many viruses such as **measles, mumps, rubella,** and **parvovirus B19** enter through the respiratory tract but produce multisystem involvement. They undergo initial replication in the mucosal epithelium and travel to regional lymph nodes and then, via the blood, to other organs, including the skin, conjunctiva, placenta, testicles, and respiratory tract.

Viruses may enter the gastrointestinal tract through the mouth (see Fig. 1–5). Using contaminated food or water as their vehicle, **Norwalk virus, enteric adenoviruses, rotavirus,** and others make their way through the stomach and into the small intestine. Here viruses damage epithelial cells lining the small intestine, resulting in blunting of absorptive villi, decreased sodium absorption, and electrolyte imbalance. Decreased action of disaccharidases leads to increased carbohydrates in the intestine, which stimulates osmosis of water and electrolytes into the intestine [7]. The end result is diarrhea.

Hepatitis A virus, the **enteroviruses,** and others also enter the body through the mouth and eventually travel through the stomach and into the intestine. **Enteroviruses** replicate in epithelial cells and lymphoid tissues in the pharynx and intestine and are excreted in large numbers in the feces. Then these viruses can enter the blood and travel to distant target organs such as the central nervous system and pleura. In target organs some enteroviruses such as **poliovirus** produce lytic

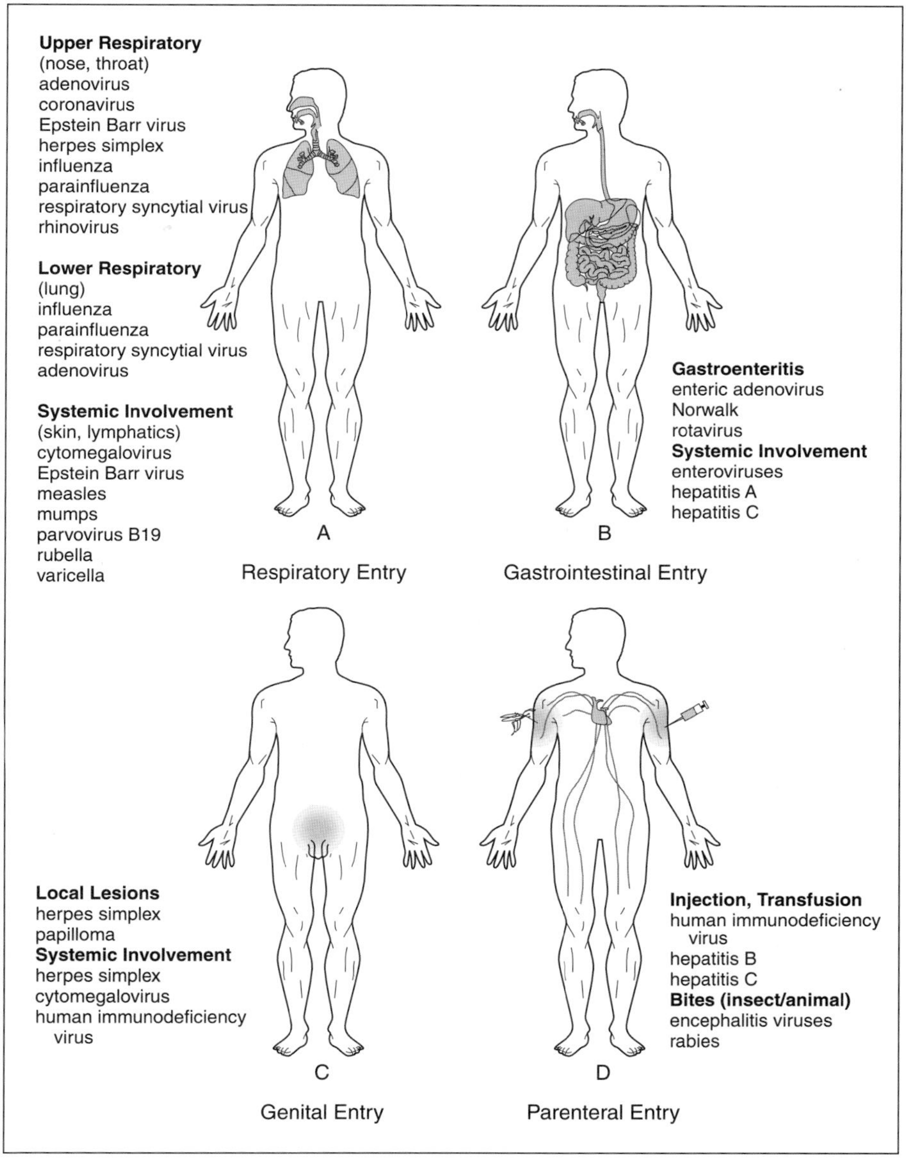

Upper Respiratory
(nose, throat)
adenovirus
coronavirus
Epstein Barr virus
herpes simplex
influenza
parainfluenza
respiratory syncytial virus
rhinovirus

Lower Respiratory
(lung)
influenza
parainfluenza
respiratory syncytial virus
adenovirus

Systemic Involvement
(skin, lymphatics)
cytomegalovirus
Epstein Barr virus
measles
mumps
parvovirus B19
rubella
varicella

A

Respiratory Entry

Gastroenteritis
enteric adenovirus
Norwalk
rotavirus
Systemic Involvement
enteroviruses
hepatitis A
hepatitis C

B

Gastrointestinal Entry

Local Lesions
herpes simplex
papilloma
Systemic Involvement
herpes simplex
cytomegalovirus
human immunodeficiency
  virus

C

Genital Entry

Injection, Transfusion
human immunodeficiency
  virus
hepatitis B
hepatitis C
Bites (insect/animal)
encephalitis viruses
rabies

D

Parenteral Entry

· · · · · · · · · · · · ·
FIGURE 1–5 ROUTES OF TRANSMISSION AND PATHOGENESIS OF VIRUSES.
Viruses may enter through the respiratory tract (A), the gastrointestinal tract (B), or the genital tract (C) or by penetrating the skin (D). After entry into the body, viruses may produce symptoms at the site of infection or may replicate at the site but move to other nearby areas or distant organs to produce disease.

infections that destroy the target tissues. Other enteroviruses produce infections that result in damage that is thought to be related to the body's immune response. In **coxsackie B** myocarditis, the coxsackie B virus infection stimulates production of antibodies that cross-react with host tissues; the action of the antibodies results in myocarditis. **Hepatitis A virus** replicates initially in the enteric mucosa and enters the blood. It reaches the liver, where it replicates, resulting in necrosis.

Other viruses are frequently transmitted in contaminated fluids that enter through mucous membranes or abraded skin in oral and genital areas (see Fig. 1–5). Some of these viruses may also enter through the respiratory or gastrointestinal route. These viruses include **herpes simplex,**

cytomegalovirus, varicella-zoster, papilloma viruses, Epstein-Barr virus, and **human immunodeficiency virus (HIV). Herpes simplex virus** may cause oral or genital lesions at sites where virus infects epithelial cells. These viruses infect local sensory nerve endings and are then transported to nearby ganglia, where they establish latency. On reactivation, the virus migrates via peripheral sensory nerves to mucosal and skin surfaces, and, in severe disseminated disease, other organs are involved [7]. **Varicella-zoster** acts similarly by infecting the skin after an initial replication period at an unknown site. As skin lesions heal, the virus establishes latency in dorsal root ganglia. **Cytomegalovirus** infects lymphocytes and epithelial cells and is carried to the salivary glands, respiratory tract, and kidneys. **Epstein-Barr virus** acts similarly. In contrast, **papilloma viruses** remain near the site of contact to produce epithelial tumors and warts. **HIV** infects lymphocytes, depressing their function to allow immunodeficiency that results in acquired immunodeficiency syndrome (AIDS).

Some viral infections result after entry of the virus by penetration of the skin (see Fig. 1–5). Insect bites may transmit various **encephalitis viruses,** animal bites may transmit **rabies,** and administration of contaminated blood and blood products may transmit several of the **hepatitis viruses, HIV,** and **other retroviruses.** Viruses may enter the blood and lymphatic vessels directly and travel to target organs where they replicate, or, as in the case of rabies, the virus replicates in muscle at the site of the bite before traveling through the nerves to the central nervous system.

Production of obvious disease symptoms in the host such as those just described is one possible outcome of viral infection. Other viral infections may be subclinical with no obvious symptoms at all. Infecting viruses such as **herpes simplex, cytomegalovirus,** and **parvovirus B19** may produce disease not only in the host but in the fetus in pregnant hosts. Viruses such as **Epstein-Barr virus** may transform the cells to eventually produce malignant cells.

The manifestations of viral infections are numerous, and mechanisms for disease transmission are constantly being studied to identify approaches for treatment and prevention. The disease associations and approaches for laboratory diagnosis of each of the more common viruses are described in Chapters 8 and 9.

VIRAL RESPONSE TO INTERFERON AND ANTIMICROBIAL AGENTS

When a virus infects a cell, the process either directly or indirectly results in the appearance of double-stranded RNAs, which stimulate production of a factor that interferes either directly or indirectly with viral replication; this factor is called **interferon.** Interferons are a family of proteins. Interferon-α is produced by B lymphocytes, monocytes, and macrophages, and interferon-β is made by fibroblasts and other cells. Interferon-γ is produced later in infection, acts in a manner distinct from that of interferon-α and interferon-β, and is known as macrophage activation factor [8]. Interferon-α and interferon-β can be induced, produced, and released within hours of infection. When excreted outside the infected cells, interferon acts on the cell that produced it as well as on surrounding cells of the same type to induce production of enzymes that interfere with viral replication. Interferon induces an antiviral state that lasts for 2 to 3 days, during which the cell and host defenses may be able to eliminate the virus. Interferon acts most effectively in cells of the species in which it was originally produced. It acts to block infection by all viruses, not just by the virus that stimulated its production. Interferons are not virus specific. Most interferons are not inactivated by low pH (pH = 2) or by heat (1 hour at 50°C) [9].

True antibiotics are chemical substances produced by microorganisms, whereas other types of antimicrobial agents are chemically synthesized. These substances have the capacity to inhibit or kill various bacteria, fungi, chlamydiae, rickettsiae, and parasites. The goal of antimicrobial therapy is to selectively inhibit or kill the infecting organism without harming the host cell. Each agent has a specific site of action, usually the organismal cell walls, cell membranes, or protein-synthesizing processes, sites at which the microorganisms differ significantly from the host cell. Because viruses are devoid of such structures and processes, antimicrobial agents are not active against viruses. Because viral replication is dependent on host cell genes, it is difficult to develop agents that can inhibit viruses without affecting host cells. Some therapeutic antiviral agents have been developed and are now being used in the treatment of certain viral infections. These act by interfering with viral attachment, penetration, replication, and assembly. Antivirals and antiviral susceptibility testing are discussed in Chapter 10.

Antibacterial and antifungal agents are added to viral culture media. These substances inhibit growth of any bacteria, fungi, and so on in the culture but do not affect replication of viruses. This practice ensures that other microorganisms do not overgrow the culture before the viruses have time to replicate.

APPROACHES FOR LABORATORY DIAGNOSIS OF VIRAL INFECTIONS

Because electron microscopes are not routinely available in most clinical virology laboratories, the clinical virologist cannot rely on observing viruses to classify or identify them. Because viruses do not replicate on artificial media, the virologist cannot use agar or broth media for virus isolation. How does the clinical laboratory virologist approach virus detection and identification? Clinical diagnostic virology relies on three traditional approaches for virus detection: virus isolation in living systems, viral antigen detection, and viral serology. A fourth, more contemporary approach is the use of molecular biology technology in viral diagnoses.

1. **Virus isolation.** The clinical virologist provides living systems in which viruses will proliferate. Cell cultures are the living system used in most clinical laboratories (see Chapter 3). Although the viral particles cannot be seen as they replicate in cell cultures, their presence is signaled by changes in the appearance of the virus-infected cells. These changes, called the cytopathogenic effect (CPE), can be detected when cells are viewed with an ordinary light microscope. CPE may be detectable in 24 to 48 hours with viruses such as herpes simplex virus and some of the enteroviruses; however, many viruses require 7 to 10 days or more for detection. Several modified cell culture systems have been developed that facilitate rapid isolation of certain viruses (see Chapter 4). Some viruses will not proliferate in standard cell cultures.

2. **Viral antigen detection.** The clinical virologist uses immunological techniques, which rely on the specific reactivity of known viral antibodies with their antigens, to demonstrate that viral antigens are present (see Chapter 5). The binding of antibodies and antigens is signaled to the clinical virologist through reactions such as agglutination, fluorescence, or color change, which can be observed visually or can be measured with laboratory instruments such as a spectrophotometer. Viral antigens present within infected cells in viral cultures or in samples taken directly from the infected individual can be detected and identified. Viral antigen detection methods usually require only a few hours to complete.

3. **Viral serology.** The clinical virologist uses standard serological methods to detect specific antibodies that have been produced by the host in response to viral infection or exposure. By demonstrating that antibodies are present or that there is a change in antibody level, the virologist can provide valuable information concerning viral disease status (see Chapter 6). Antibody detection methods are available in most clinical laboratories. This approach is especially useful in circumstances in which the virus cannot be conveniently isolated in cell culture nor its antigens detected by routine viral antigen detection methods.

4. **Molecular diagnostics.** Scientists are using molecular biology as a tool for viral disease diagnosis. Through application of molecular "probes," which are labeled DNA sequences that are complementary to unique portions of viral DNA, viral nucleic acids within infected cells can be detected and identified. This technology paired with polymerase chain reaction (PCR), a method for the amplification of specific pieces of DNA *in vitro,* allows detection of minuscule quantities of viral nucleic acids that may be missed by traditional viral assays. Molecular diagnostic technology may not yet be a part of the routine test offerings of many clinical diagnostic virology laboratories, but the molecular approach will eventually have a dramatic

effect on how viral diagnostic testing is approached. Molecular techniques are described in Chapter 2, and the clinical applications of PCR are presented in Chapter 10.

Viral disease diagnosis is not restricted to the four approaches just presented. Virus-infected cells scraped from the base of infected lesions or collected from other infected sites may be smeared on a microscope slide and stained with Giemsa, hematoxylin and eosin, or Papanicolaou stain and observed with the light microscope for the presence of virus-induced inclusions. These inclusions may be located in the nucleus or cytoplasm and are either large aggregates of viral nucleoproteins or combinations of assembled virions and cellular breakdown products. Some of these inclusions have a characteristic appearance that allows presumptive identification of the virus. When material from vesicular lesions is stained in this manner, the procedure is called the **Tzanck test.** If the vesicle is the result of herpes simplex or varicella infection, characteristic multinucleated giant cells can be seen. These cells are typical of both herpes simplex and varicella and cannot be differentiated. Other viruses such as adenoviruses, papovaviruses, and respiratory syncytial virus also produce inclusions.

Characteristic viral inclusions can also be seen in stained histological sections of paraffin-embedded tissue. Enlarged cells with basophilic nuclear inclusions surrounded by a clear halo and described as "owl's eye" cells may be observed in tissue infected with cytomegalovirus. Other viruses produce various types of viral inclusions, most of which are not characteristic of a specific virus but suggest viral origin for the infection.

If an electron microscope is available, clinical samples and infected cell cultures can be examined. Electron microscopy may be especially helpful in the diagnosis of viral infections produced by viruses such as Norwalk virus that fail to proliferate in standard cell cultures. Electron microscopes are not available in many clinical virology laboratories, so this technique is primarily a research tool. Viral detection via cytological, histological, and electron microscopic analyses does not provide the sensitivity and specificity offered by the four major viral diagnostic approaches (described previously), which are the focus of this text.

Although all of the techniques for the laboratory diagnosis of viral infection were slower to develop than laboratory methods for identification of other microorganisms, they are now becoming standardized, and many are available to laboratorians for routine use. Many viral laboratory techniques are very similar to those used by clinical microbiologists who study bacteria and fungi. The virologist inoculates patients' samples into various types of cell cultures, whereas the bacteriologist uses a variety of selective and nonselective agars and broths. The virologist examines cells for production of CPE to indicate that virus is present, whereas the bacteriologist watches for bacterial colonies to appear on the surface of the agar plates or in broth. For both the virologist and the bacteriologist, the final identification of the organisms may involve reacting the organism with specific antibodies. In addition, microbiologists are familiar with sterile technique and the general concepts of diagnostic microbiology. Most microbiologists are able to perform diagnostic virology laboratory assays with minimal additional training.

LABORATORY DIAGNOSIS OF VIRAL INFECTIONS—WHY BOTHER?

Before the early 1970s there was little demand for laboratory confirmation of viral infections. Physicians involved in the diagnosis of viral infections often thought that the signs and symptoms of viral illnesses were sufficiently characteristic that the diagnosis was obvious. This was especially true of epidemic viral infections encountered in individuals of appropriate age and accompanied by a characteristic rash and so on. For example, laboratory diagnosis of measles in a child was of no interest. The diagnosis was routine and obvious on clinical grounds alone. For cases in which the diagnosis was less obvious, supportive laboratory evidence such as normal or low white cell counts or lymphocytosis with atypical lymphocytes was relied on to implicate a viral rather than a bacterial cause [10]. Additionally, clinical laboratory virology identification, which depended largely on virus isolation, was simply too slow to provide information that would be helpful in patient management. After waiting 7 to 10 days for identification of the infecting virus, it was too late for the physician to do much to help the patient; also, there were no antiviral agents available for treatment. Because viral laboratory services were not widely available and required technical expertise and unusual reagents, the cost for testing was higher than that of most other laboratory tests. So why is it important to provide definitive laboratory evidence to confirm virus identification?

There are many reasons why a definitive viral diagnosis is helpful. Although typical uncomplicated viral infections may be diagnosed on clinical grounds alone, the more complicated and less characteristic infections encountered in contemporary settings, especially in immuno-compromised individuals, present a greater challenge. In immunocompromised individuals, signs and symptoms may not be characteristic. Likewise, many viral infections that were common in the past have now been largely eradicated through immunization programs. Now when these infections occur, they may not be readily recognized because they are rare and physicians are no longer familiar with them. They may also occur in a partially immunized individual whose symptoms will not be typical. Laboratory confirmation may be the only avenue for definitive identification of the infecting virus in these situations.

When a viral cause for an illness can be confirmed, any unnecessary therapy can be discontinued and appropriate treatment initiated. For example, in cases involving pharyngoton-sillitis presumed to be due to group A streptococci and treated with antibiotics, a lack of response to therapy may signal a viral infection. Such pharyngotonsillitis is often seen in young adults infected with herpes simplex type 2 [11]. Discontinuation of antibiotic therapy reduces cost and eliminates undesirable side effects of the antibiotics. If the infection is caused by a virus for which specific antiviral therapy is available, this therapy can be implemented. At this writing, antiviral therapy is available for treatment of infections resulting from herpes simplex, cytomegalovirus, influenza A, varicella-zoster, HIV-1, and respiratory syncytial virus. Most antiviral agents have a very narrow spectrum of activity; therefore, the infecting virus must be precisely identified before treatment is initiated [11].

Viral identification in cell culture, although still an essential component in the virology laboratory, has been modified and improved to yield more rapid viral identification. Many viral isolates are identified within a few days, with an average viral detection time of 3 to 4 days; more than 70% of viral isolates can be reported within 5 days [11]. Newer viral antigen detection methods can detect and identify many infecting viruses in a few hours. With viral diagnostic testing services becoming more widely available, the cost of these procedures is comparable to that of many other laboratory assays, allowing cost-effective viral diagnosis.

A definitive viral diagnosis may also be important from an infection control standpoint. If a hospitalized patient, hospital staff member, or visitor to the hospital can be shown to have chickenpox (varicella), measles, or rubella, the entire hospital staff and patient population will be evaluated for immunity. This follow-up is essential to prevent the transmission of these diseases within the hospital. Likewise, infection control involving viral infections such as influenza can be important in the entire community and worldwide as epidemics and pandemics are monitored and mass immunizations are made available.

Definitive confirmation of viral causes is also important in education and research. By studying viral infections, virologists may obtain the information required for the development of new and improved antiviral agents and therapies as well as new viral vaccines. Processes and sequelae of viral disease syndromes can be more carefully evaluated, and previously unknown or undetected viruses can be identified and studied. New diagnostic tests can be developed.

When the viral identification is known, the physician can provide the patient with an answer to the question, "What's wrong with me?" The physician can also provide information concerning the expected course of the illness and any anticipated sequelae.

In the chapters that follow, the methods and approaches for laboratory diagnosis of viral infections are presented. In addition, the disease associations and avenues for diagnosis of infections of common viruses are addressed.

R E F E R E N C E S

1. Preston R. The Hot Zone. New York: Random House, 1994.
2. Dulbecco R, Ginsberg HS. The nature of viruses. In Davis BD, Dulbecco R, Eisen HM, Ginsberg HS (eds), Microbiology, 3rd ed. New York: Harper & Row, 1980, pp 854–884.
3. Black JG. Viruses. In Microbiology Principles and Applications, 2nd ed. Englewood Cliffs, NJ: Prentice Hall, 1993, pp 264–291.
4. Boyd RF, Hoerl BG. Basic Medical Microbiology, 3rd ed. Boston: Little, Brown, 1986.
5. Roizman B. Multiplication of viruses: an overview. In Fields BN, McKnipe D, Chanock RM, et al (eds), Virology, 2nd ed. New York: Raven Press, 1990, pp 87–94.
6. Volk WA, Benjamin DC, Kadner RJ, Parsons JT. Structure and classification of animal viruses and growth, purification, and characterization of animal viruses. In Essentials of Medical Microbiology, 4th ed. Philadelphia: JB Lippincott, 1991, pp 573–601.
7. Ellner PD, Neu HC. Understanding Infectious Disease. St. Louis: Mosby-Year Book, 1992.
8. Rosenthal K. Virology. In Murray PR, Kobayashi GS, Pfaller MA, Rosenthal KS (eds), Medical Microbiology, 2nd ed. St. Louis: CV Mosby, 1994, pp 526–723.
9. Dulbecco R. Interference with viral multiplication. In Davis BD, Dulbecco R, Eisen HM, Ginsberg HS (eds), Microbiology, 3rd ed. New York: Harper & Row, 1980, pp 1002–1015.
10. Evans AS. Epidemiologic concepts and methods. In Evans AS (ed), Viral Infections of Humans, Epidemiology and Control, 3rd ed. New York: Plenum, 1989, pp 3–49.
11. Drew WL. Controversies in viral diagnosis. Rev Infect Dis 1986;8:814–824.

R E V I E W Q U E S T I O N S

1. Number the following microscopic entities in order according to their size ("1" represents smallest entity and "4" represents the largest):

_____ staphylococcus

_____ poxvirus

_____ herpes simplex virus

_____ polio virus

2. Indicate which kind of microscope (light vs. electron) is needed to observe the following entities:

herpes simplex virus _____

staphylococcus _____

erythrocyte _____

poliovirus _____

3. Which of the following phrases characterize icosahedral viruses?
  a. Are rod shaped
  b. Have 20 triangle-shaped facets
  c. Are described as "complex" in configuration
  d. Can have only DNA, never RNA

4. Which of the following phrases characterize helical viruses?
  a. Have both DNA and RNA
  b. Are often described as cubic
  c. Have a cylindrical capsid
  d. Resemble crystals

5. Match the description in Column B with the viral component it describes in Column A.

A		B
_____ Capsid		a. Nonrigid outer coat consisting of protein and lipid
_____ Capsomere		b. Glycoproteins that protrude and appear as projections or spikes
_____ Envelope		c. A rigid protein coat that surrounds the nucleic acid
_____ Matrix protein		d. Nonglycosylated proteins that form a layer that connects other viral components
_____ Peplomers		e. Identical repeating protein subunits

6. Provide the classification data for the following viruses:

Virus	DNA or RNA?	Family
herpes simplex	_____	_____
hepatitis B virus	_____	_____
cytomegalovirus	_____	_____
human immunodeficiency virus	_____	_____

7. Which of the following statements provides the best overview of viral replication?
   a. The parent virus divides into two identical daughter virions.
   b. Each parent virus produces one offspring via budding.
   c. A replicative endospore is formed in which new virions grow and mature.
   d. Nucleic acid and capsid are replicated separately and then new virions are assembled.

8. Viral replication is best described by which of the following statements?
   a. Occurs exclusively in the nucleus of the infected cell
   b. Involves "viropexis," which is the doubling of nucleic acids just before division by binary fission
   c. Ends with release of virions by budding or cell lysis
   d. Includes an eclipse phase in which intact virions are attached to the cell membrane

9. Viruses have various ways of entering the human body and producing disease. Which of the following descriptions accurately describe the route and mechanism for the virus indicated?
   a. Mumps virus enters through abraded skin in the genital area and moves into the testicles of males to produce swelling and sterility.
   b. Coronaviruses enter the gastrointestinal tract through the mouth and move into the stomach, where they proliferate within mucosal cells to produce peptic ulcers.
   c. Enteroviruses enter through the mouth, replicate in the pharynx and bowel, and move via the blood to distant target organs such as the central nervous system.
   d. Influenza viruses enter through the respiratory tract, replicate within lymphocytes in the lung, and move via the lymphatic vessels to joints and the central nervous system to produce muscle aches, stiff joints, and fever.

10. Interferons, which are involved in the body's response to viral infections, are characterized by which of the following?
    a. Composed of double-stranded RNA
    b. Released early on in viral infection to stimulate production of enzymes that interfere with viral replication
    c. Virus specific; act against only the virus that stimulated their production
    d. Induce a permanent antiviral state

11. Four major approaches for providing viral disease diagnosis are described in this chapter. Which of the following is **not** one of the diagnostic approaches that provides definitive identification of viruses?
    a. Identification of virus isolated in cell culture
    b. Tzanck preparation
    c. Molecular probe
    d. Viral antigen identification

12. All of the following are benefits associated with definitive viral diagnoses **except**
    a. Proper patient therapy
    b. Management of nosocomial infections in the hospital and the community
    c. Improved concept of prognosis of illness for the physician and the patient
    d. Reduced emphasis on disease prevention because viral diagnosis can be confirmed

Concepts of Immunoserological and Molecular Techniques

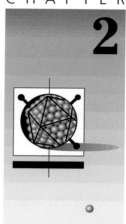

OBJECTIVES

At the completion of this unit of study, the student will be able to do the following:

1. List general factors that affect *in vitro* immunoserological assays.

2. For the following immunoserological principles, describe the antigen, give an overview of the procedural steps (including a diagram for those principles that are widely used in clinical virology), and describe the appearance of "positive" and "negative" results: precipitation, flocculation, direct (hem)agglutination, passive (hem)agglutination, viral hemagglutination, hemagglutination inhibition, direct immunofluorescence, indirect immunofluorescence, complement fixation, enzyme immunoassay (competitive and noncompetitive), immunoblotting, and virus neutralization.

3. Compare the basic concepts of immunoserological assays with those of molecular diagnostic techniques.

4. Diagram and describe *in situ* hybridization and polymerase chain reaction.

5. Define and provide formulas for calculation of sensitivity, specificity, and predictive values, and, when provided with data, calculate these values.

INTRODUCTION

The purpose of the clinical diagnostic virology laboratory is to aid the physician in the diagnosis of viral infections through identification of viruses isolated in cell culture, detection of viral antigens in clinical samples, identification and quantitation of viral antibodies in serum, and detection of viral nucleic acids. In this chapter the generic concepts of various testing principles are introduced and described, and examples of applications of these principles in clinical virology are presented in the text and summarized in Table 2–1. The methods are divided into two broad categories: (1) **immunoserological assays,** which depend on the reactivity of antibodies with their corresponding antigens, and (2) **molecular diagnostic techniques,** which involve the detection of unique nucleic acid sequences to confirm the identity of the virus.

This chapter does not include descriptions of all known or accepted immunoserological or molecular methods; only those that are important in the diagnosis of the viral infections discussed in this volume are included. Among the assays not included is radioimmunoassay. This methodology has numerous applications in many laboratory areas; however, use of radioactive reagents such as those required in radioimmunoassays is becoming less popular because of the associated hazards, and these methods are being replaced by other assays.

IMMUNOSEROLOGICAL ASSAYS *IN VITRO*

Factors Affecting Immunoserological Assays *In Vitro*

In diagnostic virology many of the methodologies used for identification of viruses, detection of viral antigens, and identification of viral antibodies rely on the specific reactivity of antibodies with their antigens. Various immunological principles are involved in these assays, and the manipulations required for mixing reactants, observing the final result, and interpreting the significance of reactivity may differ from method to method. However, the basic concept involved in each of these reactions is that antibodies will specifically bind to only their corresponding antigens. If the virologist is attempting to detect and identify an unknown virus or unknown viral antigen, he or she uses antibody of known specificity in the test system. Conversely, if the virologist is attempting to identify viral antibodies, he or she uses known virus or viral antigen in the test system.

Regardless of specific methodology or type of antigen or antibody being detected or identified, there are several concepts that are essential for successful immunoserological assays *in vitro*.

1. **Electrolyte dependency.** Electrolytes are the charged molecules that are present in most biological fluids. These include sodium (Na^+), potassium (K^+), calcium (Ca^{2+}), chloride (Cl^-), and many others. Immunological reactions cannot go to completion unless electrolytes are present because electrolytes are important in antigen-antibody binding. The necessary electrolytes can be supplied in the test system in a diluent solution, in one of the reagents used, or in human serum that is being tested [1].

2. **Time and temperature.** Immunological reactivity is influenced by the length of the reaction time or incubation period and by the temperature. Proper temperature and length of incubation will vary from assay to assay. Times and temperatures other than those specified for a given assay may result in poor performance of the assay [1].

3. **pH.** Forces of attraction that bind antigens and antibodies are weaker in an acid environment (below pH 4) and in alkaline environments (above pH 10) [2]. Most immunoserological assays are performed at neutral pH.

4. **Reagent quality.** The capacity of a given immunoserological assay to measure or to detect the substances it is designed to measure or detect depends heavily on the quality of reactants used in the test system. When a pure whole virus or viral antigen suspension is used in an antibody detection system, the likelihood of detecting only the appropriate viral antibodies is improved. This is in contrast to the use of crude viral culture extracts or lysates that contain bits of cell culture-related antigens; presence of such extraneous debris and antigens may allow the test system to show reactivity with antibodies other than the viral antibodies it is designed to detect. Many newer test systems include antigens that are artificially engineered through molecular cloning. Such antigens represent the purest antigens available

. . . .

TABLE 2–1 APPLICATIONS OF IMMUNOSEROLOGICAL AND MOLECULAR PRINCIPLES IN THE CLINICAL DIAGNOSTIC VIROLOGY LABORATORY

PRINCIPLE	APPLICATION IN DIAGNOSTIC VIROLOGY
Passive agglutination	Detect antibodies of rubella, cytomegalovirus, and varicella; detect rotavirus antigen
Passive hemagglutination	Detect antibodies of rubella
Viral hemagglutination*	Detect and characterize hemagglutinating viruses such as influenza and parainfluenza
Hemagglutination inhibition	Detect antibodies of influenza, parainfluenza, mumps, measles, and rubella; confirm identification of the hemagglutinating viruses
Direct immunofluorescence	Detect antigens of herpes simplex types 1 and 2 and respiratory syncytial virus; detect cytomegalovirus antigens after culture amplification
Indirect immunofluorescence	Detect antigens of adenovirus, influenza, parainfluenza, respiratory syncytial virus, and cytomegalovirus (after culture amplification); detect antibodies of mumps, respiratory syncytial virus, herpes simplex, cytomegalovirus, Epstein-Barr virus, varicella
Complement fixation	Detect antibodies of influenza, parainfluenza, adenovirus, and others; can be used to identify various unknown viruses but is not widely used for this purpose
Immunoperoxidase	Detect various viral antigens
Noncompetitive solid-phase EIA, bead based	Detect antibodies of hepatitis A, B, and C, and HIV and antigens of hepatitis B, HIV, and rotavirus
Noncompetitive solid-phase EIA, microwell or tube based	Detect antibodies against herpes simplex, cytomegalovirus, rubella, measles, varicella, Epstein-Barr virus, hepatitis, HIV; detect antigens of herpes simplex, respiratory syncytial virus, rotavirus
Noncompetitive solid-phase EIA, test pack configuration	Detect antigens of herpes simplex, respiratory syncytial virus, influenza, rotavirus; detect antibodies of cytomegalovirus
Competitive solid-phase EIA	Detect various hepatitis antibodies
Immunoblotting	Used extensively in identification of HIV antibodies
Virus neutralization	Can be used to identify nearly all viruses and viral antibodies; not used widely except to identify antibodies and viruses of the enterovirus group
Nucleic acid probe	Applied for *in situ* detection of viral antigens of cytomegalovirus, Epstein-Barr virus, and papilloma virus in infected tissues and other clinical samples
Polymerase chain reaction	An amplification technique used to multiply the amount of target viral DNA in a sample; used in conjunction with molecular probes and other molecular techniques for detection of viral nucleic acids of hepatitis viruses, HIV, cytomegalovirus, and others

*Viral hemagglutination is not an immunoserological technique because antibodies are not involved in the reaction. This is a direct reaction between viral antigens and erythrocytes that results in agglutination of the erythrocytes.
EIA = enzyme immunoassay; HIV = human immunodeficiency virus.

and should contribute to superior performance of the test system regarding detection of only the viral antibodies sought.

Likewise, the use of monoclonal antibodies, which have a single unique specificity, enhances the capacity of the test system to react with only the single virus or viral antigen that it is designed to detect. Polyclonal antibody systems may yield false identifications of closely related viruses and may not accurately differentiate related types or strains.

5. **Types of immunological events.** Two classifications of immunological events *in vitro* have been described [3]: primary, involving antigen and antibody recognition and interaction, and secondary, which are based on manifestations such as precipitation or agglutination. Primary reactions include immunofluorescence, radioimmunoassay, and enzyme immunoassays. These methods involve labeled products that allow measurement of antigen-antibody complexes. Secondary reactions include precipitation, agglutination, and complement fixation. These reactions depend on the combination of antigen-antibody's combining in correct proportions to result in formation of visible product or to react with other components to ultimately signal that antigen-antibody complexes were formed.

In secondary reactions, more so than in primary reactions, the antigen-antibody ratio in the test system is very important. When antigens and antibodies are present in relatively similar quantities, immunoserological reactions go to completion most efficiently. This condition of antigen versus antibody equality is called the **equivalence zone.** If antibody is in extreme excess **(prozone)** or if antigen is in extreme excess **(postzone),** immunoserological reactions may fail to occur (Fig. 2–1). Such falsely negative reactions occur not because of an absence of test substance (unknown antibody or unknown antigen) but because too much antibody or antigen is present in the test system [1]. The excess components prevent the cross-linking that is essential for formation of large, visible aggregates. When weak or falsely negative results caused by prozone reactions are experienced in antibody detection assays, the test serum should be diluted and retested. If the reaction is stronger in the diluted serum than in the concentrated serum, the prozone reaction is confirmed. Dilution of serum should eliminate prozone reactions. Most immunological assays are carefully designed to use reactants in quantities that ensure that reactions take place in the equivalence zone.

Innumerable protocols rely on antigen-antibody reactions. Many have been important in diagnostic virology for identification of unknown viruses or viral antigen or for identification of viral antibodies. Descriptions and illustrations of several of the immunoserological concepts

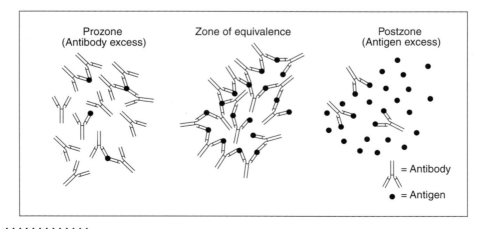

FIGURE 2–1 ANTIGEN-ANTIBODY RATIOS IN IMMUNOSEROLOGICAL REACTIONS. With excess antibody (prozone) or antigen (postzone), antibodies bind to antigens but do not cross-link to produce large complexes. When components are present in relatively similar quantities (zone of equivalence), cross-linking occurs to yield large complexes required for a visible reaction.

follow. For each illustration, both "positive" and "negative" sequences are provided to show the events that result when antigens and antibodies recognize each other and bind (i.e., "positive") or when antigens and antibodies do not recognize each other and do not bind (i.e., "negative"). In observing illustrations, one must remember that major reaction steps usually require an incubation period and are followed by thorough rinsing to eliminate unbound reactants.

Precipitation and Flocculation

Precipitation is the simplest serological method. Precipitation methods involve soluble antigens, which are usually solutions of protein or carbohydrate molecules [3]. Most precipitation assays are one-step procedures in which the soluble antigen is mixed with antibody (in patient's serum). Precipitation occurs if the antigen and antibody bind to each other to produce a visible precipitate. Precipitation reactions may be carried out on a slide (slide test), in a test tube (ring test), in a capillary tube (capillary precipitation test), or in a semisolid medium such as agar (immunodiffusion or gel diffusion test). Not all antibodies or antigens are detectable by precipitation; a more complex test system may be required.

Another type of reaction called **flocculation** is believed to be a type of precipitation reaction. In flocculation the exact nature of the antigen is somewhat questionable. The antigen may be soluble or may be in the form of very tiny insoluble particles [2]. A second substance may be involved in the reaction [1]. The reaction of this antigen with specific antibody produces loose, fluffy floccules. Neither precipitation nor flocculation is used extensively in clinical virology.

Direct and Passive (Hem)agglutination

Direct (hem)agglutination is the mechanism by which particulate or cellular antigens are clumped together by specific antibody. The antigen may be a bacterial cell or an erythrocyte (or other particulate antigen); the antigenic determinants involved in the reaction with antibody are **naturally occurring** parts of the particulate antigen. When the antigen is not an erythrocyte (i.e., a bacterium or another type of particle), the clumping reaction is called **direct agglutination.** When the antigen is an erythrocyte, the agglutination reaction is called **direct hemagglutination.** This immunoserological principle is not used extensively in clinical virology. Direct hemagglutination should not be confused with viral hemagglutination, which is also described in this chapter.

Passive (hem)agglutination is very similar to direct (hem)agglutination with the exception that in the former the antigenic substance actually involved in the reaction is **artificially attached** to the surface of a carrier particle. The carrier particle may be an erythrocyte, a latex particle, and so on. Erythrocytes can absorb various polysaccharides and, after treatment with tannic acid, can absorb many protein antigens [3]. The carrier particles are clumped by the binding of antibodies that are specific for the artificially attached antigen (Fig. 2–2). As with direct (hem)agglutination, the nature of the particle determines the naming of the passive reactions. With nonerythrocyte carriers, the reaction is called **passive agglutination,** whereas reactions involving erythrocyte carriers are referred to as **passive hemagglutination.**

The passive (hem)agglutination principle is used for detection of viruses and viral antigens. For virus and viral antigen detection, the component that is artificially attached to the carrier particle is a viral antibody of known specificity. This is sometimes called **reverse passive (hem)agglutination.** The antibody-coated particles are mixed with suspensions of virus-containing material, and, as the viral antibodies on the carrier particles recognize and bind to the viral antigens in the test sample, the carrier particles clump to signal that the binding has occurred. Passive agglutination is used in some virology laboratories for detection of rotavirus antigen in fecal samples.

Passive (hem)agglutination is also used in clinical virology for identification of viral antibodies. For this purpose, viral antigens of known type are attached to carrier particles, either

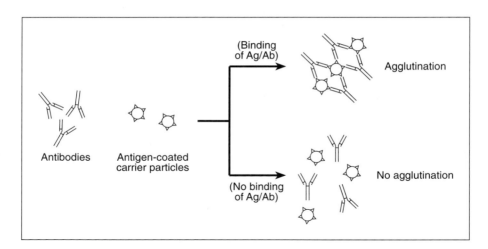

· · · · · · · · · · · · ·
FIGURE 2–2 PASSIVE (HEM)AGGLUTINATION. Antigen-coated carrier particles are mixed with antibodies. If the antibodies recognize the antigen, antibody binding produces agglutination. If the antibodies do not recognize the antigens, no binding occurs, and there is no agglutination. The term agglutination is used when the carrier particle is not an erythrocyte; the term hemagglutination is used for erythrocyte carriers. (Ag/Ab = antigen-antibody.)

latex particles or erythrocytes, and the antigen-coated particles are mixed with human serum. If viral antibodies specific for the viral antigens are present in the serum, they will bind to the viral antigens on the carrier particles and cause the particles to clump. Passive agglutination featuring virus-coated latex particles is used in some clinical virology laboratories for detection of antibodies of rubella, cytomegalovirus, and varicella. The results of a latex agglutination test for detection of cytomegalovirus antibodies are shown in Figure 2–3.

Viral Hemagglutination and Hemagglutination Inhibition

Certain viruses are capable of agglutinating various species of erythrocytes. This phenomenon is called **viral hemagglutination.** Viruses attach directly to the erythrocytes, which results in a visible clumping reaction (Fig. 2–4); thus, viral hemagglutination is not actually an immunoserological reaction because it does not involve binding of antigens and antibodies. The ability to hemagglutinate is restricted; not all viruses can hemagglutinate, and, for those that can hemag-

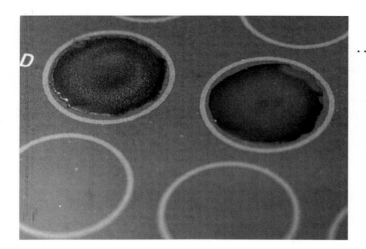

· · · · · · · · · · · ·
FIGURE 2–3 LATEX AGGLUTINATION (PASSIVE AGGLUTINATION) TEST RESULTS IN A TEST FOR CYTOMEGALOVIRUS ANTIBODIES. When antibodies recognize and bind to the antigen that is attached to the latex particles, the binding causes clumping or agglutination of the particles as shown in the left test area. If the antibodies do not recognize and bind to the antigens on the latex particles, the latex suspension remains smooth as shown in the right test area.

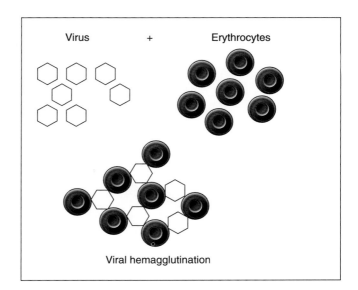

FIGURE 2–4 VIRAL HEMAG-GLUTINATION. When live hemagglutinating viruses are mixed with erythrocytes of appropriate species, viruses attach directly to the erythrocytes to produce hemagglutination.

glutinate, the species of erythrocyte is important. For example, influenza viruses hemagglutinate guinea pig, human, and chicken erythrocytes; enteroviruses hemagglutinate human erythrocytes; and cytomegalovirus is not known to have hemagglutinating ability for any type of erythrocyte. Viral hemagglutination is used in the virology laboratory for detecting hemagglutinating viruses. It is also the basis for an immunological method called hemagglutination inhibition.

In **hemagglutination inhibition,** the hemagglutinating capacity of a virus is blocked when the virus is reacted with specific antibody. Hemagglutination inhibition assays are two-stage assays (Fig. 2–5). In stage one, the live hemagglutinating virus is mixed with antibody. If this antibody is specific for the virus, the antibody attaches to the virus and inhibits it so that it is unable to hemagglutinate. In stage two, erythrocytes are added to the stage one mixture; the antibody-coated (inhibited) viruses are unable to hemagglutinate the erythrocytes. When the antibodies in stage one are not specific for the virus, there is no binding, and the virus remains active and uninhibited. When erythrocytes are added in stage two, the active (uninhibited) virus hemagglutinates the erythrocytes. This technique is, of course, applicable only to viruses with hemagglutinating ability. For antibody identification, known hemagglutinating virus is mixed with the patient's serum. If the serum inhibits hemagglutination of the virus, the antibodies in the serum are identified. The most common application of hemagglutination inhibition is in the identification of viral antibodies, including measles, mumps, and rubella antibodies.

Hemagglutination inhibition can be used by the virologist in the identification of unknown viruses. The unknown virus is mixed with antibodies of known specificity; if the antibodies inhibit hemagglutination, the virus is identified.

Immunofluorescence

Immunofluorescence techniques use antibodies labeled with fluorescent dyes. Labeled antibodies are often called **conjugates** because they are labeled, conjugated, or joined together with dyes. The fluorescent dye used most often in clinical virology is fluorescein-isothiocyanate (FITC), which produces apple-green fluorescence. A counterstain such as Evans blue, which masks weak nonspecific staining by FITC and stains background tissues a red-orange color, is often included in the conjugate preparation.

Direct immunofluorescence methods are used for identification of many viral antigens. In direct immunofluorescence, a conjugate of known specificity is reacted with a virus-infected cell preparation fixed on a microscope slide (Fig. 2–6). If the antibodies are specific for the antigen,

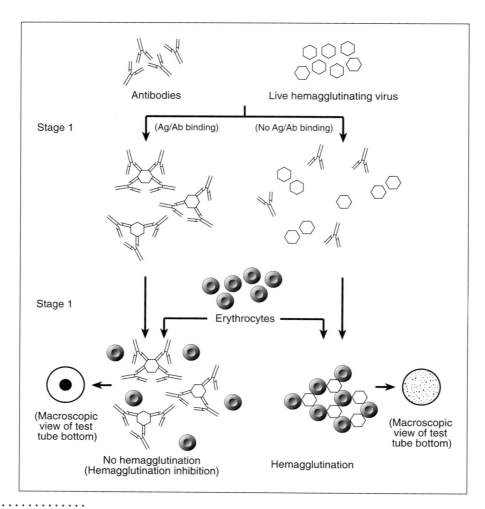

FIGURE 2–5 HEMAGGLUTINATION INHIBITION TESTING is performed in two stages. In stage one hemagglutinating viruses and antibodies are mixed. In stage two erythrocytes are added. If the antibodies bind to the virus in stage one, the virus is inhibited and fails to hemagglutinate the erythrocytes. If the antibodies do not bind to the virus in stage one, the virus remains active and hemagglutinates the erythrocytes in stage two. Hemagglutination appears as a layer or "shield" of tiny aggregates in the bottom of the tube. Unagglutinated cells settle into a button in the center of the bottom of the tube. (Ag/Ab = antigen-antibody.)

antigen-antibody complexes form, and, after unbound conjugate is washed away, fluorescence is seen when the preparation is observed with a fluorescence microscope. If the conjugate is not specific for the antigen, antigen-antibody complexes do not form, and no fluorescence is seen when the test is read. Most direct immunofluorescence methods require only 30 to 40 minutes to complete. Unfortunately, direct immunofluorescence cannot be used for detection or identification of all viruses. However, several clinically significant human pathogens, including herpes simplex types 1 and 2 and respiratory syncytial virus, can be identified by direct immunofluorescence. High-quality monoclonal antibodies are used in most of the direct immunofluorescence methods marketed commercially.

Indirect immunofluorescence techniques are used in the virology laboratory for identification of both antigens and antibodies. Indirect immunofluorescence assays are performed in two stages (Fig. 2–7). In stage one, unlabeled antibodies are reacted with infected cells that are fixed to a glass microscope slide. After an incubation period, smears are rinsed to wash away any unbound antibodies. In stage two of the assay, fluorescein-labeled antispecies

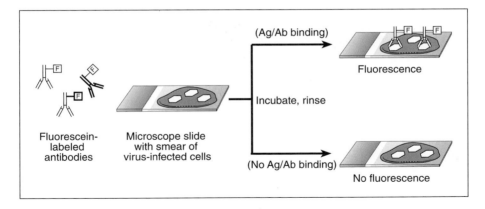

....
FIGURE 2–6 DIRECT IMMUNOFLUORESCENCE. Fluorescein-labeled antibodies are applied to material fixed on a microscope slide. If the antibodies bind to the viral antigens in the material, fluorescence will be visible when the smear is observed with a fluorescence microscope. If the antibodies do not recognize and bind to the antigens in the material fixed on the slide, the antibodies will be rinsed away, and no fluorescence will be seen. (Ag/Ab = antigen-antibody.)

globulin ("conjugate"), usually with counterstain included, is added. The type of conjugate is determined by the species of the antibodies used in stage one. For example, if mouse monoclonal antibodies are used in stage one, then FITC-labeled antimouse globulin is used in stage two. If human serum (antibodies) are used in stage one, then FITC-labeled antihuman globulin is used in stage two. After an incubation period and rinsing, the smear is viewed with a fluorescence microscope. If the antibodies added in stage one attach to the antigen,

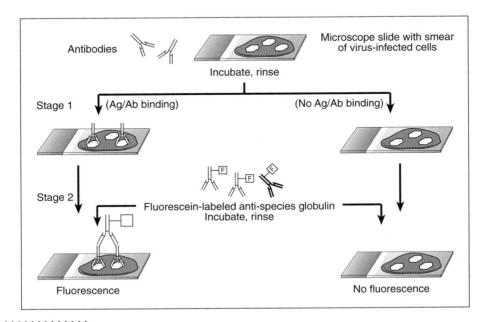

....
FIGURE 2–7 INDIRECT IMMUNOFLUORESCENCE. Testing is performed in two stages. In stage one unlabeled antibodies are applied to material fixed on a microscope slide. In stage two fluorescein-labeled antispecies globulin is added. If the unlabeled antibodies bind to viral antigens in stage one, the antispecies globulin binds to those bound antibodies during stage two, and fluorescence is seen when the smear is examined with the fluorescence microscope. If no antibodies bind in stage one, the fluorescein-labeled antispecies globulin is unable to bind in stage two, and no fluorescence is seen. (Ag/Ab = antigen-antibody.)

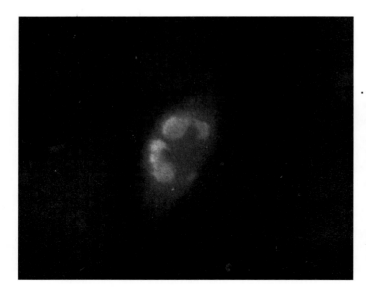

. . . .
FIGURE 2–8 RESULTS OF AN INDIRECT IMMUNOFLUORESCENCE TEST FOR DETECTION OF CYTOMEGALOVIRUS (CMV) IMMUNOGLOBULIN M (IGM). In the first staining step, CMV IgM in the patient's serum bound to CMV inclusions in the infected cells. In the second step, fluorescein-labeled antihuman IgM was added. The labeled antihuman IgM bound to the CMV IgM that had bound to the CMV antigen in the first staining step, and fluorescence is seen.

the labeled antispecies globulin binds to those bound antibodies in stage two, and fluorescence is seen when the antigen smear is observed. If the antibodies in stage one are not specific for the antigen and do not attach, the labeled antispecies globulin does not bind in stage two, and fluorescence is not observed. Indirect immunofluorescence methods usually require 1.5 to 2.0 hours to complete.

Indirect immunofluorescence is the testing principle used for detection of several types of respiratory viral antigens, including influenza and parainfluenza virus antigens. When indirect immunofluorescence is used for identification of unknown viral antigens, a preparation of virus-infected material is fixed to the microscope slide. The antibodies that are added in the first stage of testing are viral antibodies, usually mouse monoclonal antibodies, of known specificity. For example, if the unknown virus antigen in the sample is thought to be influenza type A virus, then monoclonal antibodies against influenza A will be used in stage one. After incubation and rinsing, fluorescein-labeled antimouse globulin is added.

Indirect immunofluorescence is also used for identification of viral antibodies in human serum. For identification of viral antibodies, a preparation of cells or tissue known to be infected with a certain virus is used to make the antigen smear that is fixed to the microscope slide. In stage one of the assay, the patient's serum is added to the antigen smear. After incubation and rinsing, fluorescein-labeled antihuman globulin, usually antihuman immunoglobulin (Ig) G, is added. The specificity of the conjugate can be varied to aid in detection of antibodies of other classes, for example, IgM and IgA (see Chapter 6). Figure 2–8 shows the typical fluorescence observed in an indirect immunofluorescence test for cytomegalovirus IgM. Indirect immunofluorescence is the test principle used in identification of viral antibodies such as Epstein-Barr virus antibodies and respiratory syncytial virus antibodies.

The hallmark advantage of the immunofluorescence methods is that the fluorescence can be visually correlated to antigenic structures in virus-infected cells. In Chapter 5 the characteristic distribution of fluorescence in cells infected with various viruses is described. The visual examination required in immunofluorescence methods allows the investigator to differentiate fluorescence caused by nonspecific binding from that of virus-specific binding. Nonspecific binding may be seen in clinical samples that contain mucus or lymphocytes. False fluorescence may also result from clumps of unbound, precipitated conjugate. In addition, nonspecific binding is sometimes seen in cells infected by members of the Herpesviridae family. These viruses produce Fc binding receptors in the cytoplasm of infected cells; these receptors may bind antibodies nonspecifically by their Fc pieces, which results in nonspecific fluorescence. Other chapters in this text provide additional information about immunofluorescence testing in viral antigen detection (Chapter 5) and in viral antibody testing (Chapter 6).

Complement Fixation

Complement fixation is a versatile system that can be used to identify either viral antigens or viral antibodies. The complement fixation assay is based on the principle that complement, a lytic agent, is bound (fixed) by antigen-antibody complexes. Complement fixation is a two-stage examination (Fig. 2–9). In stage one, antibody, antigen, and complement are mixed and incubated for 18 to 24 hours. If the antibody is specific for the antigen, antigen-antibody complexes form, and the complement is fixed. In stage two, antibody-coated erythrocytes, which serve as antigen-antibody complexes, are added to the stage one mixture and incubated for 1 to 2 hours. If the complement was fixed by antigen-antibody complexes in stage one, it is no longer active or available to act on the antibody-coated erythrocytes, and the erythrocytes remain intact and are not hemolyzed. Therefore, an absence of hemolysis indicates that the antigen and antibody of stage one were specific for each other.

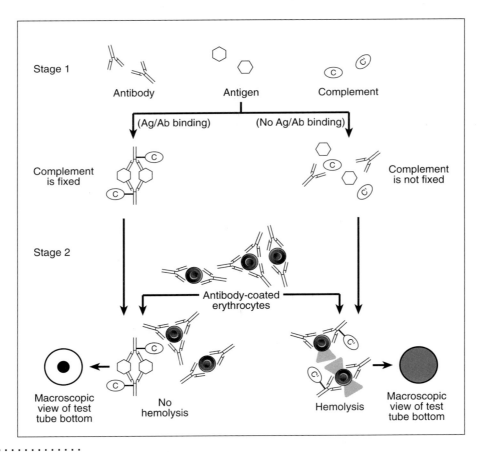

. . . .
FIGURE 2–9 COMPLEMENT FIXATION TESTING. Antigen, antibody, and complement are mixed in stage one. If the antigen and antibody bind, complement is fixed and will be unable to act on antibody-coated erythrocytes added in stage two. The final reaction appears as an absence of hemolysis. If the antigen and antibody do not bind in stage one, complement is not fixed and remains free to act on the antibody-coated erythrocytes added in stage two. The final result appears as hemolysis of the erythrocytes. Unhemolyzed cells settle into a button in the center of the bottom of the test tube, whereas hemolyzed cells produce a reddish discoloration of fluid with very few if any cells settled in the center of the bottom of the tube. (Ag/Ab = antigen-antibody.)

In stage one, if the antibody is not specific for the antigen, no antigen-antibody complexes form; thus, complement is not fixed and remains free and active. When the antibody-coated erythrocytes are added in stage two, the active complement recognizes the coated erythrocytes as antigen-antibody complexes, to which it fixes or binds; it is then triggered through its cascade, resulting in hemolysis of the erythrocytes. Hemolysis signals that the antigen and antibody in stage one were not specific for each other.

The complement fixation testing procedure is lengthy and requires careful quantitation of all test components and rigid adherence to detailed procedures. When complement fixation is used for identification of an unknown virus, the antigen in stage one is a suspension of cells infected with virus of unknown type, and the antibody in stage one is a known viral antibody. At present, complement fixation is seldom used for identification of unknown viruses because newer, less cumbersome methods are available. When complement fixation is used for identification of unknown antibodies, the antigen in stage one is a suspension of known virus, and the antibody is supplied by adding the patient's serum. Complement fixation is commonly used for measurement of antibodies against influenza viruses and parainfluenza viruses.

Enzyme Immunoassay

Enzyme immunoassay is the basis for many assays that can be used for identification of either antibodies or antigens. The detection system involves antibodies conjugated with active enzymes. The test result is determined by observing or measuring the color change produced through the action of the active enzyme on its substrate.

One very simple qualitative application of enzyme immunoassay is **immunoperoxidase staining** of materials, such as patients' clinical samples or cells from virus-infected cell cultures, fixed on microscope slides. Immunoperoxidase staining involves the use of antibodies that are conjugated with the enzyme peroxidase. The staining may be direct or indirect and is performed in sequences that are comparable to those of direct and indirect immunofluorescence staining. The immunoperoxidase techniques require one additional step: the addition of a substrate solution. Then, in areas of the smears to which the peroxidase-labeled antibodies have bound, a color change occurs because of the action of the peroxidase enzyme on the substrate solution. Finally, the preparation is viewed with a standard light microscope. An alteration in color will be seen in the areas to which the peroxidase-labeled antibodies have bound.

Immunoperoxidase staining has been applied in the clinical laboratory for detection of many viral antigens and antibodies, although this staining is not used as frequently as immunofluorescence. The obvious advantage of immunoperoxidase over immunofluorescence is that no fluorescence microscope is required for evaluation of immunoperoxidase stains; a standard light microscope is all that is necessary. Disadvantages of immunoperoxidase methods include the additional time required for color development during the staining process and nonspecific staining that may be due to indigenous peroxidases in some types of clinical specimens.

One additional type of enzyme immunoassay that is similar to immunoperoxidase staining is called immunoblotting and is described later in this chapter.

NONCOMPETITIVE SOLID-PHASE ENZYME IMMUNOASSAY. This is the type used most commonly in clinical virology laboratories. Although the configuration may vary from assay to assay, the basic concepts are consistent for most of these systems. Either the antigens or antibodies in the test system are bound to a solid phase. This solid phase may be the surface of a test tube, the wall of a microwell, or the surface of a plastic bead. In immunoassays for antibody identification, a known viral antigen is usually bound to the solid phase, whereas in immunoassays for antigen identification, a known viral antibody is bound to the solid phase. Then the solid phase is exposed to the unknown or test material. In immunoassays for antibody identification, the test material is the patient's serum, and in immunoassays for antigen identification, the test material is a clinical sample (e.g., from the throat, a lesion, or the genital area) collected from the patient or a suspension of virus-infected cells from a cell culture. After the test material is allowed to react with the solid phase and the unbound reactants are rinsed away, a preparation of enzyme-labeled antibodies is added. After incubation and rinsing, a substrate solution is added; the enzyme (attached to the antibodies) acts on this substrate to produce a color change. The substrate solution in the tube is observed for a change in color. The color change may be measured visually but is most often quantitated spectrophotometrically.

A diagram of an enzyme immunoassay for identification of antibodies is provided in Figure 2–10. In this assay system, the solid phase is the wall of a test tube; known viral antigen is bound to this surface. Initially, the patient's serum is added to the test tube. After incubation and rinsing, a preparation of enzyme-labeled antihuman IgG is added. If the patient's serum contains viral antibodies specific for the viral antigens bound on the wall of the tube, the patient's antibodies bind in step 1. The bound antibodies are recognized and bound by the enzyme-labeled antihuman IgG conjugate added in the next step. If the patient's serum does not contain viral antibodies, no binding of the patient's antibodies occurs, and the enzyme-labeled antihuman IgG conjugate is unable to bind.

In the next step of the enzyme immunoassay, a substrate solution is added to the reactants, incubated, and observed for a change in color. A color change indicates that the enzyme-labeled antihuman IgG conjugate has bound to the patient's antibodies that were bound to antigen in the first step. The color change results from the action of the active enzyme on the substrate solution. A lack of color change indicates that the enzyme-labeled antihuman IgG conjugate failed to bind because there were no patient antibodies bound in the first step. Therefore, enzyme-labeled antibodies are absent, and there is no enzyme to act on the substrate to produce the color change. Enzyme immunoassays that use coated test tubes or microwells are available for detection of a variety of viral antibodies.

In Figure 2–11 another configuration for an enzyme immunoassay for antibody identification is shown. This system uses a plastic bead as the solid-phase surface to which known viral antigen is bound. In the system, the first step involves placing the antigen-coated bead in a dilution of the patient's serum. If the patient's serum contains specific viral antibodies, they will bind to the antigens on the bead. If specific viral antibodies are not present, no binding of patient's antibodies will take place. After an incubation period and rinsing, the bead is transferred to a solution containing enzyme-labeled antihuman IgG conjugate. If antibodies were bound in step one, the enzyme-labeled antihuman IgG conjugate will bind to the bound antibodies. If no antibodies were bound in step one, the enzyme-labeled antihuman antibodies will not be able to bind. After incubation and rinsing, the bead is transferred to a substrate solution. If bound enzyme-labeled antihuman IgG conjugate is present, the enzyme will act on the substrate to produce a color change. If the enzyme-labeled antihuman IgG conjugate was not able to bind, no enzyme will be present, and no color change will occur. The bead-type enzyme system is often used for detection of human immunodeficiency virus type 1 (HIV-1) antibodies as well as other viral antibodies such as hepatitis A and B.

When enzyme immunoassay is used for detection of viral antigens, the component of the system that is attached to the solid phase is an antiviral antibody of known specificity. In antigen detection enzyme immunoassays, the patient's clinical sample (a fecal sample, throat sample, lesion sample, or serum) or a suspension of virus-infected cells from a cell culture tube is exposed to the antibody-coated solid phase. The antibodies on the solid phase function in "capturing" any viral antigen that is present in the sample. In some enzyme immunoassays, enzyme-conjugated antiviral antibodies are added in the first step along with the patient's sample (Fig. 2–12), whereas in other immunoassays the enzyme-labeled antibodies are not added until the initial reactants have been incubated and carefully rinsed. The enzyme-labeled antibodies bind to the viral antigen that was captured by the antibodies on the solid phase. After incubation and rinsing, a substrate solution is added, and the enzyme attached to the bound antibodies acts on the substrate to produce a color change. Both microwell- and bead-based enzyme immunoassays are used for viral antigen detection. Antigens of HIV-1, rotavirus, respiratory syncytial virus, and herpes simplex virus may be detected in these systems.

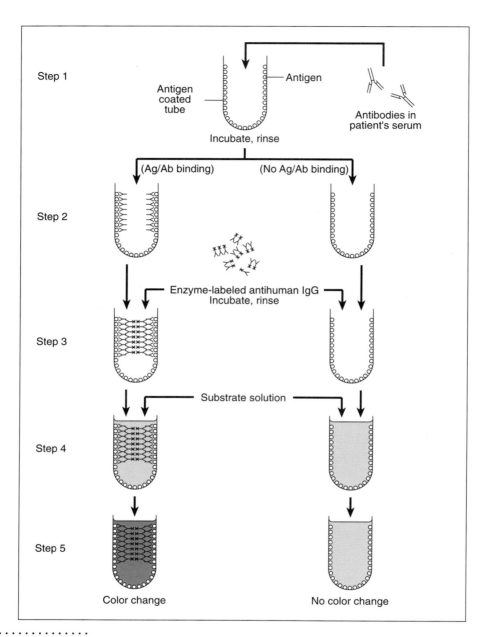

- - - - - - - - - - - - - -
FIGURE 2–10 SOLID-PHASE ENZYME IMMUNOASSAY FOR ANTIBODY DETEC-TION. In step one the patient's serum is added to a tube or microwell that is coated with known antigen. In step two, if the antibodies recognize the antigen, they will bind. In step three, enzyme-labeled antihuman immunoglobulin G (IgG) is added, and the bound antibodies will be recognized and bound. In step four, when a substrate solution is added, the enzymes on the bound enzyme-labeled antihuman IgG will act on the substrate to produce a color change (shown in step five). Conversely, if the patient's antibodies do not bind to antigens on the tube surface in step one, the enzyme-labeled antihuman IgG is unable to bind. When substrate is added, there is no enzyme to act on the substrate, and there is no color change. (Ag/Ab = antigen-antibody.)

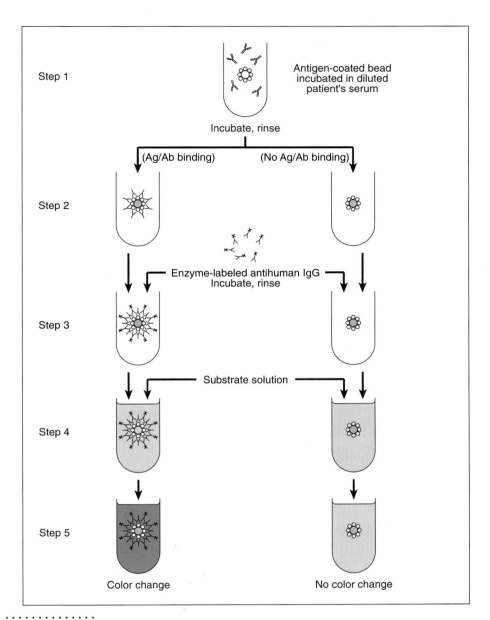

FIGURE 2–11 SOLID-PHASE BEAD ENZYME IMMUNOASSAY FOR IDENTIFICA-TION OF ANTIBODIES. In this configuration, the known antigen is attached to the surface of a bead. This bead is exposed to various solutions, starting with unknown antibodies in the patient's serum (steps one and two), then enzyme-labeled antihuman immunoglobulin G (IgG) (step three), and then substrate solution (step four). Color change (shown in step five) will be seen if antibodies are bound to the antigen on the bead in step two. If the antibodies do not recognize and bind to the antigen in step two, the enzyme-labeled antihuman IgG will not bind, and no color change will result after addition of substrate. (Ag/Ab = antigen-antibody.)

COMPETITIVE SOLID-PHASE ENZYME IMMUNOASSAY. This is another type of solid-phase enzyme immunoassay used in clinical virology. In competitive solid-phase systems, as in noncompetitive solid-phase systems, either an antigen or antibody is bound to the solid phase. In contrast, in the competitive system a measured amount of known enzyme-labeled component (of the same specificity as the component being detected in the assay) is added along with the

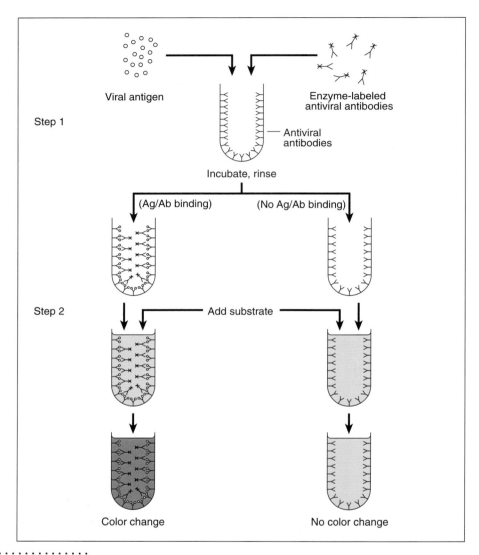

. . . .
FIGURE 2–12 MODIFIED ENZYME IMMUNOASSAY FOR ANTIGEN DETECTION. In step one, known antibodies (attached to a solid phase), the test material, which may contain antigen, and enzyme-labeled antiviral antibodies are mixed. If the antibodies on the solid phase recognize and bind antigen in the test material, the labeled antibodies bind to the bound antigen. When substrate is added in step two, a color change occurs. If the antibodies on the solid phase do not recognize and bind antigen in the test material, the enzyme-labeled antibodies cannot bind, and no color change occurs when substrate is added. (Ag/Ab = antigen-antibody.)

patient's sample (Fig. 2–13). For example, in a hepatitis B core (HBc) antibody (anti-HBc) detection competitive enzyme immunoassay, a bead coated with HBc antigen is used. The antigen-coated bead is incubated in a mixture of patient's serum (possibly containing anti-HBc) and enzyme-labeled anti-HBc. The enzyme-labeled anti-HBc "competes" against the unlabeled anti-HBc from the patient's sample to bind to the antigens on the bead. After incubation and rinsing, the bead is incubated in a substrate solution. If the patient's sample contains anti-HBc, the patient's unlabeled anti-HBc and little, if any, of the labeled anti-HBc will bind to the bead; the color of the substrate will probably change only slightly or not at all when the bead is incubated in the substrate solution. If the patient's sample does not contain anti-HBc, the labeled anti-HBc will bind to the antigens on the bead, and color change will be obvious when the bead

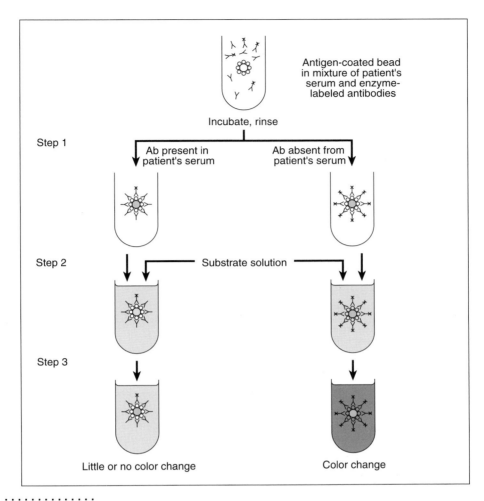

Step 1

Antigen-coated bead
in mixture of patient's
serum and enzyme-
labeled antibodies

Incubate, rinse

Ab present in
patient's serum

Ab absent from
patient's serum

Step 2 ——— Substrate solution ———

Step 3

Little or no color change

Color change

············
**FIGURE 2–13 COMPETITIVE SOLID-PHASE ENZYME IMMUNOASSAY FOR IDEN-
TIFICATION OF ANTIBODY (Ab).** The known antigen is attached to the surface of a bead.
The bead is incubated in a mixture of the patient's sample (possibly containing the antibody)
and enzyme-labeled antibody. The labeled antibody competes with unlabeled antibodies in
the patient's sample to bind to antigen on the bead. If many antibodies are present in the
patient's sample, many unlabeled patient's antibodies and few labeled antibodies bind to
antigen on the bead. When substrate is added, slight or no color change is seen. If few or no
antibodies are present in the patient's sample, labeled antibodies will bind to the antigen on
the bead. When substrate is added, the color changes.

is incubated in the substrate solution. Therefore, in the competitive immunoassays, the expected
results are the reverse of those expected in noncompetitive systems. A color change signals
presence or positivity in noncompetitive systems, whereas color change indicates absence or
negativity in a competitive immunoassay system.

Solid-phase enzyme immunoassays, in general, are becoming very popular in clinical
laboratories because they are suitable for testing large numbers of samples and they generally
require little technical expertise to perform. Because the color change reactions are objectively
measured by a spectrophotometer, the technologist is not required to make subjective
assessments. The results are produced in the form of continuous-scale numerical readings. With
enzyme immunoassays, as with immunofluorescence testing for antibody detection, the
specificity of the conjugate can be adjusted to aid in making the assay specific for IgM or IgA
(i.e., antihuman IgM conjugate will detect IgM and antihuman IgA will detect IgA; IgA detection
is often performed on saliva).

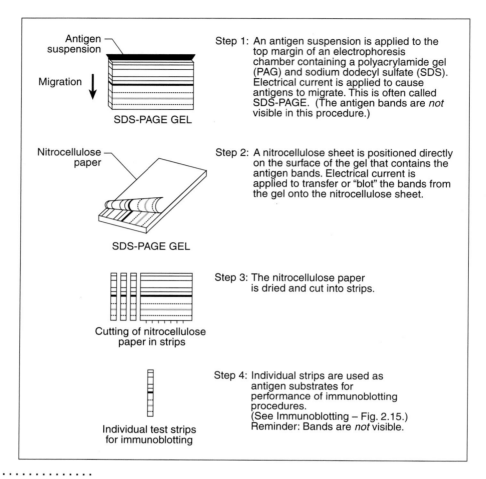

Step 1: An antigen suspension is applied to the top margin of an electrophoresis chamber containing a polyacrylamide gel (PAG) and sodium dodecyl sulfate (SDS). Electrical current is applied to cause antigens to migrate. This is often called SDS-PAGE. (The antigen bands are *not* visible in this procedure.)

Step 2: A nitrocellulose sheet is positioned directly on the surface of the gel that contains the antigen bands. Electrical current is applied to transfer or "blot" the bands from the gel onto the nitrocellulose sheet.

Step 3: The nitrocellulose paper is dried and cut into strips.

Step 4: Individual strips are used as antigen substrates for performance of immunoblotting procedures.
(See Immunoblotting – Fig. 2.15.)
Reminder: Bands are *not* visible.

FIGURE 2–14 WESTERN BLOTTING. This technique uses electrophoresis to separate protein antigen suspensions into distinct bands on the basis of molecular weight.

Many enzyme immunoassays, especially those for viral antibody measurement, have been successfully automated. The technologist prepares the samples and the instrument and can then walk away to perform other duties while the automated enzyme immunoassay instrument performs all dilution, mixing, timing, and rinsing steps and adds reagents as needed. The major drawback of the solid-phase enzyme immunoassays is that patterns of reactivity cannot be evaluated to differentiate specific from nonspecific antibody binding, as is done in the evaluation of immunofluorescence results.

Several new, rapid (10–20 minutes) enzyme immunoassay systems are available in which the test system is a self-contained unit assembled in a test packet format. In one such system, the test packet contains a membrane on which viral antibody is attached. After extraction or filtration of the patient's clinical sample, the sample is poured onto the membrane, and viral antigen in the sample is captured by the viral antibodies bound to the membrane. Then enzyme-labeled viral antibodies are added; these bind to bound viral antigens. After rinsing to remove unattached antibodies, a substrate solution is added, and color develops on the membrane in the area, usually a triangular or X-shaped area, at which the original viral antibodies were attached.

In a second type of packet enzyme immunoassay system, a pretreatment of the patient's clinical sample is required. This includes filtering and then mixing the sample in a tube with microparticles coated with viral antibodies and with biotin-labeled viral antibodies. This mixture is poured through the test packet, and enzyme-labeled antibiotin antibodies are added followed by substrate. Color development occurs on the pad in the packet. Packet systems are available for detection of rotavirus and respiratory syncytial virus. These systems are expensive but are useful when a rapid result is needed and trained virologists are not available.

Immunoblotting

Immunoblotting is another application of enzyme immunoassay used in the clinical virology laboratory. Immunoblotting combines electrophoretic separation techniques with antibody detection methods. Blotting, which refers to the transfer of DNA, RNA, or protein from electrophoretic gels to a membrane, is used to prepare the antigen, and an immunoassay method is used to react antibodies with the blotted antigen to identify or characterize either the blotted antigen or the antibodies [4]. Immunoblotting is often casually referred to as Western blotting because the antigen used in the test system is usually a protein antigen that has been blotted using the Western blotting technique (Fig. 2–14). In the Western blotting procedure, a viral extract is separated using sodium dodecyl sulfate–polyacrylamide gel electrophoresis (SDS-PAGE). Then the resulting (invisible) bands are electrophoretically blotted onto nitrocellulose

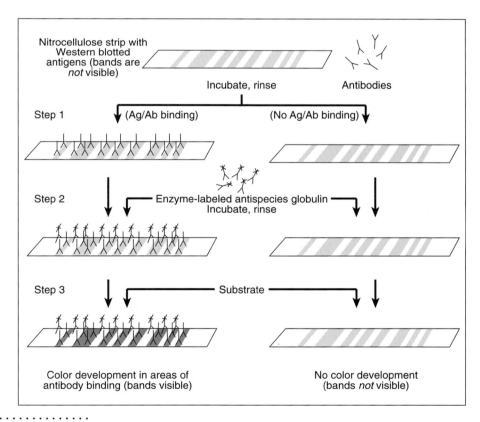

FIGURE 2–15 IMMUNOBLOTTING. The antigen system is a strip containing antigens that have been electrophoretically separated and blotted on nitrocellulose paper (see Fig. 2–14, Western blot). In step one antibodies are added to the strip; the antibodies will bind to the strip in areas where they recognize antigenic components. In step two enzyme-labeled antispecies globulin is added and binds to antibodies bound in step one. When a substrate solution is added, color develops in the areas where the antibodies bound in the initial staining steps. If the antibodies in step one do not recognize any components in the antigen preparation, they do not bind, enzyme-labeled antispecies globulin does not bind in step two, no color development occurs after addition of substrate, and no bands are seen. (Ag/Ab = antigen-antibody.)

paper, which is dried and cut into strips; each strip serves as the antigen substrate for one immunoblotting test. Each of the invisible antigen bands on the strip is related to the structure of the intact virus. This relationship is important in determining the outcome of the immunoblotting assay.

The steps in the immunoblotting test proper for identification of serum antibodies are shown in Figure 2–15. The testing is performed much like an indirect immunoperoxidase stain except that the antigen is the Western blot strip rather than infected cells fixed to a microscope slide. The sequence of staining steps involves flooding the immunoblot antigen strip with antibodies. Then, after incubating and rinsing, the appropriate enzyme-labeled conjugate is added followed by substrate. The immunoblot result is not evaluated microscopically to determine color change; rather, the test strip is observed grossly. Reactivity is signaled by the presence of colored bands at appropriate positions and of sufficient intensity on the strip. The test bands are compared with bands produced by positive control samples to characterize the bands. The immunoblotting technique is used extensively in clinical virology in the confirmatory testing for HIV-1 antibodies. Figure 2–16 shows control and patients' immunoblot results from HIV-1 antibody immunoblotting assay.

Virus Neutralization

The neutralization test is based on the principle that a live virus, when acted on by its specific antibody, will be neutralized and thus incapable of infecting susceptible cells. The neutralization procedure is performed in two stages (Fig. 2–17). In the first stage, live virus and antibodies are reacted. In stage two, aliquots of the stage one mixture are inoculated into susceptible cell cultures. After a suitable incubation period of 5 to 7 days, the host tissue is examined for the presence of cytopathogenic effect. If antibodies bind to the virus in stage one, the virus is neutralized and prevented from infecting the susceptible cell culture to produce a cytopathogenic effect. If antibodies do not bind to the virus in stage one, the virus remains active and infects the susceptible cells to produce a cytopathogenic effect.

Neutralization can be used for identification of either unknown virus or viral antibodies. When an unknown virus is to be identified, a suspension of the unknown virus is mixed with antibodies of known specificity in stage one of testing. If unknown antibodies are to be identified, a suspension of known virus is mixed with the patient's serum that contains the antibodies of unknown specificity.

In all virus neutralization testing, the virus must be carefully quantitated before the actual

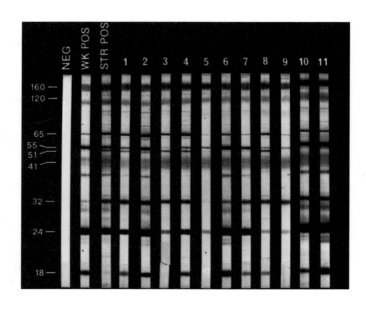

FIGURE 2–16 HUMAN IMMUNODEFICIENCY VIRUS TYPE 1 (HIV-1) IMMUNOBLOTS. Western blotted antigen strips (molecular weights in kilodaltons for antigen bands are shown on the left) were immunoblotted with control or patients' serum. (Multiple bands, indicating antibody binding, are present on all strips except the negative control. Neg = negative control serum; WK POS = weak positive control serum; STR POS = strong positive control serum, 1–11 = 11 sera positive for HIV-1 antibodies.)

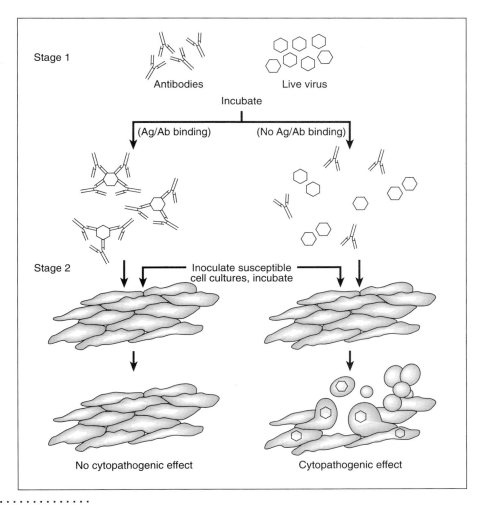

. . . .
FIGURE 2–17   VIRAL NEUTRALIZATION. This testing is performed in two stages. In the first stage, live virus and antibodies are mixed. Susceptible cell cultures are inoculated with the mixtures in stage two. If the antibodies bind to the virus in stage one, the virus is neutralized and unable to infect the susceptible cells. If the antibodies do not bind to the virus in stage one, the virus remains active and infects the susceptible cells to produce cytopathogenic effect. (Ag/Ab = antigen-antibody.)

neutralization test is performed. A procedure called a viral titration (see Appendix) is used to quantitate the virus. Virus neutralization procedures provide the most accurate results and are the reference standard against which viral identification methods are compared. Groups of viruses, such as the enteroviruses, which include many closely related serotypes, can be differentiated only by neutralization testing. A procedure for enterovirus identification by neutralization is provided in the Appendix.

MOLECULAR DIAGNOSTIC TECHNIQUES

Several contemporary viral identification techniques are not immunological and do not depend on binding of antibodies and antigens. These technologies are based on the molecular biology of the viruses, specifically on identification of unique sequences within the nucleic acid of the virus. This type of identification should be the most specific identification possible because of the nature of the detection method. Through detection of unique amino acid sequences in the nucleic acid of the virus, the unknown viruses can be identified with certainty. These methods are not widely available in clinical virology at this writing; however, their concepts are essential for understanding the technology that likely will soon be a part of the diagnostic clinical virology laboratory.

Unique regions have been identified in the nucleic acid sequences of most viruses. Enzyme-labeled or radiolabeled nucleic acid sequences complementary to these unique regions are now manufactured commercially; these labeled complementary sequences are called **nucleic acid probes** and are capable of hybridizing to (attaching to) complementary nucleic acid strands of DNA or RNA to form stable double strands. Specimens containing viral nucleic acid can be treated (usually by heating) to cause the double strands of nucleic acids to separate and thus become susceptible to hybridization with the nucleic acid probe. During the process of hybridization, any single-stranded nucleic acid will attempt to pair up with (hybridize to) any complementary strand. In this process, the labeled probe competes with complementary strands in the mixture for binding to the target [5]. The hybridized nucleic acid is harvested and subjected to a detection process that confirms that the labeled probe was hybridized. The detection process will vary depending on the type of label attached to the probe. Probes labeled with radioactive labels such as phosphorus (^{32}P) or iodine (^{125}I) are detected through the use of x-ray film or radioactive counting. Nonradioactive labels such as enzymes or fluorescent dyes are detected through observation or measurement of either color change reactions or fluorescence.

The probing process may be carried out on clinical samples collected from the patient or on material from virus-infected cell cultures. The material may be fixed to a microscope slide and "probed" in a process termed *in situ* nucleic acid probing (described later), or the material may be denatured in suspension and probed. Because viral nucleic acid may be in very small quantities in infected material collected from the patient, the probing process is sometimes preceded by a technique called polymerase chain reaction (PCR), which amplifies the amount of nucleic acid present.

In Situ Hybridization

In *in situ* **hybridization** methods, cells or tissue specimens are fixed on a glass microscope slide. The slide is treated, often by heating, to denature the target viral DNA, causing the double strands to separate. Then labeled DNA probe is added. The probe will hybridize to complementary sequences in the denatured target viral DNA. Nonhybridized probe is rinsed away, and a substrate solution is applied. The smear is examined microscopically to determine whether or not probe was hybridized. The steps in one *in situ* DNA probe technique are shown in Figure 2–18.

The visual microscopic assessment of the *in situ* probing results allows the virologist to determine which cells are infected and provides relatively sensitive detection in samples with many infected cells. Samples with few infected cells may be misidentified as uninfected [5].

Polymerase Chain Reaction

PCR is an amplification technique used for *in vitro* synthesis of specific DNA sequences [6]. Initially, a target nucleic acid (DNA or RNA) is isolated from tissue or fluids from the patient or from infected cell cultures. If the target nucleic acid is RNA, it must be converted to DNA before the process can begin. Then the DNA is amplified enzymatically by PCR. PCR is a cyclical process requiring a DNA template (the target viral DNA), a buffer system, the four deoxynucleotide triphosphates (deoxyadenosine triphosphate, deoxythymidine triphosphate, deoxycytidine triphosphate, and deoxyguanosine triphosphate), primers, and DNA polymerase. Primers are oligonucleotides with sequences that are complementary to specific sequences that flank the target segment of DNA that will be amplified. The primers determine the specificity and size of the product. When the primers anneal to the DNA, the DNA polymerase, using the

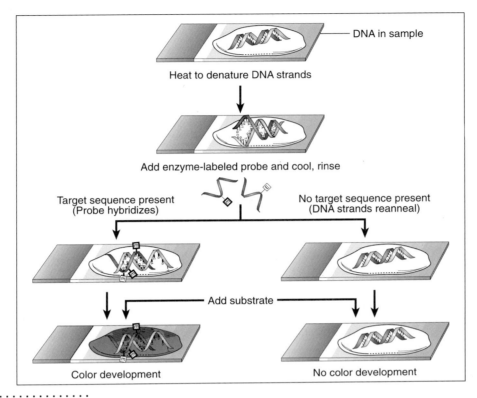

DNA in sample

Heat to denature DNA strands

Add enzyme-labeled probe and cool, rinse

Target sequence present
(Probe hybridizes)

No target sequence present
(DNA strands reanneal)

Add substrate

Color development

No color development

FIGURE 2–18 *IN SITU* **HYBRIDIZATION METHOD.** The specimen is fixed to a microscope slide. The slide is heated to cause DNA strands to denature and separate; then enzyme-labeled probe is added, and the slide is cooled to allow the probe to hybridize to target sequences. Substrate is added. If the probe has hybridized, color will develop in the area where the hybridized probe is located. If the sample does not contain target sequences, the probe does not hybridize, and no color develops when substrate is added.

deoxynucleotide triphosphates as substrates, initiates replication of the target sequence. The buffer system provides the optimal environment for polymerase activity.

Each cycle of PCR involves three steps [6] (Fig. 2–19): (1) Target DNA is denatured by heating the reaction mixture to 94°C for approximately 1 minute; this results in separation of the DNA strands; (2) reactants are cooled to 25 to 60°C to allow the primers to anneal to the template at complementary sites near areas of unique nucleotide sequences; and (3) the temperature is increased to allow optimal polymerase activity. The DNA polymerase in the reaction mixture will add deoxyribonucleotide bases, resulting in duplication of the target sequence. This cyclical process is repeated up to 40 times to amplify the original DNA in an exponential fashion. The cyclic process can be carried out by an instrument called a thermocycler, which increases and lowers temperature as needed to facilitate the PCR reaction.

The amplified product is called the amplicon [7]. The amplicon can be detected by either hybridization with a probe or visualization after electrophoresis and staining. With proper technique, even a single target molecule can be amplified by PCR and then detected.

There are several major advantages of PCR: (1) only a small amount of clinical material is required, (2) viruses that cannot be isolated in standard cell culture systems can be detected, and (3) nonviable viruses can be identified. Also, by the use of PCR, the waiting period required for viral proliferation in culture is eliminated. PCR is often used in conjunction with nucleic acid probe technology to enhance the quantity of target nucleic acid.

At this writing, PCR is still too cumbersome, expensive, and nonstandardized for most clinical diagnostic virology laboratories. With additional modifications and technical improvements,

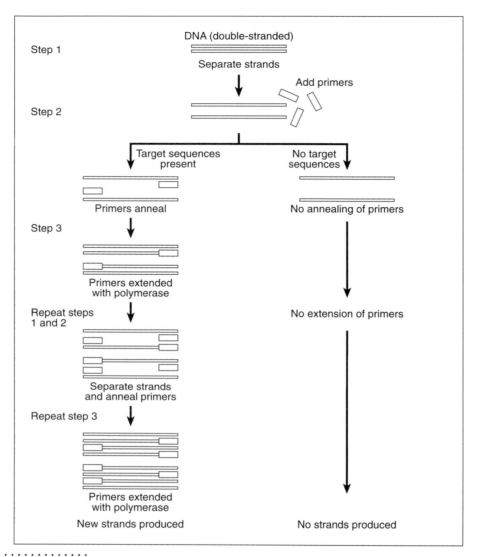

FIGURE 2–19 POLYMERASE CHAIN REACTION (PCR). PCR is a DNA amplification technique involving three steps. In step one samples are treated to cause separation of DNA strands. In step two primers are added, which should anneal to strands containing target sequences. In step three primers extend with polymerase to produce new complementary DNA strands. The same steps are repeated to produce more new strands. If the sample does not contain target sequences, the primers fail to anneal, there is no extension of the primers, and no new DNA strands are produced.

PCR will become an important tool in the diagnostic virology laboratory. Applications of PCR in clinical virology are described in Chapter 10.

SENSITIVITY, SPECIFICITY, AND PREDICTIVE VALUES

For all laboratory methods, terms are applied to describe or quantify how effectively the method performs or to determine to what extent a test can be relied on to confirm or exclude the presence of the analyte (antigen or antibody) in question [8]. **Sensitivity** refers to the ability of the test to detect positive or abnormal results. A **100% sensitive** method will detect **all** positives, even when the test substance is present in very small quantities. An **insensitive** method will detect fewer positives and may be **falsely negative,** especially when only a small quantity of test substance is present. To evaluate test sensitivity, known **positive** samples are tested. Then a numerical value for test sensitivity is calculated using the equation shown in Table 2–2.

Specificity is the term used as a measure of the capacity of a given testing procedure to remain negative when the proper test substance is absent or, conversely, to yield positive results only when the proper test substance is present. A **100% specific** method will yield positive results only when the desired antibody (or antigen) is present. A method with **low specificity** may yield **falsely positive** results in the absence of the appropriate test substance. This false positivity is found most often in the presence of antibodies (or antigens) that are closely related to the desired product (this is called cross-reactivity). To evaluate test specificity, known **negative** samples are tested. Then a numerical value for test specificity is calculated using the equation shown in Table 2–2.

Both terms, sensitivity and specificity, may be used to describe the capacity of a given test method to confirm or support disease diagnoses. The sensitivity or specificity of a test in disease diagnosis may differ from that of the test in detecting a particular test substance, especially in cases in which the test substance may be found in individuals who do not have the disease in question.

For example, in syphilis, an antibody called reagin is produced. Laboratory methods are both sensitive and specific in detection of reagin. Reagin, however, is produced occasionally by individuals with infectious mononucleosis, leprosy, pregnancy, and so on. Such individuals may have positive reagin test results, but they do not have syphilis. Therefore, reagin tests have high specificity for reagin antibody, but they do not have high specificity in confirming a diagnosis of syphilis. In systems such as this, the positive reagin test result in patients who do not have syphilis is described as a **biologic false positive.** Such false-positive results do not represent a technical failure of the testing method; this situation simply represents the complexity of diagnosis of diseases in which individuals may produce unusual antibodies.

Although the sensitivity and specificity of the test method are valuable in evaluating how well the test will perform in the laboratory, another factor, the **predictive value** of the result, may give even more helpful information about test results. The predictive value is dependent on sensitivity, specificity, and prevalence or frequency of appearance of the result in question. Predictive values for positive and negative results can be calculated according to the equations shown in Table 2–2.

Table 2–3 provides an example demonstrating the importance of predictive values. This example involves a test for detection of influenza virus type A antigen in throat swab samples, which has demonstrated a sensitivity of 90% and a specificity of 95%. These sensitivity and

TABLE 2–2 EQUATIONS FOR CALCULATING SENSITIVITY, SPECIFICITY, AND PREDICTIVE VALUES

TERM	EQUATION
Sensitivity	$\dfrac{\text{No. of true positives}}{\text{No. of true positives + no. of false negatives}} \times 100$
Specificity	$\dfrac{\text{No. of true negatives}}{\text{No. of true negatives + no. of false positives}} \times 100$
Predictive value of a positive result	$\dfrac{\text{No. of true positives}}{\text{No. of true positives + no. of false positives}} \times 100$
Predictive value of a negative result	$\dfrac{\text{No. of true negatives}}{\text{No. of true negatives + no. of false negatives}} \times 100$

True positives are positive samples that are correctly identified as positive. False negatives are samples that are known to be positive but have been misidentified as negative. True negatives are negative samples that are correctly identified as negative. False positives are samples that are known to be negative but have been misidentified as positive.

TABLE 2–3 CALCULATION OF PREDICTIVE VALUES FOR AN INFLUENZA VIRUS DETECTION ASSAY WITH 90% SENSITIVITY AND 95% SPECIFICITY AT 4% AND 25% PREVALENCE

90% SENSITIVITY	95% SPECIFICITY	PREDICTIVE VALUE OF POSITIVE RESULT	PREDICTIVE VALUE OF NEGATIVE RESULT
For 4% prevalence, of 100 samples, 4 will have influenza A and 96 will not have influenza A.			
.90 × 4 = 3.6 true positives	.95 × 96 = 91 true negatives	3.6 true positives	91 true negatives
4 − 3.6 = 0.4 false negatives	96 − 91 = 5 false positives	3.6 true positives + 5 false positives	91 true negatives + 0.4 false negatives
		$\dfrac{3.6}{8.6} \times 100 = 42\%$	$\dfrac{91}{91.4} \times 100 = 99\%$
For 25% prevalence, of 100 samples, 25 will have influenza A and 75 will not have influenza A.			
.90 × 25 = 22.5 true positives	.95 × 75 = 71 true negatives	22.5 true positives	71 true negatives
25 − 22.5 = 2.5 false negatives	75 − 71 = 4 false positives	22.5 true positives + 4 false positives	71 true negatives + 2.5 false negatives
		$\dfrac{22.5}{26.5} \times 100 = 85\%$	$\dfrac{71}{73.5} \times 100 = 97\%$

specificity values are both high and would generally be acceptable for tests used in the clinical laboratory. However, the predictive values of results obtained by this method differ substantially depending on the prevalence of the virus. In the example, predictive values are calculated for prevalences of 4% and 25%.

By comparing the predictive values for the two rates of prevalence of influenza A, 4% versus 25%, the substantial difference between the actual meanings of positive and negative results is clearly shown. In the low-prevalence population, the predictive value of a positive result is very low, whereas in the higher prevalence population, the predictive value of a positive result is in an acceptable range.

REFERENCES

1. Delaat ANC. Primer of Serology. Hagerstown, MD: Harper & Row, 1976.
2. Hyde RM, Patnode RA. Immunology. Reston, VA: Reston Publishing Co, 1978.
3. Bryant NJ. Antigen-antibody reactions in vitro. In Laboratory Immunology and Serology, 3rd ed. Philadelphia: WB Saunders, 1992, pp 88–105.
4. Lee HH, Canavaggio M, Burczak JD. Immunoblotting. In Lennette EH (ed), Laboratory Diagnosis of Viral Infections, 2nd ed. New York: Marcel Dekker, 1992, pp 195–210.
5. Cone RW. Assays for viral nucleic acids. In Lennette EH (ed), Laboratory Diagnosis of Viral Infections, 2nd ed. New York: Marcel Dekker, 1992, pp 175–194.
6. Williams SD, Kwok S. Polymerase chain reaction: applications for viral detection. In Lennette EH (ed), Laboratory Diagnosis of Viral Infections, 2nd ed. New York: Marcel Dekker, 1992, pp 147–173.
7. Campbell SH, Fiedler PN, Persing DH. Nucleic acid amplification techniques in clinical diagnostics. In Rose NR, DeMacario EC, Fahey JL, et al (eds), Manual of Clinical Laboratory Immunology, 4th ed. Washington, DC: American Society for Microbiology, 1992, pp 27–36.
8. Strongin W. Sensitivity, specificity, and predictive value of diagnostic tests: definitions and clinical applications. In Lennette EH (ed), Laboratory Diagnosis of Viral Infections, 2nd ed. New York: Marcel Dekker, 1992.

REVIEW QUESTIONS

1. Which of the following is generally identified as important in successful function of immunoserological assays?
   a. pH above 10
   b. Electrolyte-free environment
   c. High-quality reagents
   d. Extreme antibody excess
2. Prozone reactions can be expected in serum that contains
   a. Excess antigen
   b. Bacterial or fungal contaminants
   c. Very high titers of antibody
   d. Cross-reacting antibodies
3. The prozone reaction may be eliminated by
   a. Incubation
   b. Refrigeration
   c. Dilution
   d. Centrifugation
4. A postzone reaction giving a falsely negative result may occur when
   a. The quantity of antigen is excessive
   b. There is more antibody than antigen
   c. Serum has not been heat inactivated before titering
   d. Antigens are very closely related

5. In direct immunofluorescence testing for detection of viral antigens,
   a. The component fixed on the microscope slide is antiviral antibodies
   b. Fluorescein-labeled antiviral antibodies bind to antigens
   c. A positive (antigen present) result appears as absence of fluorescence
   d. The test is performed in two stages, the second of which involves application of labeled antihuman globulin

6. All of the following phrases describe indirect immunofluorescence testing for identification of antibody **except**
   a. A known antigen is fixed on a slide
   b. A positive (antibody present) result appears as yellow-green fluorescence
   c. Staining is performed in two stages
   d. Fluorescein-labeled antihuman globulin attaches to known antigen used in the test system

7. In the blank to the left of the items in Column A, write the letter of the serological method from Column B with which the item is associated. Methods in Column B may be used more than once.

A	B
___ 1. Antigen-antibody complexes fix one of the test components	a. Complement fixation
___ 2. Soluble antigen plus specific antibody	b. Direct (hem)agglutination
___ 3. Form of antigen is questionable (soluble vs. tiny insoluble)	c. Direct immunofluorescence
___ 4. Antigen is natural part of particulate or cellular antigen	d. Enzyme immunoassay
___ 5. Bacterial cells clumped by antibody	e. Flocculation
___ 6. Antigen-coated particulate carrier	f. Indirect immuno-fluorescence
___ 7. Immunodiffusion	g. Passive (hem)agglutination
___ 8. Virus-specific antibody labeled with fluorescein	h. Precipitation
___ 9. Fluorescein-labeled antispecies globulin	i. Viral hemagglutination
___ 10. Enzyme-labeled antispecies globulin	
___ 11. Live virus is the antigen	

8. All noncompetitive solid-phase enzyme immunoassays have several features in common. One of these is
   a. One of the test components is labeled with fluorescein-isothiocyanate
   b. A color change is produced by the action of complement on erythrocytes
   c. An enzyme label is bound to a solid phase in the system
   d. Bound enzyme acts on a substrate to produce a color change

9. In competitive enzyme immunoassays for detection of antigen,
   a. A positive (antigen present) result appears as a color change
   b. The antibodies on the solid phase are labeled with enzyme
   c. Enzyme-labeled antigens of the same type as those being detected in the assay are incubated with the patient's sample
   d. A simple one-step procedure is all that is required

10. Molecular diagnostics is based on which of the following concepts?
    a. All viruses have unique antigens.
    b. Unique amino acid sequences are found in the DNA of each virus.
    c. Antibodies react specifically with unique determinants on the viral capsid.
    d. Viral replication involves unique enzymes.

11. Which of the following phrases describes the polymerase chain reaction technique?
   a. Is an *in vitro* technique for replicating viral DNA
   b. Is performed by inoculating viruses into susceptible hosts to permit viral replication
   c. Facilitates virus detection by attaching lengthy chains of polymers to viral surface antigens
   d. Initiates a chemical chain reaction that results in production of viral enzymes that can be detected and used to identify the virus

12. A test that is very sensitive
   a. Yields positive results only when the appropriate antibody (or antigen) is present
   b. Is very delicate and requires careful quality control
   c. Uses sensitized (antibody- or antigen-coated) erythrocytes as part of the indicator system
   d. Detects even a very small quantity of the unknown antigen or antibody

13. In testing 100 serum samples that were known to be positive for antibody A, method 1 identified 50 samples as positive and method 2 identified 98 samples as positive. In testing 100 serum samples that were known to be negative for antibody A, method 1 identified 100 samples as negative and method 2 identified 88 samples as negative. Which of the following is true?
   a. Method 1 is more sensitive than method 2.
   b. Method 1 is more specific than method 2.
   c. Method 2 is more sensitive and more specific than method 1.
   d. Method 1 is more sensitive and more specific than method 2.

Virus Isolation in Traditional Cell Cultures

OBJECTIVES

At the completion of this unit of study, the student will be able to do the following:

1. Identify the preferred clinical specimens for viral isolation in various disease syndromes and for isolation of common human viral pathogens.

2. Provide instructions for collection of the various types of clinical samples for virus isolation, including urine, peripheral blood, throat swab, rectal swab, stool, cerebrospinal fluid, sputum, and lesion or vesicle samples. Describe proper containers for specimen collection and transport, and indicate whether viral transport medium should be used.

3. Give directions for short- and long-term storage and for transport of clinical samples for virus isolation studies to both in-house laboratories and off-site reference facilities.

4. Describe viral transport media, listing components and their purposes.

5. Characterize the major categories of cell cultures used in clinical virology, providing origin of cells, ploidy, and potential for successive generations. Give one example of a cell type or line that is included in each category.

6. List the basic steps in the processing of clinical samples for inoculation into cell cultures and explain the purpose of each step.

7. Define cytopathogenic effect (CPE) and give three examples of how CPE may appear.

8. Explain how traditional cell cultures are examined for evidence of viral CPE.

9. Explain the procedure and underlying biological features that are important in hemadsorption, interference challenge, and hemagglutination.

10. Provide examples of viruses that can be definitively identified by immunofluorescence and neutralization techniques.

11. Describe viral neutralization testing, including test principle, viral titration, and viral back titration.

12. List the more common sources and types of cell culture contaminants and possible methods of dealing with these contaminants when they are encountered.

INTRODUCTION

Isolation of viruses in cell cultures is the hallmark of diagnostic virology and has long been the standard against which most other methods are judged. Although the commercial availability of high-quality cell cultures has simplified and streamlined virus isolation, this approach is still the most challenging and technically demanding of the common viral diagnostic avenues.

The sequence of events involved in traditional virus isolation and identification, beginning with selection of appropriate specimens and ending with reporting of results, is diagrammed in Figure 3–1, and each phase of the process is described in this chapter. Although the procedural details may vary at each point depending on the virus in question, the general sequence is uniform for all human viral pathogens that can be isolated in standard cell culture systems. Viruses that are commonly isolated in standard cultures include adenovirus; cytomegalovirus; many of the enteroviruses (Coxsackie B, echovirus, and poliovirus types 1, 2, and 3); herpes simplex virus types 1 and 2; influenza A and B; measles; mumps; parainfluenza types 1, 2, 3, and 4; respiratory syncytial virus; and varicella. Unfortunately, neither all strains of the "culturable" viruses listed nor all human viral pathogens proliferate in standard cell cultures. The names and numbers of viruses isolated during a 2-year period at a large, full-service clinical virology laboratory are shown in Table 3–1.

SELECTING, COLLECTING, STORING, AND TRANSPORTING CLINICAL SPECIMENS FOR VIRUS ISOLATION

The more virus contained in a specimen, the more successful and rapid will be its isolation [1]. Virus shedding is greatest during the acute stage of illness; therefore, specimens should be collected as soon as possible after the onset of illness. The chance of viral recovery is best during the first 3 days after onset and is greatly reduced with many viruses beyond 5 days [2]. Successful isolation and identification of a viral agent from clinical material depend on proper care in selecting, collecting, and transporting the specimen to the laboratory. The importance of proper specimen selection, collection, and transport is summed up as follows [3]:

> No matter where it is done, who it is done by, or what technique(s) are used, it will be wasted time, effort, and resources if the specimens taken are poor, ill timed, or incorrectly handled between the time of collection and the time laboratory procedures are begun.

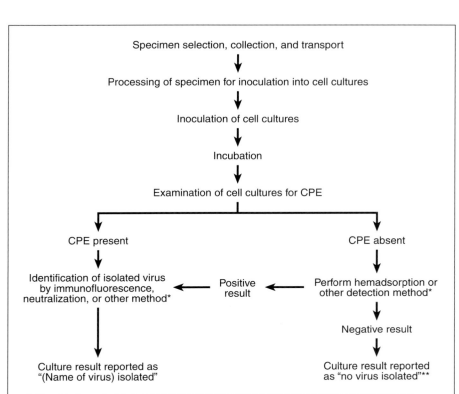

Specimen selection, collection, and transport

↓

Processing of specimen for inoculation into cell cultures

↓

Inoculation of cell cultures

↓

Incubation

↓

Examination of cell cultures for CPE

CPE present		CPE absent
↓		↓
Identification of isolated virus by immunofluorescence, neutralization, or other method*	← Positive result ←	Perform hemadsorption or other detection method*
		↓
		Negative result
↓		↓
Culture result reported as "(Name of virus) isolated"		Culture result reported as "no virus isolated"**

* Other detection methods include interference challenge, plaquing, and hemagglutination; other identification methods include enzyme immunoassay, nucleic acid probe, complement fixation, and hemagglutination inhibition.

** If viruses that do not proliferate in standard cell cultures are suspected, the original specimen can be used as inoculum for alternative culture systems such as eggs or animals.

FIGURE 3–1 SEQUENCE OF VIRUS ISOLATION PROCEDURES (CPE = CYTO-PATHOGENIC EFFECT).

TABLE 3–1 VIRUSES ISOLATED IN STANDARD CELL CULTURES AT THE INDIANA UNIVERSITY VIROLOGY LABORATORY*

VIRUS ISOLATED	NUMBER (%)
Herpes simplex, types 1 and 2	1103(47)
Cytomegalovirus	603(26)
Respiratory syncytial	210 (9)
Adenovirus	156 (7)
Enteroviruses†	103 (4)
Parainfluenza 3	53 (2)
Influenza B	32 (1)
Parainfluenza 1	25 (1)
Influenza A	23 (1)
Parainfluenza 2	14(<1)
Varicella-zoster	6(<1)
Rhinovirus	4(<1)
Parainfluenza 4	3(<1)
Total	2335

*A total of 15,100 samples were cultured during a 2-year period from September 1992 through August 1994.
†Enteroviruses include Coxsackie A and B, echovirus, and poliovirus.

The selection of the specimen is based on the site of infection or clinical syndrome or the virus suspected (Table 3–2). Specimens such as blood, throat swabs, spinal fluid, stools, vesicle fluid, lesion scrapings, and urine are usually submitted for virus isolation.

Swabs are used for collection of many types of samples, especially those from the nose or throat or from skin or genital lesions. Many commercially marketed swabs are suitable for collection of samples for viral culturing. Those with tips made of rayon, Dacron, cotton, or polyester are acceptable for use; however, calcium alginate–tipped swabs have been shown to be toxic for herpes simplex virus [4, 5] and should not be used. For collection of most types of specimens, the swab is used to collect the sample and is then inserted into a liquid medium. The shaft of the swab is broken off, and the swab tip is transported in the liquid medium to the laboratory.

Instructions for proper specimen collection are given in Table 3–3. Clinical samples collected from body sites that are routinely contaminated with usual bacterial and fungal flora should be placed in an antibiotic-containing transport medium. These specimens include throat and genital swabs, lesion samples, sputum, and others. Specimens such as cerebrospinal fluid that are

TABLE 3–2　SELECTION OF SPECIMENS FOR ISOLATION OF VIRUSES IN STANDARD CELL CULTURES*

CLINICAL SYNDROMES: RELATED VIRUSES	CLINICAL SPECIMENS FOR VIRUS ISOLATION							
	Blood	Throat, N/P Swab	Sputum	Vesicle, Lesion	Urine	Stool, Rectal	CSF	Other
Respiratory Tract Infection								
Adenovirus		X	X		O			
Cytomegalovirus	X	X	X		X			BAL
Enteroviruses		X	X			X		
Herpes simplex		X	X					
Influenza		X	X					BAL
Mumps		X			X			
Parainfluenza		X	X					BAL
RSV		X	X					
Exanthem								
Enteroviruses		X		X		X		
Herpes simplex				X				
Measles	X	X			O			Serol
Rubella		X			O		O	Serol
Varicella-zoster	O	O		X				
Gastroenteritis†								
Enteroviruses		X				X		
CNS Infection‡								
Enteroviruses		X				X	X	Brain
Herpes simplex		O		X			X	Brain
Measles	X						X	Serol
Mumps		X			X		X	Serol
Congenital								
Cytomegalovirus	X	X			X			
Enteroviruses		X				X		
Herpes simplex		X		X	O		O	
Rubella		X			O		O	IgM
Infectious Mononucleosis§								
Cytomegalovirus	O	X			X			

*In all syndromes, appropriate biopsy or autopsy tissue may be helpful. Febrile illnesses such as tick, dengue, or yellow fevers are diagnosed through serology.

†Most viral gastroenteritis is caused by unculturable agents: rotavirus and adenovirus types 40, 41 can be detected by enzyme immunoassay; Norwalk virus can be observed with the electron microscope.

‡Rabies and arthropod-borne encephalitis including western equine, eastern equine, St. Louis, and California must be confirmed serologically.

§Mononucleosis symptoms are also associated with Epstein-Barr virus and hepatitis viruses A, B, and C, which must be confirmed serologically.

X = preferred specimen types; O = specimen may be helpful; BAL = bronchoalveolar lavage; Serol = serological testing; IgM = IgM-specific serological testing is recommended; CNS = central nervous system; CSF = cerebrospinal fluid; RSV = respiratory syncytial virus.

....

TABLE 3–3   COLLECTION OF SPECIMENS FOR VIRAL CULTURE*

Autopsy tissue: Collect samples as soon as possible after death. Place cubes of 1 cm³ or less in viral transport medium. **Do not place tissue in formalin.**

Blood (anticoagulated): Collect whole blood in heparin, EDTA, or sodium citrate. Sample should arrive in the laboratory within 2 hours of collection.

Eye exudate: Rub corneal or conjunctival ulcers with a sterile swab moistened with Hanks medium. Place swab in transport medium.†

Genital, cervical: Lesions of the external genitalia should be sampled as any other lesion (see lesions, ulcers, and vesicles). Cervical specimens should be collected after the cervix has been cleared of mucus and pus. Then any lesions should be swabbed; if no lesions are present, the swab should be inserted 1 cm into the cervical canal and rotated. Place swab in transport medium.†

Lesions, ulcers, and vesicles: Collect specimens within 3 days of eruption. Aspirate vesicle fluid with a syringe with a 26- or 27-gauge needle. Place aspirated fluid in transport medium. Rub lesion, ulcer, or opened vesicle with a swab, being sure to obtain cells from the base of the lesion or active edge (rather than necrotic center) of the ulcer. Place swab in transport medium.† Swabs from vesicles may be placed in transport medium already containing the vesicle fluid.

Nasal swab: Sample turbinates, not anterior nares. Insert dry cotton swab gently into nose. Leave the swab in the nose for a few seconds so that secretions can be absorbed. Sample both nasal passages. Place swabs in transport medium.†

Rectal swab: Insert dry cotton swab 4 to 6 cm into the anal orifice and rotate it against the mucosa. Place swab in transport medium.†

Spinal fluid: Collect at least 1.0 ml of CSF; 2 to 3 ml is preferred. Collect in a sterile screw-capped container. Do not place fluid in transport medium.

Sputum: Collect expectorated sputum in a sterile screw-capped container.

Stool: Collect a 2- to 4-g specimen in a sterile container.

Throat swab: Collect the sample by vigorously rubbing the posterior pharyngeal wall and posterior nasal passages with a dry cotton swab. Place swab in transport medium.†

Tissue (biopsy): Remove tissue surgically from the site of infection. Place intact specimen in transport medium. **Do not place tissue in formalin.**

Urine: Collect 10 to 50 ml of freshly voided urine in a sterile container. Sample should arrive in the laboratory within 2 to 4 hours of collection. Keep sample at room or refrigerator temperature. **Do not freeze.**

Washings (throat, nasal): Infuse 10 to 15 ml of saline or viral transport medium into nasal passages. Use suction device to collect washings. Place washings in a sterile, screw-capped container.

---

*A suitable transport medium (use 3 ml per tube) is composed of Hanks balanced salt solution with 2% fetal bovine serum, 100 µg/ml gentamicin, and 0.5 µg/ml amphotericin B.
†Break off swab above tip by pressing it against the inside of the transport medium tube.
CSF = cerebrospinal fluid.

generally free of usual flora organisms should not be placed in transport medium. The purpose of viral transport medium is to prevent drying of the sample, to maintain viability of the virus, and to inhibit the growth of microbial contaminants [2].

Many types of transport media are available commercially; these are marketed in a variety of containers and often in combination with various collection devices. Two collection systems, the Culturette (Becton Dickinson, Cockeysville, MD) and the Virocult (Medical Wire and Equipment Co., Victory Gardens, NY), have been evaluated in comparison studies of collection and transport of samples for virus isolation. The Culturette apparatus is a plastic tube that holds a sterile rayon-tipped swab that can be withdrawn, used to collect the sample, and reinserted into the tube. After the sample is collected and the swab reinserted, an ampule containing modified Stuart transport medium, which is installed in the bottom of the plastic tube, is crushed to release the medium and keep the swab moist. The Virocult system includes a sterile collection swab and a plastic transport tube that holds a sponge containing a balanced salt solution, glucose, lactalbumin hydrolysate, chloramphenicol, and cycloheximide. Both of these systems have been shown to be satisfactory for collection and transport of samples for virus isolation [6–8]. The commercially marketed collection systems are convenient but may be expensive. Swabs received in containers that do not contain at least 2 ml of fluid must be transferred in the virology laboratory to a tube containing approximately 2 ml of transport medium (described later). During the transfer process, some of the clinical sample may adhere to the inside of the transport container and be left behind.

Many simple liquid media are suitable for use as transport media. These may be prepared in house, aliquoted into sterile screw-capped tubes, and provided to appropriate areas of the hospital or directly to physicians or hospital staff when requested. Conical centrifuge tubes are convenient as transport containers because they can be used both in transport and in processing of samples. Hanks balanced salt solution (BSS) or other buffered broth is used to control pH. Bovine serum albumin, fetal calf serum, gelatin, or other proteinaceous supplement is added to stabilize the viruses. The use of bovine serum rather than fetal bovine serum is discouraged because bovine sera may contain antibodies that will inactivate some viruses.

Antibiotics are also included in transport media. Gentamicin and amphotericin B are the most popular, but others may be substituted. Antibiotics inhibit growth of bacteria and fungi that may be present in the clinical sample. They do not inhibit viruses. A procedure for in-house preparation of one simple, inexpensive, and effective viral transport medium is provided in the Appendix.

When clinical samples for virus isolation are received in the laboratory, the samples and accompanying test request information should be examined. Each sample must be labeled with the patient's name or identifying number, and this information must "match" the information on the test request. The virology laboratory should provide a test request form or a computer order format that encourages or forces the ordering physician to provide the information needed in processing the specimen appropriately. This includes source of specimen, time of collection, virus suspected, and any additional information, such as date of onset of disease, disease symptoms, travel history, and so on, which may be of use in determining proper culture conditions.

Because viruses are labile, it is best to process specimens as soon as possible after collection. As the time between collection of a specimen and its inoculation into cell cultures increases, chances for virus isolation decrease. If the specimen cannot be processed immediately but will be processed and inoculated within 3 to 5 days after collection, it should be refrigerated at 2 to 8°C. Although this refrigerator storage is acceptable for almost all types of specimens, it is not acceptable for anticoagulated blood samples. These cannot be stored and must be processed within 2 to 6 hours after collection.

If a swab is received in a container that does not include liquid transport medium, the virologist transfers the swab into a tube containing transport medium, mixes the tube contents thoroughly with a vortex mixer, removes the swab and discards it, and stores the transport medium, which now contains the specimen material. For swabs received in transport medium, the tube contents are mixed thoroughly with a vortex mixer, the swab is removed, and the transport medium is stored at 2 to 8°C.

Specimens that must be held for longer than 3 to 5 days before processing should be frozen at −70°C or colder. Freezing has been shown to decrease the infectivity of viruses, especially of respiratory syncytial virus and cytomegalovirus [9]. Therefore, if the viral suspect is respiratory syncytial virus or cytomegalovirus, **the specimen should not be frozen;** it should be stored at 2 to 8°C and processed as soon as possible. Storing specimens in a standard freezer (−20 to −25°C) decreases the infectivity of some viruses within a short time and is not recommended [2].

If the sample must be shipped to another location for culturing, it must be shipped on wet ice or coolant packs if it will reach its destination within 3 to 5 days. If shipping requires more than 5 days, the sample should be frozen at −70°C or colder and shipped in dry ice. For dry ice shipment, flame-sealed ampules or screw-capped vials stored in plastic bags impervious to carbon dioxide (CO_2) should be used to protect the sample against subliming CO_2, which may inactivate some viruses [10].

PROCESSING CLINICAL SPECIMENS FOR INOCULATION INTO CELL CULTURES

Before clinical specimens can be inoculated into cell cultures, they must be treated to remove contaminating organisms and other agents that may be toxic or infective for the cell cultures. The treatment procedure usually includes centrifugation and the addition of antibiotics. Centrifugation sediments contaminating bacteria and fungi and bits of cell debris into the bottom of the tube. Because viruses are so small, the centrifugal force generated by standard laboratory centrifuges is not adequate to cause them to be concentrated into the bottom of the tube. They remain in the supernatant fluid. The supernatant fluid is used for inoculation of the cell cultures. Antibiotics are added to inhibit the growth of any contaminating bacteria or fungi. If specimens are placed in an antibiotic-containing transport medium, the addition of supplemental antibiotics to the specimen itself is usually not warranted. Reminder: in the virology laboratory, as in any area of the microbiology laboratory, all potentially infectious materials must be manipulated only in the proper biological safety cabinet (laminar flow hood). These cabinets are described in Chapter 7.

If a swab sample is received in transport medium, the medium is mixed with a vortex mixer, and the swab is removed; then the liquid transport medium, which now contains the specimen material, is treated for culture inoculation. If a swab is received in a container that does not include liquid transport medium, the swab must be transferred into a tube containing transport medium and treated as described previously.

Before initiating the processing steps, the virologist evaluates (or re-evaluates for stored samples) the patient's information, labeling of the sample, tests requested, source of the sample, viral suspects, and any other pertinent information. The virologist then follows the guidelines provided for each specimen type in Table 3–4. For processing of anticoagulated peripheral blood samples for inoculation into cell cultures, a separation procedure is used that separates the leukocytes from the samples; the leukocytes are used as inoculum for the cell cultures. A detailed procedure for processing of anticoagulated blood is provided in the Appendix.

. . . .

TABLE 3–4   GUIDELINES FOR PROCESSING CLINICAL SAMPLES FOR INOCULATION INTO CELL CULTURES FOR VIRUS ISOLATION*

Blood (anticoagulated): Process to separate leukocytes (see Procedure in Appendix).

Rectal swabs: Follow directions for swab specimens through the centrifugation step. Then draw up the supernatant into a sterile syringe, attach a sterile 0.45-μm syringe-top filter, and depress the plunger of the syringe to force the fluid through the filter. Use the filtered fluid to inoculate cell cultures.

Swabs (e.g., eye, genital, lesions, throat, nose): If the swab is not received in transport medium, place it in a tube containing 3 ml of transport medium. Mix with a vortex mixer for 30 seconds. Express fluid by pressing the swab against the side of the tube; discard the swab. Spin the fluid at 1500g for 10 min. Use the clear supernatant fluid to inoculate cell cultures.

Spinal fluid and other sterile body fluids: If fluid is clear, no processing is necessary. If fluid is turbid or bloody, spin at 1500g for 10 min. Use the clear supernatant fluid to inoculate cell cultures.

Sputum: Most sputum samples are turbid and mucoid and should be diluted 1:4 in viral transport medium and mixed with a vortex mixer. Spin at 1500g for 10 min, and use supernatant fluid to inoculate cell cultures. If excessive mucus is present, remove mucus and discard.

Stool: In a centrifuge tube, mix a pea-sized portion of sample in 3 ml of transport medium. Mix well and spin at 1500g for 10 min. Draw up the supernatant into a sterile syringe, attach a sterile 0.45-μm syringe-top filter, and depress the plunger of the syringe to force the fluid through the filter. Use of several filters may be required before sufficient fluid is obtained. Use the filtered fluid to inoculate cell cultures.

Tissue (autopsy, biopsy): With a sterile tissue grinder, grind tissue in transport medium. Place ground mixture in a sterile centrifuge tube, and spin at 1500g for 10 min. Use supernatant to inoculate cell cultures. If the supernatant appears turbid or is contaminated, draw it up in a sterile syringe, attach a sterile 0.45-μm syringe-top filter, and depress the plunger of the syringe to force the fluid through the filter. Use the filtered fluid to inoculate cell cultures.

Urine:† Mix the urine by inversion or by mixing with a vortex mixer. Use the well-mixed urine as inoculum for cell culture.

Washings (throat, nasal): Transfer washings to a sterile centrifuge tube. If the washing is turbid or mucoid, dilute the sample in an equal volume of viral transport medium, mix thoroughly with a vortex mixer, and spin at 1500g for 10 min. Use clear supernatant fluid to inoculate cell cultures. If excessive mucus is present, remove mucus and discard.

*Transport medium composed of Hanks balanced salt solution with 2% fetal bovine serum, 100 μg/ml gentamicin, and 0.5 μg/ml amphotericin B is suitable.

†Addition of antibiotics and centrifugation may be useful with urine that is contaminated with bacteria or fungi.

The "finished" product after specimen processing should be a fluid that contains viruses and is free of contaminating organisms and debris. This fluid is used for inoculation of cell cultures.

CELL CULTURES AND CELL CULTURE MEDIA IN CLINICAL VIROLOGY

Cell cultures, rather than eggs or animals, are the most important host system in the clinical virology laboratory. Cell cultures of various types provide suitable environments for proliferation of many human viral pathogens, and they are convenient to maintain in the laboratory. The purpose of cell cultures in virology is to provide an economical system of actively metabolizing cells that will support virus replication.

Cell cultures are prepared using a standardized suspension of cells that have been dissociated from the tissue of origin by the action of proteolytic enzymes or chelating agents. The evenly dispersed cells adhere to the surface of culture vessels and replicate to form a confluent layer of single cells called a monolayer [11].

Three types of cell cultures are recommended for viral isolation studies: primary, diploid, and established (heteroploid).

1. **Primary cells** are the "first generation" of cells that grow directly from the animal and are not subcultured. Consisting mostly of epithelial cells, they have paired (diploid) chromosomes. Primary monkey kidney cells are probably the most commonly used primary cells. Primary cell cultures may occasionally have "indigenous" viral contaminants that were harbored by the host animal. These agents may produce visible (microscopically) signs of their presence, such as rounding of cells or a "foamy" appearance.

2. **Diploid cell lines** are usually derived from fetal tissues and are composed of fibroblast cells, which are immature cells that produce collagen and other fibers [12]. Fibroblasts maintain their characteristic diploid chromosomal configuration, which is the normal configuration of chromosomes in cells of human origin. Examples of diploid cell lines are fibroblasts from human lung or human foreskin. These cells tend to die out after the 50th generation.

3. **Established (heteroploid) cells** usually originate from malignancies. When transferred, they lose their resemblance to the parent tissue and may become heteroploid or aneuploid in chromosome number (i.e., have altered numbers of chromosomes). These cells grow rapidly and may be propagated for many generations, perhaps indefinitely [12]. Some common established cell lines are human cervical carcinoma (HeLa) and human laryngeal carcinoma (HEp-2).

It is difficult for most busy clinical laboratories to prepare cell cultures in house because cell culture preparation is time consuming, requires technical expertise and dedicated facilities, and must be carefully monitored and standardized. Most clinical virology laboratories depend on commercial suppliers for their cell culture tubes. Cell cultures can be ordered to fit the needs of the laboratory and are delivered ready to use to the laboratory once or twice each week. Cell culture monolayers are usually prepared in 16×125-mm screw-capped tubes. The monolayer covers one side of the lower half of the tube (Fig. 3–2). Most manufacturers mark the side of the tube opposite the monolayer with an insignia or label. This orients the virologist to the positioning of the monolayer; this helps in examining the monolayer and in positioning the tube for incubation. The cell culture label indicates the type of cells and their production lot number. A round stick-on label may be affixed to the lid of the screw-capped culture tubes to identify the tube. The patient's name or the laboratory number for the culture can be written on the label. Also, colored labels may be used to differentiate the various types of cell cultures; this allows the virologist to determine at a glance which tube contains which specimen and which type of cells.

Culture media are classified as either outgrowth or maintenance media. Both types include BSS, which aids in the control of physiological conditions such as pH, osmotic pressure, and inorganic ion concentration. BSS contains a CO_2-bicarbonate buffering system for maintaining

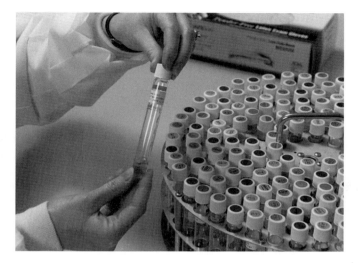

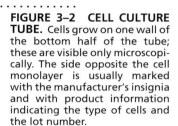

FIGURE 3–2 CELL CULTURE TUBE. Cells grow on one wall of the bottom half of the tube; these are visible only microscopically. The side opposite the cell monolayer is usually marked with the manufacturer's insignia and with product information indicating the type of cells and the lot number.

pH within suitable ranges. Amino acids, vitamins, and other nutrients are added to BSS. These media are marketed commercially in liquid form in various formulations. Some common media are Minimal Essential Medium, Medium 199, RPMI, and Dulbecco's medium. The basic cell culture media serve as the basis for outgrowth and maintenance media.

Outgrowth media are used for initial growth of a newly seeded culture. They are enriched with serum, yeast extract, or peptones, which promote rapid cellular proliferation. The serum component is important because it promotes attachment and spreading of cells on the surface of culture vessels [11]. Some outgrowth media contain up to 10% serum. Only a small amount of bicarbonate buffer is present in outgrowth media because few cells are present to produce CO_2, which ultimately joins with hydrogen to form acid. Outgrowth media are important in the clinical virology laboratory if cell cultures are prepared and transferred in house. When cell culture tubes are purchased from biological supply houses, they have already been seeded and nourished with outgrowth medium until their monolayers are nearly confluent; then their outgrowth medium has been replaced with maintenance medium before delivery to the laboratory.

Maintenance media are designed for maintaining cultures in a slow, steady state of metabolism that is suitable for viral proliferation. Maintenance media have fewer growth-stimulating substances than outgrowth media; most contain only 2% serum [13]. Because many actively metabolizing cells are present in mature cultures, maintenance media contain a large amount of bicarbonate in the buffering system.

A phenol red pH indicator is included in most cell culture media. Media containing phenol red are red-orange in color at the desired pH of 6.8 to 7.6 [14]. If the pH increases as a result of exposure to air (cap not tightly closed), cellular toxicity (specimens may contain substances that are toxic to the cells), or viral proliferation, which destroys the cells, the color of the medium changes to bright magenta-pink. If the pH decreases as a result of bacterial or fungal contamination or excessive cellular metabolism, the color changes to bright yellow. Bacterial and fungal contaminants may also cause turbidity of the media. A change in color of the cell culture medium indicates a change in the condition of the monolayer; it does not necessarily signal that a virus is proliferating. Viral proliferation is detected through microscopic examination of the monolayer, not by gross observation of the color of the medium.

Antibiotics are added to most cell culture media. This allows cell monolayers to be bathed continuously in antibiotics. The antibiotics do not interfere with cellular or viral proliferation but should inhibit bacterial or fungal growth.

Most media are commercially available in liquid form. Usually serum and antibiotics must be added before use. A procedure is provided in the Appendix (see Preparation of Transport Medium and Cell Culture Media) for adding serum and antibiotics to commercially prepared cell culture media. To prepare cell culture media for daily use, Minimum Essential Medium Eagle with Earle's BSS with L-glutamine medium or other suitable medium is used and serum and antibiotics are added.

SELECTING AND INOCULATING CELL CULTURES FOR VIRUS ISOLATION

Processed clinical specimen material may be inoculated into cell culture tubes without removing the culture medium from the cell culture tube. For standard inoculation, the processed specimen, usually 0.2 ml per cell culture tube, must be added to the medium in the culture tube [13]. However, some processed samples are more effectively inoculated by an adsorption-type inoculation in which the cell culture medium is removed from the tube, and 0.3 ml of the processed specimen is applied directly to the monolayer. The inoculated tube is incubated in a horizontal position in a slant rack for 1 hour at 35°C [13]. Then excess inoculum is removed and discarded, and fresh cell culture medium is added to the culture tube.

Processed clinical specimen material is usually inoculated into several types of cell cultures. Cell cultures are selected on the basis of the source of the clinical specimen and on the viruses suspected. Viral suspects may be specifically noted by the physician as suspects in a particular sample or may be those viruses that are commonly associated with infections at the site involved. If a suspect virus has been named by the physician, the virologist selects cell cultures that are suitable for proliferation of the virus named. If no suspect virus is named, the virologist selects an array of cell cultures that are susceptible to a variety of human viral pathogens, especially those frequently associated with infections of the anatomical site from which the specimen was collected. For example, cytomegalovirus is the most likely viral pathogen in urine and in blood; therefore, all urine and blood samples should be inoculated into human diploid fibroblast cultures, which are optimal for cytomegalovirus isolation. Also shell vials should be inoculated for testing for cytomegalovirus early antigen (see Chapter 4). For isolation of the respiratory viruses, virologists inoculate multiple tubes of primary monkey kidney cells by adsorption-type inoculation. If rubella virus is suspected, primary African green monkey kidney cells are inoculated using adsorption-type inoculation. For varicella-zoster, additional tubes of diploid lung fibroblasts should be inoculated. If only the herpes simplex viruses are of interest to the physician, cells that are very susceptible to herpes infection, such as rabbit kidney, human embryonic kidney, A549, or HEp-2 cells, should be inoculated. Examples of combinations of types of cell cultures that may be used for specific types of viruses and various types of clinical samples are shown in Table 3–5.

When appropriate cell cultures have been inoculated, if processed material has not been used up, the remaining sample should be frozen at −70°C or colder. A preservative such as 5% glycerol or 2 SP (0.2 mol sucrose in 0.02 mol sodium phosphate buffer at pH 7.2) should be added to the specimen vial before freezing [15]. This portion of the sample will then be available for follow-up studies or in case of laboratory failures that necessitate repeat culturing.

INCUBATING AND EXAMINING INOCULATED CELL CULTURES

Inoculated cell culture tubes are incubated at 35°C, although rhinoviruses and a few others may proliferate more efficiently at 33°C. A rotating rack called a roller drum (Fig. 3–3) is preferred for incubation of viral cultures. The roller drum consists of a motor that is contained in a low, square base platform with an arm that extends upward at the back of the base. The arm has a retaining pin that accommodates the large circular rack. Most standard racks hold 164 viral

TABLE 3–5 CELL CULTURE SELECTION AND INOCULATION*

| SPECIMEN SOURCE | VIRAL SUSPECT | TUBE CELL CULTURES | | | | | | | | SHELL VIAL CULTURES† | |
| | | Diploid Cell Lines | | Established Cell Lines | | | Primary Cells | | | Diploid Cell Lines | |
		MRC-5	MRHF	A549	HEp-2	RK	HNK	PMK	AGMK	MRC-5	MRHF
Blood	Cytomegalovirus	1 (ads)	1 (ads)								3
Urine	Cytomegalovirus	1 (ads)		1						2	
Spinal fluid	None indicated	1 (ads)		1				1, 1 (ads)			
Body fluid, stool, swab, or unidentified source	None indicated	1		1		1		1			
Tissue, BAL, all‡ specimens other than blood or urine	Cytomegalovirus	1 (ads)	1 (ads)	1				1		2	
All‡ specimens	Respiratory virus	1 (ads)		1	1 (ads)			2 (ads)			
All‡ specimens	Varicella-zoster	2 (ads)		1			1 (ads)				
All‡ specimens	Herpes simplex only			1		1					
All‡ specimens	Rubella	2				1 (ads)			1 (ads)	1 (ads)	

*If viral suspect is other than those named, consult a reference text to determine appropriate cell types. Use 0.2 ml of processed sample per cell culture tube and vial for standard inoculation. Use 0.3 ml of processed sample per cell culture tube for adsorption-type inoculation (see text for details).

†See Appendix for procedure for inoculation of shell vials.

‡Anticoagulated blood and urine should be inoculated as indicated in their individual listings to facilitate isolation of cytomegalovirus. The term "all specimens" excludes urine and blood.

A549 = established line of human epithelioid carcinoma; AGMK = primary African green monkey kidney cells; BAL = bronchoalveolar lavage; HEp-2 = established line of human laryngeal carcinoma; HNK = primary human neonatal kidney; MRC-5 = Medical Research human lung fibroblasts; MRHF = Medical Research human foreskin; PMK = primary Rhesus monkey kidney; RK = rabbit kidney; ads = adsorption-type inoculation.

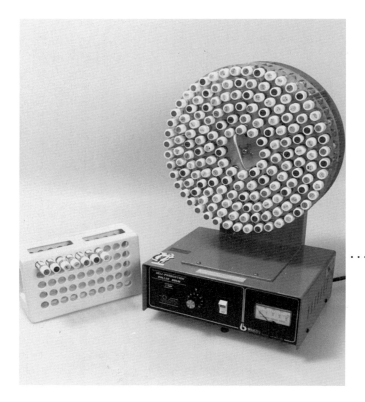

. . . .
FIGURE 3–3 RACKS FOR IN-CUBATION OF VIRAL CUL-TURE TUBES. The circular ro-tating rack (roller drum) holds tubes at an angle to keep cell culture medium in the bottom of the tube; racks usually rotate at 0.2 to 2 revolutions per minute. The stationary racks hold tubes at an angle and do not provide for movement of tubes.

culture tubes (16 mm), although racks that hold up to 350 or more tubes can be purchased. The circular rack is held at a slight angle of 5 to 7 degrees to keep the top (lid) of the tubes higher than the bottom. This keeps the cell culture medium in the bottom half of the tube, where it is needed for nourishing the cell monolayer. The angled position also keeps the cell culture medium from collecting in or near the cap of the tube [13]; this is important because medium at the top of the tube provides a convenient route for entry of contaminants into the tubes. The roller drum motor slowly rotates the rack at the desired speed. Rotation speeds of 0.2 to 2 revolutions per minute have been shown to be acceptable [13, 16]. The rotation bathes the cell monolayers in cell culture medium. Viruses have been shown to proliferate more rapidly in cell culture tubes that are rotated in this manner. This is especially helpful with samples containing only a small quantity of virus [16].

Stationary slanted racks may be used for cell culture incubation if roller drums are not available (see Fig. 3–3). Like the rotating rack of the roller drum, the stationary rack is slanted to keep the cell culture medium in the bottom half of the tubes. When stationary racks are used, it is important for the virologist to position the cell culture tubes carefully in the rack with the cell monolayer on the lower surface of the tube. The cell culture medium covers and nourishes the cells only when the monolayer is positioned on the lower surface. If the tube accidentally is positioned so that the cell monolayer is on the upper surface, the monolayer will not be covered by medium, and the cells will dry out and die. Commercially purchased cell culture tubes bear an insignia or label on the side of the tube opposite the monolayer. When tubes are positioned in the slanted racks, the insignia should be on the top surface of the tube and should be visible when the rack is observed from above. This provides a convenient mechanism for ensuring that the cell monolayer is in the correct position and will be covered with medium.

Inoculated cell cultures are routinely incubated for a period of 14 days, although the time period may vary if a specific virus is being sought. For example, with culture protocols targeting isolation of herpes simplex virus only, tubes can be incubated for a shorter period of 7 days. Herpes simplex virus proliferates rapidly, and culture results can be reported with confidence after

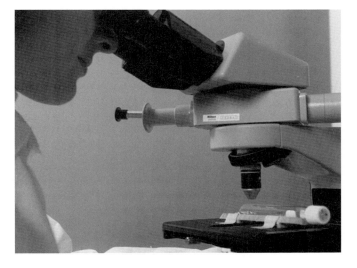

....
**FIGURE 3–4 VIRAL CUL-
TURE TUBES ARE EXAMINED
WITH A STANDARD LIGHT
MICROSCOPE.** The tube is held
in position on the microscope
stage, and the cell monolayer is
viewed through the wall of the
tube using the 10× microscope
objective.

only 7 days of incubation. Cytomegalovirus represents the opposite end of the spectrum of incubation times, often requiring 18 to 21 days or longer to proliferate. Because of this slow proliferation time, an extended incubation period of 30 days is recommended for viral cultures for cytomegalovirus.

During the incubation period, cell cultures are examined periodically using the light microscope. The observation schedule can be customized to fit the needs of the laboratorians and the types of viruses being targeted for isolation. Herpes simplex cultures that are incubated for only 7 days should be examined daily, whereas cytomegalovirus cultures that are incubated for

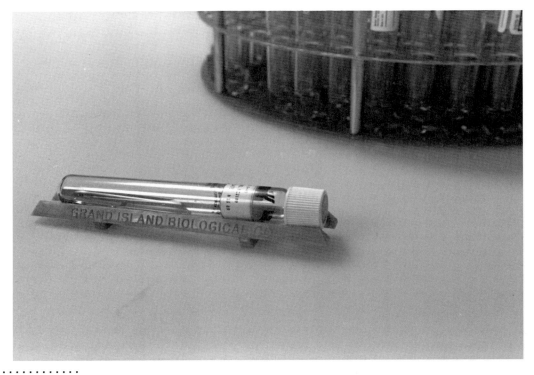

....
**FIGURE 3–5 "RAILROAD TRACK" TEST TUBE HOLDER FOR POSITIONING VIRAL CULTURE
TUBES ON THE STAGE OF THE MICROSCOPE.** Tubes are held at an angle to keep the cell culture
medium in the bottom of the tube.

(Front)

VIROLOGY LABORATORY

CALL RESULTS TO EXT/PAGE: *2447*				PATIENT INFORMATION:	LOG NUMBER:
REQUESTED BY: *Jones M.D.*				Smith,	*832*
COLLECTION TIME: DATE *1-8-95* HOUR *10:30 a.m.*				Julia L.	
x	Viral Culture/Suspect: *CMV*			628435 Q.	SPECIMEN SOURCE:
	Herpes Only Culture				*Throat*

	Respiratory Antigen Profile		RESULTS			
	Respiratory Pool	POS	NEG	ND		
	Adenovirus Ag – IF	POS	NEG	ND	CULTURE RESULTS	
	Parainfluenza Type 1 Ag – IF	POS	NEG	ND	ISOLATE 1:	TECH: *TM*
	Parainfluenza Type 2 Ag – IF	POS	NEG	ND	*Adenovirus isolated*	CALLED TO: *Jones*
	Parainfluenza Type 3 Ag – IF	POS	NEG	ND		TIME: *11:00 a.m.*
	Influenza Group A Ag – IF	POS	NEG	ND	DATE: *1-11-95*	COMPUTER ✓: ✓
	Influenza Group B Ag – IF	POS	NEG	ND	ISOLATE 2:	TECH:
	RSV Ag – IF	POS	NEG	ND		CALLED TO:
	Herpes Type 1 Ag – IF	POS	NEG			TIME:
	Herpes Type 2 Ag – IF	POS	NEG		DATE:	COMPUTER ✓:
	Varicella Ag – IF	POS	NEG		POSITIVE CULTURE FINAL	TECH:
	Rotavirus Ag – EIA	POS	NEG			COMPUTER ✓:
	OTHER (Specify)				DATE:	
	DIRECT ANTIGEN REPORT				☐ NO VIRUS ISOLATED FINAL	TECH:
TECH	CALLED/TIME		DATE	✓		COMPUTER ✓:
					DATE:	☺ HAVE A NICE DAY ☺

(Back)

Log # _*832*_

CELL TYPE	DATES OBSERVED/TECHNOLOGIST									
	1 – 9	1 – 11	1 – 13	1 – 15	1 – 17	1 – 19	1 – 21	1 – 23		
MRHF	N	N	N	N	N	N	? round	2–3+ adeno		
MRC–5	N	N	N	N	N	N	1+ adeno	3+ adeno		
A549	N	1+ round①					ANTIGEN IDENTIFICATION			TECH
							HSV 1 ○ Neg			TM
PM	N	N	N	N	focal round adeno	2+ adeno	4+ adeno	HSV 2 ○ Neg		TM
								ADENO ○ 3–4+		TM
	TM	TM	TM	LL	LL	LL	G	PARA 1		
								PARA 2		
Shell Vial/24h	Neg^PS							PARA 3		
								FLU A		
Shell Vial/48H		Neg^PS						FLU B		
								RSV		
HEMADSORPTION TESTING								RESP. POOL		
RMK	HAD NEG			HAD POS				VARICELLA ZOSTER		
								OTHER (SPECIFY)		

∙∙∙∙∙∙∙∙∙∙∙∙

FIGURE 3–6   VIROLOGY LABORATORY WORK CARD. This card provides a record of the patient's identifying information, the physician's name, the source of the sample, the date and time of collection, laboratory identification number, a list of cell culture tubes inoculated, and results of cell culture observations and follow-up testing.

30 days may be examined on alternate days during weeks 1 and 2 and only once per week for weeks 3 and 4 of incubation. Cell culture maintenance media are replaced periodically during long incubation periods so that the cells remain viable. For routine cultures that are incubated for 14 days, examination 1 day after inoculation and on alternate days thereafter may be satisfactory.

To examine cell cultures by light microscopy, the cell culture tube is positioned on the microscope stage and the unstained cell monolayer examined through the wall of the tube (Fig. 3–4). Although an ordinary light microscope is satisfactory for making the examination, the microscope must be a model that allows sufficient distance between the microscope objectives and the surface of the stage to accommodate a cell culture tube. Microscopes with adjustable stages are ideal for this purpose. A plastic tube holder, casually identified as a "railroad track" in some virology laboratories (Fig. 3–5), is positioned on the stage of the microscope; this holds the cell culture tube in a horizontal position and keeps it from rolling off the microscope stage.

The railroad track is slightly elevated at one end to keep the cell culture medium from collecting in the cap of the tube during the microscopic examination. The culture tube is placed on the railroad track and rotated until the monolayer is positioned on the surface of the tube that is nearer the objective. The low-power (10×) dry objective is the best objective to use for examining cell monolayers, and the light should be reduced by lowering the condenser and partially closing the iris diaphragm if cellular changes are to be seen clearly [17].

For each culture, a work card or sheet must be maintained to record the activities involving the culture. A sample work card is shown in Figure 3–6. This particular card is part of a three-part requisition used by hospital personnel to order viral testing. The desired testing is indicated on the top copy, along with the patient's identifying information, physician's name, source of the sample, date and time of collection, and viral suspects. When the specimen is received in the laboratory, the top copies are separated and used for billing and administrative purposes, and the back of the last copy (the work card) is used to record the progress of the culture. The back of the work card has spaces for listing the types of cell culture tubes inoculated and laboratory identification numbers. Each time a cell culture is observed, the date, virologist's initials, and results of the observation are recorded. A standard set of abbreviations should be identified and agreed on by all of the virologists in the laboratory for use in describing the culture observations. Some examples of such abbreviations follow: N, no changes seen (i.e., no growth); B, bacterial contamination; C, contamination; Y, yeast; F, fungus; TO, tissue off; SL, tissue sloughing; PT, poor tissue; pH, culture medium is purple; RD, rounded cells have been seen; TOX, toxicity; C/Filter, tube is contaminated, will be filtered, and new tube inoculated; and so on.

At least one uninoculated cell culture tube from each lot of cell culture tubes should be incubated along with the inoculated cultures. These uninoculated tubes serve as "control" tubes. Any changes in the appearance of the cells in the uninoculated tubes may signal the presence of indigenous viral contaminants (see Contamination in Cell Cultures) or indicate that the lot of cell cultures is of poor quality. The uninoculated tubes also serve as negative controls for procedures such as hemadsorption.

DETECTING VIRAL PROLIFERATION IN TRADITIONAL CELL CULTURES

Cytopathogenic Effect

How does the virologist detect virus by examining cell cultures using a light microscope? Although viruses are too small to be seen with a light microscope, many viruses infect susceptible cell cultures and produce degenerative cellular changes, which can be observed microscopically. These changes are called the cytopathic or cytopathogenic effect (CPE) of the virus. CPE appears because the virus integrates itself into the cellular nucleic acid and then directs the cell to manufacture viral components rather than the cellular components needed by the cell for its own maintenance. Without the needed components, the cell degenerates, and the cellular morphology changes; these changes are the viral CPE. The rate and patterns of CPE induced by various viruses are dependent on (1) the type of cell cultures used, (2) the concentration of virus in the specimen, and (3) the properties of the individual virus [18]. The production of CPE is sometimes slow, as in the case of cytomegalovirus, which transmits itself from cell to cell, and sometimes rapid, as in the case of poliovirus, which is excreted into the medium that surrounds the cells and progresses quickly to infect all parts of the monolayer [19].

The CPE of a virus may involve all parts of the cell. Although many types of CPE can be seen in unstained monolayers of cells, some types are visible only in stained preparations. In stained preparations, inclusion bodies may be seen. These appear as areas with altered staining behavior. Each inclusion body is believed to be either a "virus factory" in which viral nucleic acid or protein is being synthesized or a crystalline aggregate of virions [17]. Inclusions may be single or multiple, large or small, round or irregular, intranuclear or

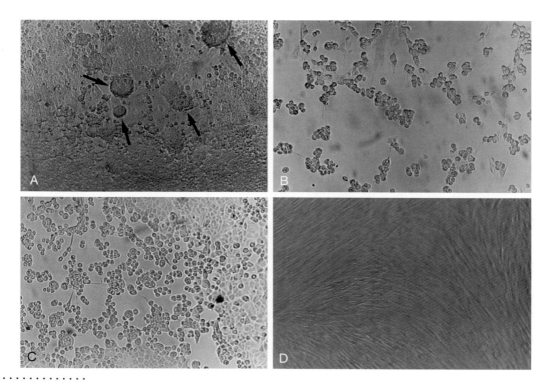

FIGURE 3–7 VIRAL CYTOPATHOGENIC EFFECT. (A) Syncytia may appear; (B) infected cells may form grapelike clusters; and (C) enlargement or swelling may be seen. (D) Uninfected cells should be used as a negative control in culture evaluation.

intracytoplasmic, and acidophilic or basophilic. Nuclear destruction may also be observed in stained preparations. Some viruses may dislocate and break up chromosomes.

Most viral cultures are observed unstained. The types of CPE described next are observed most commonly in unstained preparations.

1. **Vacuoles.** These are large, frothy, bubble-like areas usually in the cytoplasm of infected cells [17].

2. **Syncytia.** These are large cell masses that may contain up to 100 nuclei. They are sometimes called giant cells and are believed to result from fusion of virus-infected cells. The fusion may result from changes in protein synthesis in the infected cells and facilitates cell-to-cell spread of the virus.

3. **General morphological changes.** Cells may become rounded, swell, shrink, or form grapelike clusters.

4. **Loss of adherence.** Infected cells often lose their ability to adhere to the culture vessel. They may float free in the culture medium, leaving clear areas or fine prolongations [19].

5. **Cellular granulation.** Cells have a dark, rough, finely speckled appearance. This granulation may be confused with nonspecific degeneration or aging of the cell culture [20].

Several types of CPE that may be observed in unstained preparations are shown in Figure 3–7.

When cell cultures are viewed through the low-power objective of the light microscope and CPE is visible, the extent of the CPE should be estimated and scored as follows: 4+, 100% of cells in monolayer affected; 3+, 75% of cells in monolayer affected; 2+, 50% of cells in monolayer affected; 1+, 25% of cells in monolayer affected (localized areas); or the term "focal" should be used to describe CPE that is restricted to infrequent, small individual areas of involvement that represent less than 25% of the monolayer.

The CPE of a specific virus in a given type of cell culture is usually constant. The typical CPE of some of the more common viruses is described in Table 3–6. When CPE is noted and its appearance, intensity, and cell line are evaluated, a "preliminary" grouping can be identified; however, follow-up testing is required to confirm the preliminary identification. A description of tests that can be used for definitive identification of isolated viruses is provided later in this chapter.

Detecting Cytopathogenic Effect–Negative Viruses

Because some viruses may produce CPE slowly or not at all, alternative methods have been devised for detecting the presence of viruses when CPE is absent. Several of these methods are described next.

HEMADSORPTION The hemadsorption method is used most commonly for detecting non-CPE–producing viruses. During replication, some viruses may discretely alter cell surfaces. These alterations are not visible with the light microscope, but the changes cause the virus-infected cells to have an affinity for erythrocytes. Apparently, viral hemagglutinating proteins, specified by the viral genome, are expressed on the plasma membranes of virus-infected cells [17]. These same hemagglutinating proteins are present on the envelope of the infecting viruses. These viral antigens are responsible for the afffinity for erythrocytes that occurs in the infected cells. The hemadsorption procedure is used to test cell culture cells for their affinity for erythrocytes.

In hemadsorption testing, the cell culture medium is removed from infected cell cultures and replaced with a suspension of erythrocytes (usually guinea pig, but species may vary according to the virus suspected). The culture is refrigerated for 30 minutes at 4°C and observed microscopically; then the tubes are incubated at 35°C for 30 minutes and observed again [21]. If a hemadsorbing virus has altered the surface of the cells, the erythrocytes will adhere in clumps to the infected areas of the cell monolayer (Fig. 3–8). Erythrocytes will not adhere to uninfected cells. In some laboratories all cell culture tubes that have not shown CPE during the prescribed incubation period are tested for hemadsorption. The hemadsorbing capabilities of common human viral pathogens are shown in Table 3–6, and a procedure for hemadsorption testing is provided in the Appendix. The hemadsorption procedure detects only hemadsorbing viruses; nonhemadsorbing viruses are not detectable. Hemadsorbing viruses include the influenzas, parainfluenzas, measles, and mumps.

Hemadsorption is also used as a screening method for respiratory viruses such as influenza and parainfluenza during seasons when the respiratory viruses are prevalent. Although these viruses usually produce CPE, they do so very slowly, and their CPE is difficult to identify and distinguish from nonspecific degenerative changes. Because of the difficulty in observing CPE for these viruses, cell culture tubes may be tested by hemadsorption at several intervals during the routine 14-day incubation period. Hemadsorption testing at desired intervals between days 3 and 7 [22] and at 14 days has been suggested. By using hemadsorption early in the incubation period, the respiratory viruses can often be detected much sooner than if their detection depended on CPE alone.

Three additional methods—interference challenge, plaquing, and hemagglutination—are also used, although much less widely than hemadsorption, to screen for viruses that do not produce CPE.

INTERFERENCE CHALLENGE Some viruses that do not produce CPE may be detected in cell culture only by the reduced ability of the infected culture to support the replication of a second or **challenge** virus (i.e., the original virus **interferes** with infection by another virus). In interference challenge testing, a cell culture is inoculated (either with known virus or with a patient's specimen that may include a virus) and is incubated for several days. Then a standardized quantity of a known CPE-producing virus, called the **challenge** virus, is inoculated into the culture. After additional incubation, the culture is observed to determine whether or not

TABLE 3–6　DETECTION AND IDENTIFICATION OF COMMON HUMAN VIRAL PATHOGENS THAT PROLIFERATE IN STANDARD CELL CULTURES*

VIRUS	CYTOPATHOGENIC EFFECT				HAD	TESTS FOR FINAL IDENTIFICATION
	PMK	A549	Fibroblasts	Other		
Adenovirus	Some produce clusters	Grapelike clusters (5–8 days)	Some produce clusters	HNK (5–7 days) grapelike clusters	No	IF for group; neut for type
CMV	None	None	Foci of contiguous rounded cells (10–30 days)	Use shell vials for rapid detection	No	CPE alone for cell culture isolates; IF for early antigen in shell vials
Enteroviruses	Small, round cells with cytoplasmic tails (2–5 days)	Infrequent, degenerative	Some produce CPE, same as PMK (2–5 days)		No	Neut
Herpes simplex	Some produce CPE same as A549 (4–8 days)	Rounded large cells (1–4 days)	Granular, large cells (2–6 days)	HNK or RK (1–4 days) large cells	No	IF
Influenza	Undifferentiated CPE, cellular granulation (4–8 days)	None	None		GP	IF
Measles	Large syncytia (7–10 days)	None	None		Rh	IF
Mumps	Rounded cells with large syncytia (6–8 days)	None	None		GP	IF
Parainfluenza	Rounded cells, some syncytia (4–8 days)	None	None		GP	IF
RSV	Syncytia (4–10 days)	Infrequent	Infrequent, granular, degenerative	HEp-2 (4–10 days) syncytia	No	IF
Rubella	None	None	None	AGMK (8–12 days); no CPE†	No	IF
Varicella-zoster	None	Small, round cells (6–8 days)	Some CPE, small, round cells (6–8 days)	HNK (6–8 days) small, round cells	No	IF

*Rhinovirus may occasionally be isolated in standard cell cultures. It causes degeneration with some rounding in fibroblast cell lines in 7–10 days; incubate at 33°C.
†Rubella does not proliferate well in standard cell cultures; use AGMK, RK, or BSC-1, and test by interference challenge.
A549 = established line of human lung carcinoma; AGMK = primary African Green Monkey kidney; CMV = cytomegalovirus; CPE = cytopathogenic effect; GP = guinea pig erythrocytes; HAD = hemadsorption; HEp-2 = established line of human laryngeal carcinoma; HNK = human neonatal kidney cells; IF = immunofluorescence; Neut = neutralization; PMK = primary monkey kidney cells; Rh = rhesus erythrocytes; RK = rabbit kidney cells; RSV = respiratory syncytial virus.

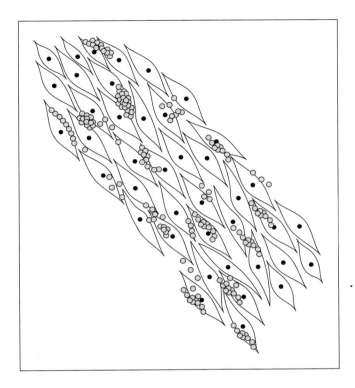

. . . .
FIGURE 3–8 HEMADSORP-TION TEST RESULT. Erythrocytes adhere to the monolayer in areas infected by virus. The erythrocytes do not float free when the cell culture tube is rotated or moved.

the challenge virus is producing CPE. If virus from the original inoculum was replicating within the cells, replication of the challenge virus is prevented because of interference by the initial virus, and no CPE will be produced. If virus from the original inoculum was not replicating within the cells, the cells remain susceptible to the challenge virus, which replicates within the susceptible cells to produce characteristic CPE. This technique was used in the past for detection of rubella virus and the rhinoviruses, both of which were thought to be incapable of producing CPE. The technique is seldom used now because cell lines have been developed in which these viruses produce CPE.

PLAQUING In the plaque method, a viral suspension (or clinical sample that may contain virus) is added to a monolayer of cultured cells. The cell culture is then covered with a nutrient agar mixture containing a vital dye, usually neutral red, which is taken up by living cells. As the virus replicates and destroys the cells, the neutral red is released by dead or dying cells, leaving cleared areas called **plaques.** The time of appearance, size, and shape of the plaques are useful in characterizing the virus. The plaquing method may also be used as a follow-up measure with cultures that have been incubated for a prescribed incubation period and have failed to demonstrate CPE. These cultures are covered with neutral red agar; areas containing dead or damaged cells will fail to take up neutral red dye, and plaques will be visible. Although plaques may have characteristic appearances, additional testing must be done to identify the virus definitively and to differentiate virus-induced plaques from those caused by nonspecific cellular degeneration. Plaquing is not widely used in the clinical virology laboratory at present but is the basis of a plaque reduction assay used for antiviral susceptibility testing (see Chapter 10).

HEMAGGLUTINATION Some viruses, or an antigen derived from them, are capable of binding to erythrocytes through complementary receptor sites on the erythrocyte surface [23]. This binding of virus and erythrocyte is called viral hemagglutination. Viral hemagglutinating antigens may occur as short projections on the viral envelope or may be distinct from the infectious particle. Viral hemagglutination is diagrammed in Chapter 2. Some viruses hemagglutinate erythrocytes from several species, whereas others hemagglutinate erythrocytes of only a single species or do not hemagglutinate at all. For example, enteroviruses hemagglutinate human O cells; influenza and parainfluenza viruses hemagglutinate human O, guinea pig, or chicken erythrocytes; and adenovirus groups 2 and 3 hemagglutinate rat cells [23].

In hemagglutination testing, a viral suspension (derived from infected cell culture medium or from disrupted infected cells) is diluted and mixed with a suspension of erythrocytes of the appropriate species. The mixture is incubated, and the erythrocytes settle to the bottom of the tube. Unagglutinated erythrocytes form a "button" or pellet in the center of the bottom of the tube; agglutinated erythrocytes make a layer of small clumps, which covers the bottom of the tube and is sometimes described as a "shield." This test is useful only with hemagglutinating viruses and, when positive, should be followed up with techniques that produce definitive viral identification.

DEFINITIVE IDENTIFICATION OF VIRAL ISOLATES

CPE, as well as the hemadsorption, interference challenge, plaquing, and hemagglutination methods, can be used as a detection method to demonstrate that viruses are proliferating within cells. The detection methods provide valuable information about the viruses detected (i.e., Is CPE characteristic of a certain virus? Is the virus capable of hemadsorbing or hemagglutinating?). However, none of these methods provides a definitive identification of the virus, and each must be followed with a test that will confirm the viral identification. Many methods can be used to provide this identification. Two of the most important of these—immunofluorescence and virus neutralization—are immunoserological methods that depend on reactivity of specific antibodies with the unknown virus. Other immunoserological and molecular techniques are also used in identification of viral isolates.

Immunofluorescence in Identification of Viral Isolates

The basic principles of direct and indirect immunofluorescence are discussed and illustrated in Chapter 2. For immunofluorescence testing, whether direct or indirect, virus-infected cells from cell cultures are fixed on a microscope slide. A procedure for preparing smears is included in the Appendix (see Preparing Antigen Smears for Immunofluorescence Testing). After the smears of infected cells are air dried and fixed in acetone, antiviral antibodies of known specificity are added to the fixed smear and allowed to incubate. Through the binding or lack thereof of the known antiviral antibodies, the unknown viral isolate in the infected cells is identified.

Because the immunofluorescence methods are so convenient and quick to perform, they are very popular. Direct immunofluorescence techniques require only 30 to 40 minutes to complete, whereas indirect immunofluorescence methods require approximately 1.5 to 2.0 hours. Fluorescein isothiocyanate–conjugated monoclonal antibodies are commercially available for use in direct immunofluorescence methods for identifying herpes simplex virus types 1 and 2, respiratory syncytial virus, varicella, influenza A and B, and adenovirus. Unlabeled monoclonal antibodies for use in indirect immunofluorescence testing are available for influenza A and B; parainfluenza 1, 2, and 3; adenovirus; and respiratory syncytial virus. Monoclonal antibodies are also available for measles and mumps identification. Procedures for performing a direct immunofluorescence test for herpes simplex virus types 1 and 2 antigen and for an indirect immunofluorescence test for parainfluenza virus 1, 2, and 3 antigen are provided in the Appendix. The viral identification provided by immunofluorescence methods is rapid, accurate, and reliable, and immunofluorescence is used widely in clinical virology laboratories. Unfortunately, immunofluorescence reagents are not available for identification of all viruses. The enteroviruses (poliovirus, coxsackieviruses, and echovirus), which are closely related antigenically, have not been effectively differentiated by immunofluorescence in the past, and their identification was achieved only through neutralization testing. At this writing, new monoclonal immunofluorescence reagents are being developed and field tested for use in identifying various enteroviruses.

Neutralization in Identification of Viral Isolates

The principle of virus neutralization is diagrammed and discussed in Chapter 2. In a neutralization test for virus identification, known specific immune serum is mixed, under carefully controlled conditions, with a suspension of live unknown virus. The serum-virus mixture is incubated, and then an aliquot of the mixture is introduced into a susceptible cell culture in which the activity or viability of the virus may be detected. If the virus fails to replicate within the susceptible host, it can be concluded that the virus was neutralized (i.e., rendered noninfectious by blockage of critical sites by antibody molecules). The antiserum used was specific for the virus, and the virus was identified. If the virus replicates within the susceptible host, the virus was not neutralized by the antibodies, the antiserum was not specific for the virus, and no viral identification can be made.

The antisera used in neutralization testing are standard reference antisera prepared against prototype strains of known viruses. These antisera are prepared and titrated so that the strength of the antibody is known and may be adjusted for use in any particular neutralization system. Because testing of viral isolates, especially enteroviruses, against individual immune sera may be difficult and time consuming, pooled immune serum may be used for screening. These sera are prepared and titered individually and then combined to make pools of controlled strength. Pools are usually designed so that a given antiserum appears in one or more pools. The unknown virus is then identified by its neutralization by the pool or pools sharing a common type-specific antiserum. This method is called the **intersecting serum schema** for viral identification [11]. A procedure for identifying the enteroviruses using the intersecting pool schema is presented in the Appendix.

Many viral identification procedures, especially neutralization, cannot be performed until the quantity or "dose" of the virus has been determined by a **titration procedure.** The titration procedure consists of preparing logarithmic or half-logarithmic dilutions of the virus suspension in a suitable diluent. Each dilution is inoculated into susceptible cell cultures. The cultures are incubated and observed for evidence of viral replication. The end point of the titration (which represents the viral dose) is the highest dilution of the viral suspension that produces a reaction in 50% of the cell cultures inoculated. In cell cultures, the dose that gives rise to CPE in 50% of the inoculated cultures is the **tissue culture infective dose (TCID$_{50}$)** [11]. The TCID$_{50}$ is used to determine the working dilution of the virus to use in the neutralization procedure. In most neutralization procedures, 100 to 1000 TCID$_{50}$ is the desired working dilution. A procedure for performing a viral titration is presented in the Appendix. If a titration cannot be performed, the test dilution may be selected empirically. Suggested dilutions include a 1:10 or 1:50 dilution for isolates that produce CPE slowly and a 1:500 or 1:1000 dilution for viruses that produce CPE rapidly [24].

Another titration procedure called a **viral back titration** is part of the quality control system used in neutralization and other techniques. This procedure is set up in conjunction with viral neutralization tests to ensure that the proper working dilution, determined in the viral titration, has been used in the test system [20]. The back titration is performed by preparing a set of 10-fold serial dilutions of the virus suspension used in the neutralization test. Then the original suspension and each of the 10-fold dilutions are inoculated into cell cultures. The cell cultures are incubated and observed for evidence of viral replication. The expected results of the titration are calculated and are then compared with the actual result. If the actual result does not resemble the predicted results, it is likely that too much or too little challenge dose of virus has been used in the test system. A procedure for performing the viral back titration is presented in the Appendix. This back titration procedure may be used to determine virus dose in any solution containing live virus; its use is not confined to the neutralization assay.

Other Methods for Identification of Viral Isolates

Immunofluorescence and neutralization are certainly not the only methods that are available and useful for making a definitive viral identification. Other immunoserological assays such as enzyme immunoassay, complement fixation, and hemagglutination inhibition as well as molecular techniques such as nucleic acid probes and polymerase chain reaction (PCR) will also provide the final identification required; each of these methods is diagrammed and discussed in Chapter 2. For each virology laboratory, the methods that are in place for other diagnostic services may dictate the methods used to identify viral isolates. For example, in a laboratory in which enzyme immunoassay is being used for detection of respiratory syncytial virus antigen in clinical samples (see Chapter 5, Viral Antigen Detection Methods), the same enzyme immunoassay can be applied to cell culture cells thought to be infected with respiratory syncytial virus. Enzyme immunoassays are also available for identification of herpes simplex and influenza A. Likewise, laboratories that use molecular diagnostic techniques, complement fixation, or hemagglutination inhibition for other purposes may well prefer to confirm viral identification using these methods.

CONTAMINATION IN CELL CULTURES

Because cell cultures are bathed in enriched media and incubated at 35°C, they provide optimal conditions for growth of bacteria and fungi. Bacterial and fungal contaminants in cell cultures present a problem in the virology laboratory. Of course, cell cultures that are overgrown with contaminants cannot effectively support viral proliferation and are usually destroyed before viruses have the opportunity to manifest their presence. Contaminants in cell cultures can be divided into two categories: those that are **indigenous** to the cells used to prepare the cell culture and those that are **introduced** into the cell culture in the diagnostic virology laboratory through inoculation and manipulation of the cell cultures.

Indigenous contaminants are usually monkey viruses that proliferate in primary monkey kidney cell culture tubes. Typical CPE for these contaminating monkey viruses is a vacuolar or "foamy" appearance or formation of syncytia. Although such contaminants may appear in only a few tubes of a given lot of cells, it is best to discontinue use of any contaminated lot immediately. Reinoculation of a stored, processed clinical sample into a different lot of cell cultures is indicated for cultures that are disrupted by appearance of indigenous contaminants. One must consult the manufacturer immediately to report any problems resulting from indigenous contaminants.

Another group of organisms that occasionally contaminate cell cultures is the mycoplasmas. Mycoplasmas grow within infected cells often without producing visible changes. Monolayers may fail to form properly or control viruses may fail to proliferate in mycoplasma-infected cells. Mycoplasma contaminants may originate from contaminated fetal bovine serum or from the tissue of origin of cell cultures. Mycoplasmal contamination may present a significant problem in laboratories in which cell cultures are prepared in house. In-house lines should be checked periodically for mycoplasmal contamination. If mycoplasma is detected, the cells (and all of the products involved in their culturing and maintenance) should be discarded. If the cells are especially valuable and cannot be discarded, antibiotics are available for treating the cells in an attempt to eliminate the contaminants. This treatment is not uniformly successful. Commercially prepared cells are monitored by their manufacturers for mycoplasmal contamination. Despite this, it is wise to perform mycoplasma testing periodically on a cell culture or two of each type of cell that is frequently purchased. The manufacturer should be consulted immediately if mycoplasmas are identified in cell cultures.

Bacterial and fungal contaminants that enter cell cultures either as flora of a clinical sample or through failures in sterile technique are far more common than the contaminants mentioned previously. What can be done with a cell culture that is overgrown with bacteria or fungi? This problem has not been resolved. Two alternatives are available: (1) The cell culture medium can be filtered from the contaminated cell culture tubes (using a 0.45-μm syringe-top filter) and the filtered fluid used to inoculate fresh cell cultures, or (2) if a stored (frozen) portion of the original processed sample is available, the contaminated cell culture tubes can be discarded and a fresh set of cultures inoculated using the stored sample; the stored material can be filtered before inoculating the fresh culture tubes [14]. There is currently no accepted protocol for "curing" bacterial or fungal infections in cell cultures by treating with antibiotics.

EVALUATING CELL CULTURES AND FOLLOWING UP

The daily routine that is followed in the diagnostic virology laboratory includes evaluating cell cultures and, on the basis of these observations, deciding on the appropriate steps to follow to produce the desired product: the final result! The information provided here is intended as a practical guide for performing the routine activities involved in isolating viruses in traditional cell cultures.

All inoculated cell cultures in their first 14 days of incubation should be viewed microscopically at least every other working day to determine whether CPE is present. Cultures that are in their 14th to 30th days of incubation should be evaluated once per week. Cultures should also be evaluated macroscopically for bacterial and fungal contamination and pH changes that may adversely affect the cell culture. All observations and follow-up actions should be recorded on the work card for each culture, and the technologist should initial each notation.

For routine observations, the cell culture tube must be first evaluated macroscopically for turbidity or media color changes that signal changes in pH. Cell culture media should be clear and orange-pink in color. If turbidity or color changes are evident, the tube must be viewed microscopically to determine the cause of the change. Using a standard light microscope, the virologist should examine the cell monolayer using 100× magnification (10× low-power objective with 10× oculars). The tube must be moved in the tube holder to examine at least 12 to 15 fields. The edges of the monolayer as well as the center areas must be examined for evidence of CPE or other changes in the cells. Observations should be noted on the work card.

If contamination resulting from bacteria or fungi is detected, a notation is made on the work card for the affected tube. An uninoculated cell culture tube of the same type is retrieved and labeled with the culture identification number of the original tube and the letter A. Subsequent passages of the same tube can be designated B, C, and so on. The cell culture fluid is treated by filtering as described previously for contaminated cell cultures. The filtered fluid can be used as inoculum for the new culture tube (labeled A). Several tubes from the same culture can be filtered with a common syringe and filter. When the filter is clogged and excess force is needed to depress the plunger on the syringe, the filter should be removed and replaced with a new one. The stored (frozen) processed original sample can be used, rather than filtered contaminated fluid, to initiate a repeat culture when contamination is severe. To inoculate a new set of cell culture tubes, the stored, processed sample is thawed and filtered and used to inoculate fresh tubes labeled with the original culture number and the letter R (R for reinoculated).

If turbidity resulting from excess clinical specimen inoculum (e.g., white cells, biopsy debris) is detected, a notation is made on the work card for the affected tube. The monolayer is rinsed two to three times by aspirating the cell culture media and adding fresh media. Then fresh medium is added, and the tube is reincubated.

If the appearance of the cell monolayer is altered as a result of pH changes, specimen toxicity, cell deterioration, or very early viral proliferation that is too weak to evaluate, a notation is made on the work card for the affected tube. Then, 0.1 to 0.5 ml of media is withdrawn from the original tube and used to inoculate a fresh tube. The smaller volume (0.1 ml) of fluid can be used for specimens thought to be toxic (e.g., stool, bile), and the larger volume (0.5 ml) can be used for specimens with possible early CPE. This procedure is referred to as "passing." The passing procedure is done to dilute toxic material so that the new cell culture will remain unaffected and to allow any virus present to infect another host. If the changes in the initial cell culture were due to viral proliferation, the CPE will recur in the new culture tube. If the changes in the initial cell culture were due to toxicity and so on, the problems may be eliminated by using the fresh tube, and the culture may now progress normally.

During routine observations when viral CPE is detected, a notation is made on the work card for the affected tube. The CPE is described (i.e., rounding, swelling, shrinking, vacuoles, clusters, syncytia) and quantitated (as described earlier in this chapter). Two technologists should evaluate CPE from positive cultures and reach agreement on the virus suspected and the follow-up actions to take.

If the virus suspected is adenovirus, herpes simplex, measles, respiratory syncytial virus, or varicella, the virologist should scrape cells from the monolayer and prepare smears for immunofluorescence testing. (See Appendix: Preparing Antigen Smears for Immunofluorescence Testing.) If another identification method is used in the laboratory, the virologist prepares the infected cell culture material for testing by that method. Then the confirmatory test procedure can be performed.

If the virus suspected is influenza, mumps, or parainfluenza, a hemadsorption procedure should be done. For cultures with positive hemadsorption test results, smears for immunofluorescence testing are prepared (or the sample is prepared for testing by another appropriate method) to identify the hemadsorption-positive virus definitively.

If the CPE is characteristic for cytomegalovirus, "CMV isolated" should be reported. If CPE is questionable, cells may be scraped from the cell culture tube and inoculated into shell vials for detection of cytomegalovirus early antigens. (See Appendix: Inoculation of Shell Vial Cultures and Cytomegalovirus Early Antigen Detection in Shell Vials.)

If the virus appears to be an enterovirus, cell culture material should be passed to a fresh cell culture tube of the same type. The fresh culture should be observed in 24 hours to determine whether evidence of viral proliferation recurs. If CPE characteristic of the enteroviruses is evident in the fresh culture tube, "entero-like virus isolated" should be reported. This is often the final report for enteroviruses because they can be accurately identified only through neutralization testing. In laboratories that perform the neutralization test for identification of enteroviruses (see Appendix for procedure for identification of enteroviruses using the Lim Benyesh-Melnick pools), enteroviral isolates from spinal fluid are usually identified. Other isolates are not identified unless the physician indicates there is a specific reason why the testing is necessary.

When the identity of the isolated virus has been determined, "(name of virus) isolated" should be reported to the physician. If viral CPE is not typical or if other problems are encountered, a fellow virologist or the virology laboratory supervisor should be consulted. Problems can be addressed more efficiently when experienced virologists are consulted.

It is helpful to preserve (frozen at −70°C or colder) viral isolates. Stored isolates are especially useful in epidemiological investigations and for antiviral susceptibility testing. To store adenovirus and enterovirus isolates, the infected cell culture tube is placed in the −70°C freezer with the cell culture medium resting on the cells. The medium should be allowed to freeze. The frozen medium can be thawed by running cold water on the culture tube. The freeze-thaw cycle should be repeated two more times. The material can be transferred to a conical centrifuge tube and spun at approximately 1600g for 10 minutes. Then the supernatant fluid is transferred to a cryovial for storage. For all other virus isolates, the cell culture medium is transferred from an infected tube into a cryovial. The cryovial is labeled with the patient's name, specimen type, log number, date collected, and virus type.

In routine evaluation of cell cultures when there is no evidence of viral CPE in any of the cell culture tubes for a clinical sample, the virologist makes a notation on the work card for the culture. If the sample is a respiratory specimen, one of the primary monkey kidney cell culture tubes from the culture should be tested by hemadsorption after 6 to 8 days of incubation (see Appendix for hemadsorption procedure). If the hemadsorption test is positive, the infected cell monolayer is prepared for testing for virus identification (by immunofluorescence or other method available in the laboratory). If the hemadsorption test is negative, the monkey kidney cell monolayer is rinsed with cell culture medium, fresh cell culture medium added, and the tube returned to the incubator. A hemadsorption test is performed routinely on all CPE-negative primary monkey kidney tubes from respiratory specimens before their disposal at the end of the routine 14-day incubation period.

If no CPE is observed during the 14-day incubation period and all additional tests such as hemadsorption fail to demonstrate that a virus is present, the culture result is reported as "no virus isolated." The incubation period for routine cultures is 14 days; for "herpes only" cultures, 7 days; and for the diploid fibroblast tubes from cultures with cytomegalovirus as the suspect, 30 days. The accompanying cell culture tubes containing other types of cells (e.g., A549, primary monkey kidney) on the cytomegalovirus cultures may be discarded after 14 days if they show no evidence of viral proliferation.

For all cell culture tubes being maintained during their 2- to 4-week incubation periods, it is necessary to provide fresh cell culture medium periodically to ensure the integrity of the monolayer. Once each week, the cell culture medium is decanted from all tubes that have been incubating for 24 hours or longer. Two milliliters of fresh cell culture medium is added to each tube. This addition can be accomplished quickly using an inexpensive, autoclavable repipettor device (see Chapter 7).

R E F E R E N C E S

1. Drew WL. Viral Infections. Philadelphia: FA Davis, 1976.
2. Leonardi GP, Gleaves CA. Selection, collection, and transport of specimens for viral and rickettsial cultures. In Isenberg HD (ed), Clinical Microbiology Procedures Handbook. Washington, DC: American Society for Microbiology, 1992, pp 8.2.1–8.2.10.
3. Madeley RC, Lennette DA, Halonen P. Specimen collection and transport. In Lennette EH, Halonen P, Murphy FA (eds), Laboratory Diagnosis of Infectious Diseases Principles and Practice, vol 2. New York: Springer-Verlag, 1988, pp 1–11.
4. Bettoli EJ, Brewer PM, Oxtoby MJ, et al. The role of temperature and swab materials in the recovery of herpes simplex virus from lesions. J Infect Dis 1982;145:399.
5. Crane LR, Gutterman PA, Chapel T, Lerner AM. Incubation of swab materials with herpes simplex virus. J Infect Dis 1980;141:531.
6. Huntoon CJ, House RF Jr, Smith TF. Recovery of viruses from three transport media incorporated into culturettes. Arch Pathol Lab Med 1981;105:436–437.
7. Johnson FB, Leavitt RW, Richards DF. Evaluation of the Virocult transport tube for isolation of herpes simplex virus from clinical specimens. J Clin Microbiol 1984;20:120–122.
8. Smith TF. Specimen requirements. In Spector S, Lancz GJ (ed), Clinical Virology Manual. New York: Elsevier, 1986, pp 22–29.
9. Chernesky MA, Ray CG, Smith TF. In Drew WL (ed), Cumitech 15, Laboratory Diagnosis of Viral Infections. Washington, DC: American Society for Microbiology, 1982.
10. Lennette EH. General principles underlying laboratory diagnosis of viral and rickettsial infections. In Lennette EH, Schmidt NJ (eds), Diagnostic Procedures for Viral and Rickettsial Infections, 4th ed. New York: American Public Health Association, 1969.
11. Schmidt NJ. Tissue culture technics for diagnostic virology. In Lennette EH, Schmidt NJ (eds), Diagnostic Procedures for Viral and Rickettsial Infections, 4th ed. New York: American Public Health Association, 1969, pp 79–178.
12. Black J. Microbiology Principles and Applications, 2nd ed. Englewood Cliffs, NJ: Prentice Hall, 1994.
13. Clarke LM, McPhee JM, Cummings RV. Isolation of viruses in conventional tube culture: selection and inoculation of cell cultures. In Isenberg HD (ed), Clinical Microbiology Procedures Handbook. Washington, DC: American Society for Microbiology, 1992, pp 8.5.1–8.5.13.
14. Aarnaes S, Daidone BJ. Observation and maintenance of inoculated cell cultures. In Isenberg HD (ed), Clinical Microbiology Procedures Handbook. Washington, DC: American Society for Microbiology, 1992, pp 8.7.1–8.7.16.
15. Lennette DA. Preparation of specimens for virological examination. In Balows A, Hausler WJ Jr, Herrman KL, et al (eds), Manual of Clinical Microbiology, 5th ed. Washington, DC: American Society for Microbiology, 1991.
16. Hughes JH. Physical and chemical methods for enhancing rapid detection of viruses and other agents. Clin Microbiol Rev 1993;6:150–175.
17. Fenner F, White DO. Medical Virology, 2nd ed. New York: Academic Press, 1976.
18. Hsiung GD. Diagnostic Virology. New Haven, CT: Yale University Press, 1973.
19. Debre R, Celers J. Clinical Virology. Philadelphia: WB Saunders, 1970.
20. Grist NR, Ross CA, Bell EJ. Diagnostic Methods in Clinical Virology, 2nd ed. Oxford, England: Blackwell Scientific Publications, 1974.
21. Swenson PD. Detection of viruses by hemadsorption. In Isenberg HD (ed), Clinical Microbiology Procedures Handbook. Washington, DC: American Society for Microbiology, 1992, pp 8.8.1–8.8.5.
22. Minnich LL, Ray GC. Early testing of cell cultures for detection of hemadsorbing viruses. J Clin Microbiol 1987;25:421–422.
23. Revozzo GC, Burke CN. A Manual of Basic Virological Techniques. Englewood Cliffs, NJ: Prentice-Hall, 1973.
24. Lipson SM. Neutralization test for the identification and typing of viral isolates. In Isenberg HD (ed), Clinical Microbiology Procedures Handbook. Washington, DC: American Society for Microbiology, 1992, pp 8.14.1–8.14.8.

REVIEW QUESTIONS

1. Match the clinical specimen of choice from Column B with the clinical manifestation from Column A:

A	B
___ Respiratory tract infection	a. Stool
___ Central nervous system infection	b. Throat or nasal swab
___ Exanthem	c. Vesicle fluid and scrapings
___ Gastroenteritis	d. Urine
	e. Cerebrospinal fluid

2. In selecting and collecting samples for viral culturing, which of the following guidelines is applicable?
   a. An anticoagulated peripheral blood sample is appropriate regardless of the virus suspected or clinical signs and symptoms.
   b. Specimens collected from normally sterile sources such as cerebrospinal fluid should be placed in an antibiotic-containing transport medium.
   c. Calcium alginate swabs are preferred for sample collection.
   d. Specimens should be collected early in the acute phase of the infection to obtain maximal virus yield.

3. Viral transport media are important in the collection process for many viral culture specimens. The purpose and content of these media are defined as follows:
   a. Contain antibiotics that suppress the growth of usual flora organisms such as bacteria and fungi
   b. Contain glucose to stimulate and nourish the virus during the transport period
   c. May contain a neutral red dye, which should be bright yellow in color if the pH of 6.9 to 7.2 is maintained
   d. Contain buffers and proteins to enhance viral replication during transport

4. Specimens for virus isolation that must be shipped to a virology laboratory and that will not be processed for 5 days or longer after collection should be shipped as follows:
   a. Use screw-capped container and ship on wet ice
   b. Lyophilize and ship at ambient temperature
   c. Freeze at $-70°C$ or colder and ship in dry ice in a container impervious to CO_2
   d. Remove from transport medium and ship at $37°C$

5. Processing of most clinical specimens is required before the specimen is inoculated into cell cultures for virus isolation. Which of the guidelines describes proper specimen processing?
   a. Centrifugation aids in concentrating the viruses into the bottom of the tube.
   b. Specimens collected from sterile sites should be filtered before inoculation into cell cultures.
   c. For most specimens, sediment is used to inoculate cell cultures.
   d. Antibiotics aid in decontamination of specimens collected from contaminated sites.

6. Which of the following phrases accurately describes cell culture media?
   a. Include a phenol red color indicator that turns bright magenta-pink when the pH of the culture medium is neutral and cells are healthy
   b. May be classified as a maintenance medium or an outgrowth medium depending on the amount of enrichments and buffers
   c. Always contain approximately 15 to 20% serum
   d. Contain T-soy broth and a reducing agent

7. Each phrase and cell line listed in Column A is in some way associated with one of the cell culture classifications given in Column B. Record the letter of each of the items in Column A in the blank to the left of the classification it describes in Column B. (Use all of the items in Column A; there will be more than one correct answer for each item in Column B.)

A		B
a. Can produce new generations indefinitely	_____	Primary cells
b. Are freshly explanted from tissue	_____	Diploid cells
c. Have altered numbers of chromosomes	_____	Established
d. Maintain diploid chromosomal configuration throughout multiple passages		(heteroploid)
e. May harbor "indigenous" viral contaminants		
f. Tend to die out after 50 generations		
g. Usually originate from malignancies		
h. MRC-5 cells		
i. Rhesus monkey kidney cells		
j. A549 and HeLa cells		

8. Observing cytopathogenic effect (CPE) is one method of detecting viral proliferation in cell cultures. Which of the following is true concerning CPE?
    a. For cytomegalovirus, CPE routinely appears within 24 to 48 hours and involves grapelike clustering of cells throughout the monolayer.
    b. CPE may appear as swelling, shrinking, syncytia formation, clustering, and so on.
    c. If typical, CPE provides a definitive identification of a virus; no additional testing is required.
    d. CPE can be observed only when stained preparations of infected cells are examined with the oil immersion objective of a light microscope.

9. Hemadsorption testing is used frequently to detect viral proliferation in cell cultures. Which of the following phrases describes the hemadsorption testing procedure, principle, or appearance of results?
    a. The hemadsorption phenomenon results from interferon production in virus-infected cells.
    b. Hemadsorption testing involves replacing the cell culture medium with a suspension of erythrocytes.
    c. In a positive hemadsorption test, large clumps of erythrocytes will be seen floating in the cell culture medium.
    d. A positive hemadsorption test confirms the identification of the virus as influenza A.

10. Which of the following procedures is suitable for making a definitive viral identification?
    a. Viral titration and back titration
    b. Immunofluorescence
    c. Interference challenge
    d. Hemadsorption

11. True or false: In collecting a specimen for virus isolation from a skin lesion, it is important to collect material from the base or active edge of the lesion rather than from necrotic material or from dry, crusty material from the top of the lesion.

12. True or false: In processing a heparinized blood specimen for viral culture, the specimen is allowed to settle for 1 hour at room temperature, and the packed red cells in the bottom of the tube are used to inoculate the cell culture tubes.

13. True or false: Syncytia are large, frothy, bubble-like clear areas, usually in the cytoplasm of virus infected cells.

14. True or false: In an interference challenge test, the suspect cell culture was challenged with echovirus. The echovirus produced characteristic CPE. Therefore, we can conclude that a virus was *not* proliferating in the suspect culture.

15. True or false: In a neutralization test, poliovirus antiserum is mixed with the unknown virus. After a sample of the virus-serum mixture is added to a cell culture tube, no CPE is seen. This result confirms that the unknown virus is *not* poliovirus.

16. True or false: One option for dealing with contaminated cell culture tubes is to filter the cell culture medium from the contaminated tube and use the filtered medium to inoculate new cell culture tubes.

Modified Virus Isolation Systems

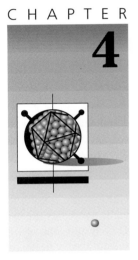

OBJECTIVES

At the completion of this unit of study, the student will be able to do the following:

1. List three reasons why modified virus isolation systems are important in virus isolation.
2. Describe the shell vial system, including proper inoculation, incubation, and staining.
3. Give specific information comparing isolation of cytomegalovirus in shell vials and in traditional cell cultures.
4. Give examples of viruses other than cytomegalovirus that can be identified in shell vials.
5. Describe virus isolation in cell cultures grown in microwell plates and indicate how this system is used for virus isolation.
6. Describe one herpes isolation and identification system and explain how this system is used in the laboratory.
7. Describe human lymphocyte suspension cultures and list viruses that require this type of system for their isolation.

INTRODUCTION

Although traditional cell cultures of adherent cells growing in tubes have long been the standard for virus isolation, the traditional system is not necessarily the best choice for all viruses and for all laboratory situations:

    1. A laboratory may wish to offer only a limited set of diagnostic virology services. Limiting of services may be required because of a lack of personnel who are trained in diagnostic virology or a lack of time or equipment for performing full-service diagnostic virology. The laboratory may want to target only one or two of the more common viruses and offer limited diagnostic services.

    2. Some viruses, most notably cytomegalovirus (CMV), may be slow and difficult to isolate in traditional cell cultures but may be more rapidly and easily detected in a modified system.

3. Some viruses do not proliferate in standard cell cultures but can be isolated when cultured in a system designed specifically to enhance their replication.

Table 3–1 lists viruses isolated in standard cell cultures at a full-service virology laboratory during a recent 2-year period. This list includes at least 10 different viruses. However, the two most frequent isolates are herpes simplex virus (HSV) and CMV, which account for more isolates than all of the other viruses combined. This list is representative of isolates from clinical virology laboratories, with many laboratories reporting even higher percentages of herpes simplex isolates [1]. Through analysis of virus isolation frequency, it is obvious that a laboratory could limit diagnostic services to detection or isolation of either HSV or CMV, or both, and still be providing a significant service. Isolation systems are needed that are efficient and cost effective for isolating the target viruses. Additionally, modified systems are required to enhance or simplify the detection of viruses that proliferate poorly or not at all in standard cell cultures.

Four types of modified cell culture systems are discussed in this chapter. The first, the **shell vial system,** involving centrifugation-enhanced inoculation of cell monolayers grown in shell vials, simplifies the task of CMV detection while dramatically improving the speed of isolation. This system has also been applied for rapid detection of other viruses. The second modified system uses cultures of adherent cells grown in **microwell plates.** This system is based on the same concepts as the shell vial system and has been used for both HSV and CMV detection. The third modified system, an **HSV isolation-identification system,** targets only HSV; the culture setup is convenient and requires little if any expertise on the part of the technologist. The fourth system, featuring **suspensions of stimulated human lymphocytes,** was developed primarily for isolation of human immunodeficiency virus (HIV), which will not proliferate in standard cell culture systems. Each modified system is designed for detection of a specific virus or group of viruses. These systems do not provide the appropriate isolation conditions or detection methods to allow them to isolate a wide range of viruses; viruses other than the target viruses will be missed by the modified systems.

SHELL VIAL CULTURES AND CENTRIFUGATION-ENHANCED INOCULATION

General Concepts

Monolayers of adherent cells grown on 12-mm round coverslips contained in 1-dram shell vials (Fig. 4–1) have provided a viral isolation system that uses centrifugation to enhance virus isolation. The shell vial technique was originally developed and has been used extensively for culturing *Chlamydia trachomatis,* which does not grow well in standard cell cultures. The vials are prepared by adding dispersed cells to sterile shell vials containing coverslips; the vials are incubated in an upright position until the cells form a monolayer on the coverslip. For vial inoculation (Fig. 4–2), the culture medium is decanted from the vial, processed clinical material is placed directly on the cell monolayer, and the vial is spun in a centrifuge at low speed for 1 hour. After centrifugation, fresh culture medium is added to each vial. The vials are then incubated for the desired time period. At the end of the incubation period, the coverslip is stained using an antigen detection method or the cells are evaluated via a molecular diagnostic technique. A procedure for shell vial inoculation is provided in the Appendix of this volume.

Shell vial inoculation, incubation, staining, and evaluation are not technically difficult. However, use of the shell vial system may require two additions to the virology laboratories' equipment list. Because the vials are spun in the centrifuge, centrifuge carriers that will safely hold the vials are needed. The vials are small and usually do not fit very well in centrifuge carriers designed for tall test tubes. Specialized carriers should be purchased for this purpose. The other device that is needed is used to aid in removing the coverslips from the bottom of the vials during the evaluation process. This process requires dexterity on the part of the virologist and is simplified when a transfer device is available. One device that can be prepared in house for this

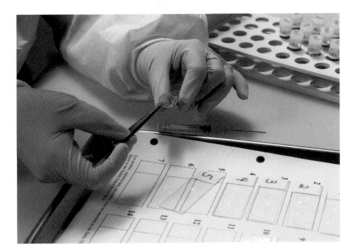

. . . .
FIGURE 4–1 THE SHELL VIAL SYSTEM features 1-dram shell vials containing cell monolayers grown on coverslips. The inoculated vial is spun in the centrifuge during the inoculation process. At the end of the incubation period, coverslips are stained and removed from the vial for microscopic examination.

purpose is made from an 18-gauge syringe needle. The tip of the needle bevel is bent with a hemostat to make a tiny hook (Fig. 4–3). When the needle is attached to a tuberculin syringe, the hook on the needle tip can be inserted under the rim of the coverslip in the shell vial, and the coverslip can be lifted up to allow it to be grasped with forceps and transferred to the microscope slide. Other types of needles may be used for the same purpose, but the one described here is inexpensive and effective.

Shell vials are used when the isolation of one particular virus (or group of viruses) is desired rather than for broad-spectrum virus isolation as with traditional cell cultures. The cell line that is grown on the coverslip, the length of the incubation period, and the type of detection method and its specificity all depend on the target virus. For example, routinely for CMV detection in shell vials, human fibroblast cell lines are grown on the coverslip, vials are incubated 24 to 48 hours or longer, and an immunofluorescent method for detection of CMV early antigen is used. For HSV detection, one of the many herpes-susceptible cell lines is grown on the coverslip, vials can be stained after a shorter incubation period (16–20 hours), and detection is by immunofluorescence, immunoperoxidase, or nucleic acid probe.

The centrifugation step in inoculation of the shell vials is an essential part of the success of the technology. The exact mechanism of centrifugation enhancement of viral infectivity is not well defined. Initially, it was assumed that centrifugal force drives bits of virus-infected material against the monolayer, which enhances viral attachment and penetration. However, a more accurate evaluation of the effects of centrifugation indicates that the centrifugation process appears to mechanically "stress" the cells in the monolayer to increase cell proliferation, decrease cell generation times, activate genes, alter cell metabolism, and increase cell longevity [2]. These effects may be beneficial for viral replication.

Shell vial cultures are not routinely examined for cytopathogenic effect (CPE) production. Instead, they are all stained or otherwise evaluated at a specified time interval to detect viral antigens within the cells. This is sometimes called **pre-CPE detection.** Because viral detection does not rely on CPE production, positive results are usually available sooner in shell vial cultures than in traditional cell cultures.

The shell vial system, when used appropriately, significantly shortens the isolation times of certain viruses, especially CMV. CMV isolation in shell vials is described later in this chapter. This system allows timely and improved isolation of CMV as well as other viruses. In addition, cell monolayers in shell vials may be less susceptible to contamination or deterioration than traditional cell culture monolayers [3].

Although the shell vial system offers considerable advantage in the speed of virus detection, there are some disadvantages of the system:

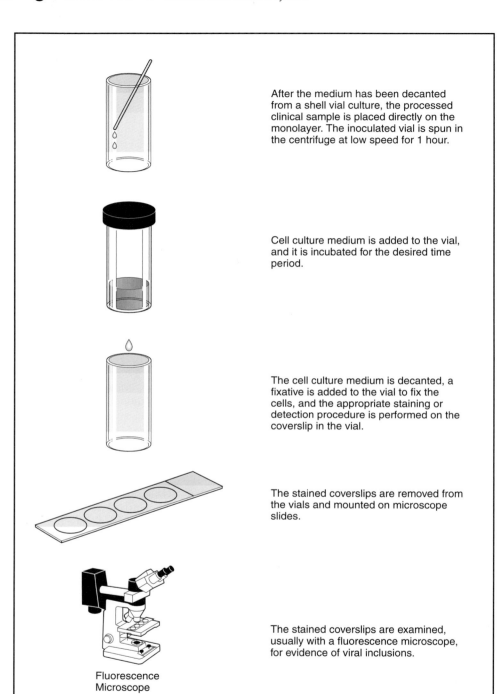

After the medium has been decanted from a shell vial culture, the processed clinical sample is placed directly on the monolayer. The inoculated vial is spun in the centrifuge at low speed for 1 hour.

Cell culture medium is added to the vial, and it is incubated for the desired time period.

The cell culture medium is decanted, a fixative is added to the vial to fix the cells, and the appropriate staining or detection procedure is performed on the coverslip in the vial.

The stained coverslips are removed from the vials and mounted on microscope slides.

The stained coverslips are examined, usually with a fluorescence microscope, for evidence of viral inclusions.

Fluorescence
Microscope

FIGURE 4–2 SHELL VIAL INOCULATION.

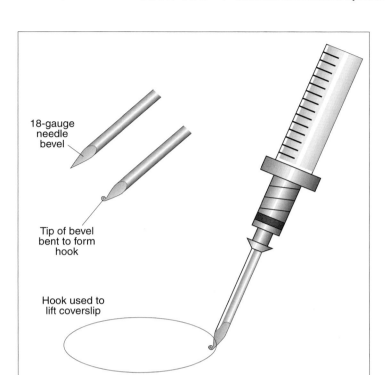

18-gauge
needle
bevel

Tip of bevel
bent to form
hook

Hook used to
lift coverslip

**FIGURE 4–3 AN 18-GAUGE NEEDLE IS USED FOR MANIPULA-
TION OF SHELL VIAL COVERSLIPS.** The tip of the bevel of the
18-gauge needle is bent to form a hook. When the needle is attached to
a syringe, the hook can be inserted under the edge of the coverslip in the
shell vial to lift the coverslip up so it can be grasped with forceps.

1. Because detection of virus in shell vials depends on the capacity of the virus to infect cells
and initiate replication, a false-negative result may be obtained with samples that are improperly
collected or transported, resulting in inactivation of the viruses. This is not simply a direct antigen
detection method; viral infectivity is required.

2. Because virus is detected through application of a specific detection method, only the virus
tested for will be identified. Any other virus that may be proliferating in the cells will be missed.

3. In the shell vial procedures that involve detection by immunofluorescence, the technologist
must devote considerable time to evaluation of each shell vial result. Each entire coverslip must
be scanned, which requires concentration and time. The tedious nature of this examination makes
the shell vial system labor intensive.

4. For isolation of most viruses, the shell vial system is not as sensitive as traditional cell
cultures. Therefore, if shell vials alone are used for virus isolation, some isolates will be missed.

5. The shell vial system may be expensive if the detection method requires monoclonal
antibody preparations. Some of the antibody preparations are expensive, and a larger volume of
reagent is required for staining of coverslips in vials than for staining of smears prepared from
cell pellets and fixed on microscope slides.

6. If shell vials are used in addition to traditional cell cultures, the added expense and time
required for the shell vial system may be significant.

Cytomegalovirus Isolation in Shell Vials

CMV was the first virus targeted for isolation in shell vials because it often requires 7 to 21 days
to produce characteristic CPE in traditional cell cultures. Routinely, when the shell vial system

is used for CMV isolation, the vials contain coverslips of fibroblast cells, which are inoculated, incubated for 24 to 48 hours, and stained by an immunofluorescence method using monoclonal antibodies against CMV immediate early antigens. Many monoclonal antibody preparations are available for this purpose. Some of the antibodies are fluorescein labeled for use in direct immunofluorescence staining, whereas others are not fluorescein labeled and must be used in indirect immunofluorescence techniques. Both direct and indirect immunofluorescence staining techniques are illustrated and described in Chapter 2, and a direct immunofluorescence staining procedure for detection of CMV immediate early antigen in shell vials is included in the Appendix. Figure 4–4 shows fluorescing CMV inclusions stained with monoclonal antibodies against CMV immediate early protein after 24 hours of incubation. The inclusions may range from few to numerous and may vary from oval to sausage shaped.

In 1984, Gleaves and colleagues [4] used shell vial cultures to study CMV isolation from urine. At 36 and 96 hours after inoculation, the coverslips were stained with a monoclonal antibody to CMV early antigen. This system yielded 100% specificity and was more sensitive than traditional cell cultures (incubated for 2 weeks) for isolation of CMV from urine specimens. Additional evaluation of this system showed that CMV early antigen could be detected as early as 16 hours after inoculation [4, 5]. This same group of investigators [6] compared this technique with standard cell culture isolation of CMV from samples other than urine (e.g., blood, throat) and found shell vial culture to be useful for CMV isolation from all types of specimens. However, culturing for CMV in conventional tube cultures as well as in shell vials was recommended by these investigators as well as others [7] to ensure optimal sensitivity of CMV isolation from sources other than urine.

Others have shown that, through the use of both shell vials and traditional cell cultures for CMV isolation, the turnaround time (time from culture inoculation until virus is identified) for detecting CMV can be reduced by half from the time required when traditional cultures alone are used. In one study [3], the turnaround time for CMV-positive urine cultures was reduced from 15 to 7 days and that for CMV-positive blood cultures was decreased from 18 to 9 days. Figure 4–5 shows the time required for CMV isolation from various types of specimens cultured in shell vials (stained at 24 to 48 hours after inoculation) and in traditional cell cultures incubated for 30 days at Indiana University School of Medicine Virology Laboratory in 1992 (unpublished data). Nearly 90% of CMV from urine specimens were identified in shell vials as well as 81% from broncho-alveolar lavage samples and 74% from peripheral blood samples. Only 50% of CMV from throat swabs was isolated in shell vials. These data demonstrate that traditional cell cultures are important for optimal CMV isolation, especially from specimens such as throat swabs.

The use of a cell line other than human fibroblasts has been reported for CMV isolation in shell vials [8]. In mink lung cells, which do not permit replication of new CMV virions, CMV enters the cells to produce early antigens that can be detected by immunofluorescent staining. The

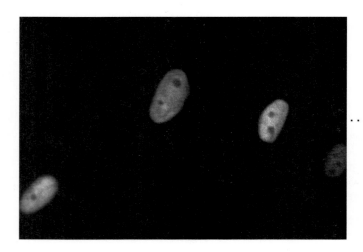

· · · · · · · · · · · · · ·
FIGURE 4–4 FLUORESCING CYTOMEGALOVIRUS (CMV) INCLUSIONS IN SHELL VIAL MONOLAYERS STAINED WITH ANTIBODIES AGAINST CMV IMMEDIATE EARLY AN-TIGENS. These inclusions range from oval to sausage shaped and produce apple-green fluorescence.

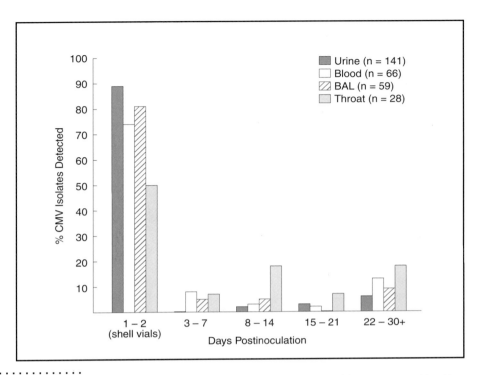

FIGURE 4–5   CYTOMEGALOVIRUS (CMV) ISOLATION TIMES. Using two fibroblast shell vials for each sample (three for blood samples), one stained at 24 hours and one (two for bloods) at 48 hours postinoculation, shell vial cultures successfully detected 89% of CMV from urine, 74% from peripheral blood, 81% from bronchoalveolar lavage (BAL) samples, and 50% from throat cultures. Other CMV isolates required from 3 to 30 days for isolation.

fluorescent foci of infection were larger and more numerous in mink lung cells than in fibroblast cultures.

Isolation of Other Viruses in Shell Vials

Another virus sometimes isolated in the shell vial system is HSV. This virus proliferates very well in traditional cell cultures; however, it was believed that it could be isolated even more quickly and effectively in shell vial cultures. When the shell vial system is applied for herpes simplex isolation, monolayers of herpes-susceptible cells such as rabbit kidney, mink lung, A549, or MRC-5 cells are used. The vials are often stained as early as 16 hours after inoculation, and an immunofluorescent or immunoperoxidase stain that detects both HSV-1 and -2 is used. This system is very effective for HSV detection. In 1985, Gleaves and associates [9] used the shell vial system for HSV isolation and found that it was as sensitive as routine tube cultures and produced results within 16 to 20 hours after inoculation.

Shell vial technology has only recently been applied for detection of the respiratory viruses (adenovirus; influenza A and B; parainfluenza types 1, 2, and 3; and respiratory syncytial virus [RSV]). Most of the respiratory viruses are slow (7–10 days) to produce CPE in traditional cell cultures or may produce CPE that is difficult to detect. RSV is the most common of the respiratory viruses, and its isolation in shell vials has been described. In one study of RSV isolation, HEp-2 shell vials incubated for 16 hours yielded more positives than antigen detection methods applied directly to the clinical sample, and it produced as many positives as conventional cell cultures [10].

Isolation of other respiratory viruses has also been achieved in shell vial cultures. Using vials of primary monkey kidney cells and of A549 cells incubated for 40 hours, 83% of adenoviruses, 94% of influenza B, and 80% of parainfluenza types 1, 2, and 3 were identified [11]. Another laboratory identified 50% of adenoviruses, 94% of influenza A, 100% of influenza B, 100% of the parainfluenzas, and 92% of RSV in shell vials of primary rhesus monkey kidney and HEp-2 cells incubated 2 to 4 days [12].

Shell Vial Purchase and Preparation

Excellent condition of the shell vial monolayer is critical for success of the shell vial technique. Shell vials are available commercially and are delivered with an intact cell monolayer growing on the coverslip. The commercial vials are routinely delivered when the monolayer is 7 days old and are used during the 7-day period between their delivery and the delivery of the next shipment. Fedorko and others [13] showed a marked drop in susceptibility of shell vials to CMV infection when monolayers reach 9 to 10 days old; therefore, the use of commercial vials may not be optimal when they pass the 10-day cutoff. Some manufacturers will provide twice-weekly deliveries of shell vials to ensure that vial monolayers are used while they are less than 10 days old and are optimally susceptible to CMV infection.

If twice-weekly delivery is not available, shell vials can be prepared in house. If virologists have time to prepare the vials from cell lines carried in house, the in-house vials are usually of higher quality than the commercial vials [14]. If carrying cell lines in house and preparing vials are too time consuming for the technical staff, kits are now available that simplify in-house preparation of vials. The shell vial preparation system includes sterile shell vials containing coverslips, outgrowth medium, and a frozen cell suspension. Vials are prepared as needed. The cell suspension is thawed as directed by the manufacturer [15], mixed with outgrowth medium, and aliquoted into the sterile vials. The vials are incubated in an upright position in a stationary rack and are ready for use 3 days after seeding.

MICROWELL CULTURES AND CENTRIFUGATION-ENHANCED INOCULATION

Another modified system, based on the same principles of centrifugation-enhanced inoculation and pre-CPE staining as the shell vial system, is prepared in a different physical configuration. Rather than using cells growing on coverslips contained in shell vials, this system features cells grown in the bottoms of wells of flat-bottomed microwell plates (Fig. 4–6). When the cell monolayer is established, the cell culture medium is discarded, and processed clinical samples are inoculated into the wells. The inoculated plate is covered and spun in the centrifuge at low speed for 1 hour. After centrifugation, fresh cell culture medium is added, and the microwell plate is incubated. At the end of the incubation period, the cell culture medium is discarded, and the reagents involved in the detection method are applied to the wells. When the staining procedure is completed, the microwell plate is positioned on the stage of a microscope. The microscope is focused to view the cells in the bottom of the plate, and the cells are examined for evidence of specific staining. Microwell plates may be prepared in house or purchased commercially.

At this writing, microwell plates for isolation of HSV and CMV are being marketed [16]. The HSV isolation plates feature African green monkey kidney cells. Inoculated plates are incubated for 24 hours; the cells are then incubated in a hybridization solution containing an alkaline phosphatase–labeled DNA probe specific for HSV-1 and -2. The results are read with a standard light microscope. The nuclei of herpes-infected cells stain purple, and uninfected cells remain unstained. This method detected 97.8% of herpes culture–positive specimens in a study of 648 clinical samples [17].

Microwell plates for CMV detection feature MRC-5 cells. After 24 to 48 hours of incubation, the cells are stained with an immunofluorescent method to detect CMV early antigen. After staining, glycerin is added to each well, the plate lid is replaced, and the stained microwells are examined on an inverted fluorescence microscope (or the plate can be inverted and examined on a standard fluorescence microscope with long working distance objectives).

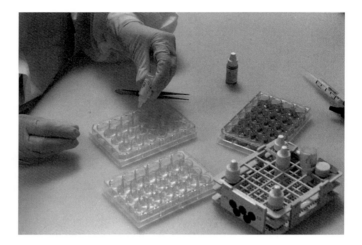

....
FIGURE 4–6 MONOLAYERS OF CELLS GROWING IN MICROWELL PLATES are featured in this modified virus isolation system. Each well is inoculated with clinical specimen material, the microwell plate is spun in the centrifuge, and viral proliferation is detected by staining with monoclonal antibodies or by molecular techniques. The plate is positioned on the stage of the microscope, and cell monolayers are observed in the bottom of the well.

The major advantage of the microwell system over shell vials is that physical manipulation of the system is simplified. There is no capping and recapping of vial tops, and there are no coverslips to manipulate. Also, the volume of expensive staining reagents is reduced because of the smaller surface area of the microwells compared with shell vials.

Because the microwell systems are newer and not widely used at this writing, there are few reports in the literature that evaluate their efficacy. Unpublished data indicate that viral detection in the microwell system is comparable to that of the shell vial system.

One disadvantage of the microwell system is the wasting of unused wells that are "left over" when there are not enough samples to fill a plate. This may make the system less cost effective. Also, the question of well-to-well contamination resulting from aerosols or condensation on the plate concerns some virologists. Although well-to-well contamination has been evaluated and shown to present no problem when careful technique is used in inoculating plates [18], this aspect of the microwell system will need further investigation.

HERPES SIMPLEX VIRUS ISOLATION AND IDENTIFICATION SYSTEMS

Because HSV-1 and -2 usually make up the majority of isolates in the clinical virology laboratory [1] and because HSV tends to proliferate rapidly and vigorously in standard cell cultures, isolation of these agents is an important laboratory service. Isolation-identification systems, designed specifically for rapid detection and identification of HSV, have been available commercially since the early 1980s. These systems include a cell culture tube or container of HSV-susceptible cells such as Vero. The cell monolayer may be grown on the flat side of a specially configured plastic tube or on a glass slide that is held against one side of the inside of a culture tube. This glass slide has a handle to facilitate its removal from the tube when the incubation period is complete. After the monolayer has been inoculated with a clinical sample and incubated for a defined period, usually 48 hours, a confirmatory test is performed on the cell monolayer. The confirmatory test is usually an immunoperoxidase staining method involving labeled antiherpes antibodies. The confirmatory test usually confirms the identification of HSV but does not differentiate HSV-1 from HSV-2.

Results obtained with these systems have varied considerably. When HSV detection at 48 hours after inoculation in an HSV isolation-identification system was compared in several studies with HSV isolation after 7 days of incubation in traditional cell cultures, the reported sensitivity of isolation in the HSV isolation-identification system ranged from 65 [19] to 92% [20]. The manufacturer of one HSV isolation-identification system currently reports 95 to 98% sensitivity for the rapid system [21].

Because HSV isolation systems rely on immunological "pre-CPE" identification of HSV antigen rather than on production of CPE, they routinely provide confirmation of HSV infection more rapidly than standard cell cultures. These systems are very useful in laboratories that do not wish to provide full-service virology. They require minimal expertise on the part of the technologist but represent an increased cost.

HUMAN LYMPHOCYTE SUSPENSION CULTURES

Viruses such as HIV-1 do not replicate within standard cultures of adherent cells. HIV-1 will replicate within lymphocytes; therefore, a modified isolation system that features laboratory cultures of human lymphocytes must be used for HIV isolation. This culture method is described as a **cocultivation culture** in which lymphocytes from the infected individual are cultured with phytohemagglutinin (PHA)-stimulated lymphocytes from an uninfected (healthy) donor [22]. The suspensions of stimulated lymphocytes are prepared in the laboratory from blood collected from HIV antibody–negative human donors. The lymphocytes are separated via Ficoll Hypaque density separation and activated for 24 hours by incubation with PHA. The stimulated human lymphocytes serve as the host cells for HIV-1 isolation. These stimulated cells can be maintained in cell culture tubes or flasks or in 24-well tissue culture plates [23].

The clinical specimen of choice for HIV-1 isolation is peripheral blood lymphocytes. Peripheral blood is collected from the patient, and the leukocytes are separated and used as inoculum for the stimulated human lymphocyte host cells. The cultures are incubated for approximately 1 month. Because human lymphocytes do not adhere to the walls of their culture vessels, the cultures are not examined microscopically for evidence of CPE production. Rather, fluorescent antibody testing, enzyme immunoassays, molecular techniques, or viral reverse transcriptase assays are used to test the lymphocyte suspension to demonstrate HIV antigen or to confirm HIV proliferation in infected cells. A detailed procedure for HIV isolation has been published previously [24].

Although HIV-1 isolation is certainly not a routine clinical virology service at this writing, the concepts of this modified virus isolation system are interesting. HIV-1 isolation may eventually become a widely requested service, and the concepts used in this system may be applicable for isolation of other viruses, such as other retroviruses or Epstein-Barr virus, that fail to proliferate in standard cell cultures.

R E F E R E N C E S

1. Moseley RC, Corey L, Benjamin D, et al. Comparison of viral isolation, direct immunofluorescence, and indirect immunoperoxidase techniques for detection of genital herpes simplex virus infection. J Clin Microbiol 1981;13:913–918.
2. Hughes JH. Physical and chemical methods for enhancing rapid detection of viruses and other agents. Clin Microbiol Rev 1993;6:150–175.
3. Leland DS, Hansing RL, French MLV. Clinical experience with cytomegalovirus isolation using both conventional cell cultures and rapid shell vial techniques. J Clin Microbiol 1989;27:1159–1162.
4. Gleaves CA, Smith TF, Shuster EA, Pearson GR. Rapid detection of cytomegalovirus in MRC-5 cells inoculated with urine specimens by using low speed centrifugation and monoclonal antibody to an early antigen. J Clin Microbiol 1984;19:917–919.
5. Gleaves CA, Smith TF, Shuster EA, Pearson GR. Comparison of standard tube and shell vial cell culture techniques for the detection of cytomegalovirus in clinical specimens. J Clin Microbiol 1985;21:217–221.
6. Paya CV, Wald AD, Smith TF. Detection of cytomegalovirus infections in specimens other than urine by the shell vial assay and conventional tube cell cultures. J Clin Microbiol 1987;25:755–757.
7. Rabella N, Drew WL. Comparison of conventional and shell vial cultures for detecting cytomegalovirus infection. J Clin Microbiol 1990;4:806–807.
8. Gleaves CA, Hursh DA, Meyers JD. Detection of human cytomegalovirus in clinical specimens by centrifugation culture with a nonhuman cell line. J Clin Microbiol 1992;30:1045–1048.
9. Gleaves CA, Wilson DJ, Wald AD, Smith TF. Detection and serotyping of herpes simplex virus in MRC-5 cells by use of centrifugation and monoclonal antibodies 16 h postinoculation. J Clin Microbiol 1985;21:29–32.
10. Smith MC, Creutz C, Huang YT. Detection of respiratory syncytial virus in nasopharyngeal secretions by shell vial technique. J Clin Microbiol 1991;29:463–465.

11. Rabalais GP, Stout GG, Ladd KL, Cost KM. Rapid diagnosis of respiratory viral infections by using a shell vial assay and monoclonal antibody pool. J Clin Microbiol 1992;30:1505–1508.
12. Olsen MA, Shuch KM, Sambol AR, et al. Isolation of seven respiratory viruses in shell vials: a practical and highly sensitive method. J Clin Microbiol 1993;31:422–425.
13. Fedorko DP, Ilstrup DM, Smith TF. Effect of age of shell vial monolayers on detection of cytomegalovirus from urine specimens. J Clin Microbiol 1989;27:2107–2109.
14. DeGirolami PC, Drew WL, Gleaves CA, et al. Procedure Manual for the Detection of CMV and HSV in Shell-Vial Cultures. Palo Alto, CA: Syva Company, 1988.
15. Diagnostic Hybrids, Inc. Product Information for FreshCells. Athens, OH: Diagnostic Hybrids, Inc., 1992.
16. Diagnostic Hybrids, Inc. Product Information for the Herpes Simplex Virus Diagnostic *In Situ* Kit (HSV Disk). Athens, OH: Diagnostic Hybrids, Inc., 1991.
17. Forman MC, Merz CS, Charache P. Detection of herpes simplex virus by a nonradiometric spin-amplified *in situ* hybridization assay. J Clin Microbiol 1992;30:581–584.
18. Yoder BL, Stamm WE, Koester CM, Alexander ER. Microtest procedure for isolation of *Chlamydia trachomatis*. J Clin Microbiol 1981;13:1036–1039.
19. Fayram SL, Aarnaes S, de la Maza LM. Comparison of CultureSet to a conventional tissue culture fluorescent-antibody technique for isolation and identification of herpes simplex virus. J Clin Microbiol 1983;18:215–216.
20. Phillips LE, Magliola RA, Stehlik ML, et al. Retrospective evaluation of the isolation and identification of herpes simplex virus with CultureSet and human fibroblasts. J Clin Microbiol 1985;22:255–258.
21. Ortho Diagnostic Systems, Inc. Product Information for CultureSet HSV System. Raritan, NJ: Ortho Diagnostic Systems, Inc., 1985 (currently marketed by Meridian Diagnostics, Cincinnati, OH).
22. Levy JA, Hoffman AD, Kramer SM, et al. Isolation of lymphocytopathic retroviruses from San Francisco patients with AIDS. Science 1984;225:840–842.
23. Erice A, Sannerud KJ, Leske VL, et al. Sensitive microculture method for isolation of human immunodeficiency virus type 1 from blood leukocytes. J Clin Microbiol 1992;30:444–448.
24. Warfield DT, Feorino PM. Isolation and identification of human immunodeficiency virus type 1. In Isenberg HD (ed), Clinical Microbiology Procedures Handbook. Washington, DC: American Society for Microbiology, 1992, pp 8.15.1–8.15.11.

REVIEW QUESTIONS ❓

1. All of the following are valid reasons to use a modified virus isolation system rather than traditional cell culture tubes **except**
   a. The laboratory needs to limit services (because of limitations in personnel, expertise, finances)
   b. Modified systems may speed up the identification of certain viruses
   c. Modified systems may provide for isolation of viruses that will not proliferate in standard cell cultures
   d. Most modified systems provide a single system with the capacity to identify a wider range of viral isolates than traditional cell cultures

2. The shell vial system has the following features **except:**
   a. Cell monolayers grow on a coverslip in the bottom of a 1-dram shell vial
   b. Monolayers are stained (or otherwise tested for viral antigens) at a designated time interval
   c. Positive shell vial cultures are detected by placing the vial on an inverted microscope and examining the monolayer for evidence of CPE
   d. The inoculation procedure involves spinning the inoculated vial in a centrifuge at low speed for 1 hour

3. All of the following statements describe the shell vial system **except:**
   a. A false-negative result may be obtained when the sample is improperly collected or transported, resulting in inactivation of viruses
   b. Only the viruses specifically tested for will be detected; any other viruses proliferating in the vial cells will be missed
   c. Examination of shell vial coverslips stained by immunofluorescence techniques is time consuming and tedious
   d. Detection in shell vials is usually slower than that of traditional cell cultures

4. The shell vial system has been applied extensively for cytomegalovirus (CMV) detection. Which of the following phrases characterizes CMV isolation in shell vials compared with isolation in traditional tube cell cultures?

    a. The turnaround time for a positive CMV can be reduced considerably when shell vials are used.

    b. Only 50 to 60% of urine samples that are CMV positive in tube cultures will be detected in shell vials.

    c. Shell vials alone are recommended for CMV isolation from all types of samples; tube cultures identify few, if any, additional positive cultures.

    d. Nearly 100% of throat samples that will be CMV positive in tube cultures will be identified as positive in shell vials.

5. Cell cultures in microwells are used for virus isolation. Which of the following features does this virus isolation system include?

    a. Monolayers of cells are grown on coverslips in the bottom of the microwells.

    b. Cells are scraped from the wells and spotted on a microscope slide for testing for viral antigens.

    c. Inoculated microwell plates are spun in the centrifuge to enhance inoculation.

    d. Cross-contamination of samples in neighboring wells is a serious flaw in the system.

6. Herpes simplex virus (HSV) isolation-identification systems target HSV only. Which of the following features do these systems have in common?

    a. They have monolayers of HSV-susceptible cells.

    b. They rely on CPE production by HSV.

    c. They are good for adenovirus and CMV detection.

    d. They have been shown to be more sensitive than traditional 7-day cell cultures.

7. Human immunodeficiency virus (HIV) can be isolated in a modified cell culture system. Which of the following is **not** a feature of this system?

    a. It involves "cocultivation" of the patient's lymphocytes with phytohemagglutinin-stimulated donor lymphocytes.

    b. Results are evaluated by observing HIV CPE in the lymphocyte monolayer.

    c. The specimen of choice is peripheral blood lymphocytes from the patient.

    d. It may be useful for isolation of other viruses such as Epstein-Barr virus or retroviruses other than HIV.

Viral Antigen Detection

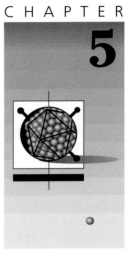

O B J E C T I V E S

At the completion of this unit of study, the student will be able to do the following:

1. List and discuss the advantages and disadvantages of viral disease diagnosis through viral antigen detection.
2. Describe proper specimen collection and antigen smear preparation for immunofluorescence testing.
3. Give an overview of the steps required in direct and in indirect immunofluorescence methods.
4. Compare virus isolation in culture with detection of viral antigen by immunofluorescence for herpes simplex virus, respiratory syncytial virus, and the other respiratory viruses.
5. Describe enzyme immunoassay for antigen detection, and profile the advantages and disadvantages of antigen detection enzyme immunoassays in detecting rotavirus, hepatitis B, respiratory syncytial virus, influenza A, and herpes simplex virus antigens.
6. Describe the latex agglutination methods for viral antigen detection, and discuss clinical applications of this technique.
7. Describe the cytomegalovirus antigenemia assay, and explain how it is used in viral antigen detection.

DIAGNOSIS OF VIRAL INFECTION THROUGH VIRAL ANTIGEN DETECTION: GENERAL CONCEPTS

One of the most frequently used approaches for laboratory diagnosis of viral infection is that of viral antigen detection. In this approach, isolation of the virus is not required. Testing is applied directly to material collected from the patient for the purpose of identifying viral antigens present in the specimen.

Many types of assays can be used for viral antigen detection, although immunoserological assays involving immunofluorescence and enzyme immunoassay are the most popular at present. Passive agglutination is also used, although less frequently. When any of these methods is used for detection of viral antigen within samples, a known antiviral antibody is used in the test system. In this way, reactivity of this antibody (i.e., binding of the antibody to target antigen) tells the virologist that the antigen in the sample is the antigen for which the known antiviral antibody is specific. This provides the identity of the unknown virus in the sample.

There are many advantages of viral antigen detection over other approaches for viral disease diagnosis. The most important advantage is that viral antigen detection methods are quick to perform, routinely producing a final answer in 30 minutes to 3 hours. Virus isolation is not required, so the lengthy incubation period is eliminated. These assays are usually well standardized; no unusual expertise is required on the part of the technologist. These assays involve laboratory equipment that is available in most clinical laboratories, so special facilities are not needed. Because assays for viral antigen do not depend on viral proliferation, the transport and handling of the sample are not as critical as they are for virus isolation. Viral antigens are still detectable even when the virus has been inactivated. Likewise, viral antigens of viruses that do not proliferate in standard cell cultures can be detected with viral antigen detection methods.

Viral antigen tests often remain positive for several days or weeks after the initial infection. This late in the infection the virus has usually been rendered nonviable or noninfectious by *in vivo* immune mechanisms and will not be isolated in culture. The antigen detection tests may still detect the inactive viruses, thus providing positive results longer than the viral culture.

The major drawback of diagnosing viral infections by viral antigen detection is that these assays usually are not as sensitive as virus isolation. Although the sensitivity of the various viral antigen detection methods is not uniform and is dependent on test methodology and target virus, none have been reported to be 100% sensitive compared with virus isolation in cell culture. However, because of the incorporation of high-quality monoclonal antibodies in the testing systems, most viral antigen detection methods produce specific results that yield a high predictive value for a positive result.

One additional disadvantage for the viral antigen detection methods is that they are usually specific for only a single virus (i.e., physicians must indicate which virus they suspect, and testing for that virus will be done). This is in contrast to viral culturing, in which appropriate cell cultures are provided to accommodate many viruses, not simply one specific virus that the physician suspects. Viral infections may be missed in viral antigen testing if the proper assay is not ordered by the physician. Because the symptoms of many viral infections may be clinically indistinguishable from those of related viruses or other microorganisms, it may often be nearly impossible for the physician to choose the best viral antigen assay to order. It is encouraged that viral antigen detection assays be accompanied or followed by viral cultures if the results of the viral antigen detection test do not confirm a viral etiology.

In some cases when viral typing, antiviral susceptibility testing, or other additional studies may be desired, virus isolation is essential to actually obtain the virus. Viral antigen detection methods do not yield viable virus as their end products and are not suitable if a viral isolate is required.

Some viruses, especially herpes simplex virus (HSV), respiratory syncytial virus (RSV), other respiratory viruses, and rotavirus, are readily detectable by antigen detection methods. Other viruses, including the enteroviruses, are seldom if ever identified by such methods.

The viral antigen detection methods may also be applied for identifying viruses isolated in cell cultures (see Chapter 3). Both immunofluorescence and enzyme immunoassay are frequently used for this purpose.

IMMUNOFLUORESCENCE

Specimen Collection and Smear Preparation

Traditionally, when immunofluorescence testing was desired, a specimen was collected from the patient's infected site, smeared on a glass microscope slide, air dried, and transported to the laboratory. The smear usually covered the entire surface of a glass microscope slide

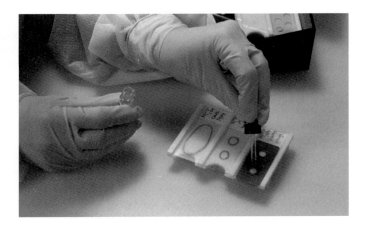

FIGURE 5–1 ANTIGEN SMEARS FOR IMMUNOFLUORESCENCE TESTING. Three smears made from clinical samples are shown. The smear (left) covers the entire slide and will require more expensive reagents to stain and much time to evaluate microscopically. The other two smears were prepared from cell pellets of clinical samples after centrifugation. Cells are concentrated into small areas that require smaller amounts of expensive reagents for staining and less time to examine. The Teflon-coated slide (right) has indented test wells that hold reagents on test areas during staining.

(Fig. 5–1) and often contained mucus, watery secretions, blood, and pus, all of which can cause nonspecific binding of antibodies and none of which is the material required for successful immunofluorescence testing. For high-quality immunofluorescence test results, the patient's sample must contain intact infected cells; it is these cells that are evaluated during the testing procedure. Samples that contain insufficient numbers of cells cannot be tested by immunofluorescence.

Because it may be difficult for the individual who collects the sample to ensure that the necessary infected cells are collected while the unnecessary and interfering components of the infection are avoided, many laboratories prefer to help in the smear preparation process [1]. These laboratories recommend that the sample for immunofluorescence testing be collected in exactly the same manner as a sample for viral culturing (see Table 3–3, Collection of Specimens for Viral Culture). The material should be placed in transport medium and transported to the laboratory. In the laboratory, mucus can be removed, and the cells in the sample can be concentrated through centrifugation of the transport medium. The cell pellet is used to prepare small antigen smears of concentrated cells (see Fig. 5–1). These smears facilitate the use of smaller volumes of expensive monoclonal antibodies in the staining process. They require less time to read because the technologist does not have to scan the surface of the entire glass microscope slide; instead, the cells are concentrated in small areas on the slide. The immunofluorescence procedure is also simplified through the use of Teflon-coated slides that have indented test areas. Because the test areas are indented, the staining reagents are retained in the proper area, and the virologist will not have to encircle the antigen smears with a ring of paint or marker to confine the liquids to the test area (see Fig. 5–1). A procedure for preparing antigen smears in the laboratory or at bedside is provided in the Appendix.

As part of the immunofluorescence testing evaluation process, the virologist must determine whether there are adequate numbers of cells present in the sample. Most manufacturers of monoclonal antibodies for use in immunofluorescence testing recommend that at least 20 cells be present in the smear if the evaluation is to be valid. If the sample has too few cells for evaluation, the virologist must indicate this on the report as "specimen unsatisfactory; insufficient cells."

General Information Concerning Immunofluorescence in Antigen Detection

Fluorescein-labeled monoclonal antibodies are available for direct immunofluorescence staining for several viral antigens. Direct immunofluorescence is discussed in Chapter 2. The direct staining process is simple, requiring only 20 to 30 minutes of incubation of the fluorescein-labeled monoclonal antibodies on the fixed antigen smears. HSV and RSV are routinely detected through direct immunofluorescence methods, and direct immunofluorescence reagents may be available for adenovirus, influenza A, influenza B, and varicella. A procedure for direct immunofluorescence staining for HSV types 1 (HSV-1) and 2 (HSV-2) is provided in the Appendix.

Indirect immunofluorescence methods are also used frequently for detection of viral antigens in clinical materials and for identification of viruses isolated in cell cultures. The mechanism of indirect immunofluorescence is discussed in Chapter 2. The assay is a two-step procedure in which unlabeled monoclonal antibodies are applied to a smear of fixed virus-infected material, either a clinical sample collected from the patient or infected cells from a viral culture. The antibodies incubate for 30 minutes, and the smear is rinsed. Then, in the second phase of the assay, fluorescein-labeled antispecies antibodies are applied. After a 30-minute incubation and rinsing, the smear is observed with a fluorescence microscope. Monoclonal antibodies for use in indirect immunofluorescence procedures are commercially available for a variety of viral antigens: adenovirus; influenza A and B; parainfluenza 1, 2, and 3; RSV; measles; and mumps. Although indirect immunofluorescence requires longer than direct immunofluorescence in the staining procedure, results are still timely. An indirect immunofluorescence staining procedure for detection of parainfluenza 1, 2, and 3 antigens is given in the Appendix.

Viruses have characteristic distribution and appearance of their antigens within the infected cells. This pattern, as well as the intensity of fluorescence, is evaluated in fluorescence testing. Although the pattern alone is not sufficient for distinguishing one virus from another, these typical patterns are the hallmark advantage of immunofluorescence over other immunoserological methods because they allow the virologist to differentiate specific from nonspecific fluorescence. Table 5–1 describes the typical appearance of fluorescence for five common viruses, and Figure 5–2 shows positive immunofluorescence stains for HSV and RSV. Notice the differences in appearance and distribution of the fluorescence of the two preparations. Nonspecific binding of antibodies may be seen in immunofluorescence testing when the clinical sample contains excess mucus, which tends to trap antibodies, or lymphocytes, to which antibodies may bind. Peripheral fluorescence alone, in the absence of virus-specific fluorescence, and fluorescence of clumps of unbound, precipitated conjugate should be ignored; these are usually an artifact of staining.

One additional type of nonspecific binding is seen in cells infected by members of the *Herpesviridae* family: HSV-1 and HSV-2, cytomegalovirus (CMV), varicella-zoster virus, and Epstein-Barr virus. These viruses produce Fc-binding receptors in the cytoplasm of infected cells. These receptors may bind antibodies nonspecifically by their Fc pieces, which results in nonspecific fluorescence. Because true viral inclusions in these cells will be found in the nucleus, the virologist is able to differentiate virus-specific fluorescence from the nonspecific fluorescence of Fc binding.

TABLE 5–1 STAINING PATTERNS IN IMMUNOFLUORESCENCE TESTING

VIRUS	APPEARANCE OF FLUORESCENCE IN INFECTED CELLS
Adenovirus	Fluorescence variable, including both nuclear and cytoplasmic staining, and often more intense staining of the periphery of infected cells; extracellular staining of soluble antigens is present with some serotypes
Herpes simplex	Fluorescence in nucleus and cytoplasm; type 1 generally produces strong perinuclear staining; type 2 produces homogeneous staining
Influenza	Fluorescence may be present in the nucleus alone, in the nucleus and the cytoplasm, or in the cytoplasm alone
Parainfluenza	Fluorescence is granular and cytoplasmic with variation from type to type; type 1 may produce rough strands; type 2 may have occasional large, single inclusions; type 3 may have irregular inclusions; type 4 may have fine particles and coarse particles, and strands may fluoresce
Respiratory syncytial virus	Fluorescence is entirely cytoplasmic; both large inclusion-like bodies and fine fluorescent particles may be present

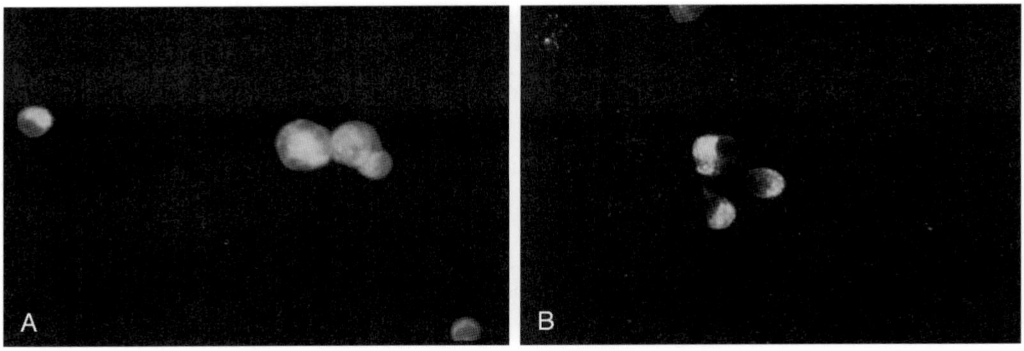

. . . .
FIGURE 5–2 POSITIVE IMMUNOFLUORESCENCE STAINS FOR ANTIGENS OF (A) HERPES SIMPLEX VIRUS (HSV) AND (B) RESPIRATORY SYNCYTIAL VIRUS (RSV). The distribution of fluorescence within infected cells is characteristic for certain viruses. Homogeneous HSV fluorescence is seen in the nucleus and cytoplasm, whereas RSV fluorescence, involving both large and small inclusions, is seen only in the cytoplasm.

Evaluation of immunofluorescence staining results requires a degree of skill and training for the virologist. However, the requirement for characteristic distribution of fluorescence in combination with the specificity of monoclonal antibodies has allowed immunofluorescence methods to provide excellent results. One drawback of extensive use of immunofluorescence for testing of large numbers of specimens is that the virologist may experience fatigue during lengthy smear evaluation sessions.

The degree to which virus isolation correlates with antigen detection by immunofluorescence is variable. Various applications of immunofluorescence testing for viral antigen detection are described next.

Applications of Immunofluorescence in Viral Antigen Detection

Direct immunofluorescence is used in many laboratories for HSV antigen detection. This may involve testing of a single smear to detect HSV group antigen or may involve staining two antigen smears from each sample; one smear is stained with HSV-1 monoclonal antibodies and the other with HSV-2 monoclonal antibodies. This approach provides for both detection and typing of the antigen. A procedure for direct immunofluorescence testing for HSV-1 and HSV-2 antigen is provided in the Appendix.

Table 5–2 compares the results of HSV cultures and immunofluorescence testing for HSV-1 and HSV-2 antigens in 163 samples (Indiana University, unpublished data). The immunofluorescence result is the same as the culture result (i.e., immunofluorescence positive and culture positive or immunofluorescence negative and culture negative) in only 80% of the samples. The sensitivity of immunofluorescence for HSV detection is low, with 11 (41%) of 27 HSV-1 culture–positive samples identified as positive by immunofluorescence and 4 (40%) of 10 HSV-2 culture–positive samples identified as positive by immunofluorescence. However, some of the lack of sensitivity probably is due to specimen quality. Specimens collected from moist lesions are often positive for HSV antigen by immunofluorescence and by culture. Samples collected from the genital tract of infected asymptomatic women may yield HSV in culture but will seldom be positive by immunofluorescence. Problems with specimen quality were obvious in Table 5–2; 12 of 163 samples contained insufficient cells for evaluation of immunofluorescence test results.

The direct immunofluorescence method is often used for detection of RSV antigen. In one evaluation comparing RSV detection by direct immunofluorescence and by virus isolation (Indiana University, unpublished data), the immunofluorescence result was the same as the viral culture result in more than 92% of the clinical samples (Table 5–3). In an additional 6% of samples, the immunofluorescence test was positive, although the viral culture was negative. This result pattern usually indicates infection in which the virus is inactivated but viral antigen persists;

. . . .

TABLE 5–2 COMPARISON OF DIRECT IMMUNOFLUORESCENCE (IF) AND VIRUS ISOLATION FOR DETECTION OF HERPES SIMPLEX VIRUS (HSV) IN 163 CLINICAL SAMPLES*

| | NO. SAMPLES WITH HSV IF RESULT SHOWN | | | |
VIRAL CULTURE RESULT	HSV-1 Positive	HSV-2 Positive	HSV-1 and HSV-2 Negative	Insufficient Cells
HSV-1 isolated	11	0	14	2
HSV-2 isolated	0	4	6	0
No HSV isolated	0	1	115†	10

*Unpublished data generated during a 25-month period (9/91–10/93) at Indiana University. For each sample, both HSV-1 and HSV-2 IF tests were performed.
†Viruses other than HSV were isolated in two samples: cytomegalovirus (n = 1) and varicella (n = 1).

. . . .

TABLE 5–3 COMPARISON OF DIRECT IMMUNOFLUORESCENCE (IF) AND VIRUS ISOLATION FOR DETECTION OF RESPIRATORY SYNCYTIAL VIRUS (RSV) IN 94 RESPIRATORY SAMPLES*

| | NO. SAMPLES WITH RSV IF RESULT SHOWN | |
VIRAL CULTURE RESULT	Negative	Positive
No RSV isolated	72†	6
RSV isolated	1	15

*Unpublished data generated during a 24-month period (1/92–12/93) at Indiana University.
†Viruses other than RSV were isolated from 11 samples: adenovirus (n = 3), cytomegalovirus (n = 1), enterovirus (n = 1), parainfluenza 1 and enterovirus (n = 1), parainfluenza 1 (n = 1), parainfluenza 2 (n = 2), parainfluenza 3 (n = 1), and parainfluenza 4 (n = 1).

this pattern is usually considered a true-positive RSV result. Table 5–3 shows that the direct immunofluorescence test for RSV antigen detection has excellent sensitivity; only 1 of the 16 RSV culture–positive samples had a false-negative immunofluorescence test result.

In a battery of indirect immunofluorescence tests designed to detect antigens of seven of the respiratory viruses, the variability in sensitivity of immunofluorescence in detecting the respiratory viral antigens is demonstrated. At the Indiana University Virology Laboratory in testing that included indirect immunofluorescence testing for antigens of adenovirus, influenza A and B, parainfluenza 1, 2, and 3, and RSV as well as viral culturing of the sample, the immunofluorescence assays overall detected 81% of the viral antigens of viruses that were isolated in culture (Table 5–4). When these same results were evaluated assuming that positive immunofluorescence results were true positives regardless of the outcome of the viral culture, the overall success of the immunofluorescence testing was 85% (see Table 5–4). When the sensitivities of the individual immunofluorescence tests are compared, percentages of RSV and influenza B virus that were identified by the immunofluorescence test were high, ranging between 87 and 94%, whereas the percentages of adenovirus and parainfluenza 2 were very low, ranging between 51 and 63%. Although the sensitivity of the immunofluorescence methods varied from virus to virus, such viral antigen detection testing is still a very important service for the virology laboratory to provide. This allows the physician to be informed of approximately 81 to 85% of the positive results within several hours of sample collection, thereby allowing efficient and informed patient management. Without the antigen detection methods, the physician would routinely wait 5 to 10 days to find out that the patient was infected with a virus; by this time, significant decisions involving patient management would already have been made without this vital information.

Notice also in Table 5–4 that viruses other than the expected respiratory viruses were isolated from some of the respiratory samples. Included were CMV, enteroviruses, HSV-1, rhino-like virus, and parainfluenza type 4. These viruses were not suspected by the physician and would have gone undetected if the respiratory viral antigen tests alone had been performed.

. . . .
TABLE 5–4 COMPARISON OF ANTIGEN DETECTION BY IMMUNOFLUORESCENCE (IF) AND VIRUS ISOLATION IN DETECTION OF SEVEN RESPIRATORY VIRUSES IN 2664 RESPIRATORY SAMPLES*

	NO. SAMPLES WITH IF AND VIRAL CULTURE RESULT PATTERN INDICATED	
VIRUS	IF Positive and Culture Positive/Culture Positive (%)†	IF Positive/Either IF or Culture Positive (%)‡
Adeno	38/74 (51)	45/81 (56)
Para 1	26/36 (72)	29/41 (71)
Para 2	12/19 (63)	12/19 (63)
Para 3	40/59 (68)	47/66 (71)
Flu A	16/26 (62)	41/51 (80)
Flu B	20/23 (87)	27/30 (90)
RSV	341/375 (91)	491/525 (94)
Total	493/612 (81)	692/813 (85)

*Unpublished data generated during a 48-month period (1/91–1/95) at the Indiana University Virology Laboratory. Forty-six samples were IF and culture negative for the respiratory viruses shown but produced cytomegalovirus (n = 16), enterovirus (n = 6), herpes simplex virus type 1 (n = 12), rhino-like virus (n = 7), or parainfluenza 4 (n = 5).
†The number of samples that were positive by IF and that grew in culture is compared with the total number of samples that grew in culture.
‡Data are re-evaluated (assuming that positive IF results are true positives regardless of culture outcome). The number of IF-positive samples is compared with the total number of samples that were positive by IF or culture, or both.
Para = parainfluenza; Flu = influenza; RSV = respiratory syncytial virus.

These findings emphasize the importance of supplementing viral antigen testing with virus isolation studies.

ENZYME IMMUNOASSAY

Enzyme immunoassays are available in a variety of configurations for detection of several viral antigens, including hepatitis B virus, rotavirus, HSV, RSV, and influenza A. The configurations and principles of various enzyme immunoassays are described in Chapter 2. Each virology laboratory must select the appropriate enzyme immunoassay to meet its own needs. The manual tube and microplate methods require approximately 2 to 4 hours to complete and are relatively inexpensive to run, whereas the test pack–style enzyme immunoassays require only 10 to 15 minutes to run and are more expensive. Test volume and technologists' time and expertise will often be the determining factors in making the selection of the best enzyme immunoassay. None of the enzyme immunoassays requires highly trained virologists because each of the assays is well standardized, and the evaluation of results depends simply on observation of a color change. Often the color change is objectively evaluated by a spectrophotometer. Most enzyme immunoassays are well suited for testing of large numbers of samples.

Although enzyme immunoassays are standardized, the testing protocols must be followed carefully. When mixing and rinsing steps are not performed as directed, test systems may become contaminated with enzyme-labeled reagents and thus yield false-positive results. Because the enzyme immunoassay systems are dependent on the action of active enzymes, all reagents must be manipulated and maintained in strict accordance with all of the manufacturers' guidelines. Enzyme solutions must be stored and handled so as to prevent any deterioration of enzyme activity. Likewise, substrate solutions must be maintained so that they are suitable for the activity of the enzyme in the test system.

The disadvantage with enzyme immunoassay is that the immunoserological reaction cannot be viewed to differentiate specific from nonspecific reactivity. The color change reaction is homogeneous and does not allow visualization of the distribution of the reactivity.

Specimen Collection

Enzyme immunoassays in various configurations are used extensively for viral antigen detection. For most enzyme immunoassays, specimens collected as described for virus isolation (see Table 3–3, Collection of Specimens for Viral Culture) are satisfactory. For several commercial enzyme immunoassay systems, the manufacturer provides a collection medium that can be distributed to physicians to use for specimen collection and transport. Other enzyme immunoassays include as part of the test system a test buffer in which technologists make suspensions of the test samples. This is frequently the case when the test sample is feces, such as in the enzyme immunoassay for rotavirus antigen detection. Manufacturers routinely specify conditions or substances that may interfere in the enzyme immunoassay.

Although the immunofluorescence testing methods require intact infected cells for a successful assay, enzyme immunoassays do not. Enzyme immunoassays have the capacity to detect viral antigens that are free in solution or are associated with other products of inflammation such as mucus. Although infected cells are still the preferred test material, their presence is not as critical in enzyme immunoassay as in immunofluorescence.

Applications of Enzyme Immunoassay in Viral Antigen Detection

Enzyme immunoassay methods for detection of rotavirus antigen are especially popular because this virus will not proliferate in standard cell cultures. Immunofluorescence techniques are not useful in identification of rotavirus. The enzyme immunoassays have been shown to produce results that are, in many cases, comparable to those of electron microscopy. The enzyme immunoassays, of course, are much less expensive and less labor intensive than electron microscopy and require little technical expertise.

The sequence of steps of one modified solid-phase immunoassay used for rotavirus antigen detection is shown in Figure 2–12. The procedure is a solid-phase manual tube method featuring antirotavirus antibodies on the wall of the test tube. These antibodies bind or "capture" rotavirus antigen in fecal samples being tested. This method is a modified immunoassay in which both the specimen and enzyme-labeled antiviral antibodies are added to the antibody-coated tube in the first step.

Another group of viruses whose presence is usually confirmed through antigen detection is the hepatitis viruses, which do not proliferate in standard cell cultures and cannot be detected through immunofluorescence. The original antigen detection methods for the hepatitis viral antigens were radioimmunoassays, which involve the same principles as enzyme immunoassays but include reagents that have radioactive labels. Because radioactive reagents present a hazard in the laboratory, most of the hepatitis antigen methods were modified, and radioactive labeling compounds were replaced by enzymes. Hepatitis B antigens are found in high titer in peripheral blood, which is the specimen of choice for hepatitis B antigen testing.

RSV is also frequently identified through antigen detection enzyme immunoassays. Although RSV proliferates well in standard cell cultures and can be identified by immunofluorescence, the rapid antigen enzyme immunoassays are popular because they easily accommodate the large volume of RSV tests performed during RSV season, and they require little of the technologist's time or expertise. Many RSV antigen detection enzyme immunoassays are available commercially; the sensitivity and specificity vary from product to product, although, in general, they are high. The sensitivities and specificities reported in evaluations of several RSV enzyme immunoassays are shown in Table 5–5.

Enzyme immunoassay reagents are available for detection of another respiratory virus: influenza A. This virus will usually proliferate in standard cell cultures, although there is variability among strains. Influenza A antigen can also be detected by immunofluorescence. The enzyme immunoassays for detection of influenza A antigen have been compared with influenza A isolation in cell cultures. Compared with virus isolation in cell cultures, one packet-type system (Directigen, Becton Dickinson) showed 86.8% sensitivity and 99.1% specificity, and one microplate system (Prima EIA, Baxter Bartels) showed 92.5% sensitivity and 90.1% specificity

····················

TABLE 5–5 COMPARISON OF THE SENSITIVITIES AND SPECIFICITIES OF VARIOUS ENZYME IMMUNOASSAY (EIA) METHODS FOR RESPIRATORY SYNCYTIAL VIRUS ANTIGEN DETECTION

METHOD (MANUFACTURER)/ DESCRIPTION	SENSITIVITY* (%)	SPECIFICITY* (%)	NO. SAMPLES TESTED	REFERENCE
Directigen (Becton Dickinson)/ packet EIA	61	95	86	2
	76	80	117	3
	83	90	583	4
	76	73	100	5
Pathfinder (Kallestad)/tube EIA	87	88	410	6
RSV EIA (Abbott)/bead EIA	71	100	117	3
RSV ELISA (Ortho)/microwell EIA	88	87	72	7
Test Pack (Abbott)/packet EIA	57	98	86	2
	94	100	117	3
	93†	90†	104	8
	87†	90†	84	8
	92	97	100	5
	91	96	152	7
	92	91	218	9
VIDAS (Vitek)/automated EIA	83†	93†	140	8
	96†	94†	87	8

*Sensitivity and specificity compared with virus isolation unless otherwise specified.
†Sensitivity and specificity relative to direct immunofluorescence.
RSV = respiratory syncytial virus.

when used to test 160 respiratory samples from geriatric patients [10]. In another study of 126 samples, the Directigen enzyme immunoassay detected 18 of 20 samples that were positive for influenza A in cell culture [11]. Because the incidence of influenza A is low in most populations, the use of an enzyme immunoassay for antigen detection may be costly and may have low yield in terms of numbers of positive results identified. However, when selected populations with a high incidence of influenza A are tested, the use of an antigen detection method becomes more cost effective.

In one additional study, 210 nasopharyngeal secretion specimens were tested by an enzyme immunoassay for influenza A and B antigens [12]. Influenza A detection by this enzyme immunoassay showed 90% sensitivity and 99% specificity. Influenza B detection showed 88% sensitivity and 100% specificity.

HSV-1 and HSV-2, which proliferate readily in standard cell cultures and can be identified by immunofluorescence, are also frequently identified by enzyme immunoassay because of the convenience of this assay system. The sensitivities and specificities reported in several evaluations of HSV enzyme immunoassays are shown in Table 5–6. These reported sensitivities are lower than those shown in Table 5–5 for the enzyme immunoassays used for RSV antigen detection. However, they are higher than those presented in Table 5–2 for immunofluorescence detection of HSV-1 and HSV-2 antigens.

LATEX AGGLUTINATION IN VIRAL ANTIGEN DETECTION

Passive agglutination is described in Chapter 2. Passive agglutination methods, often casually termed latex agglutinations, are the least technically demanding test methods. Latex particles coated with viral antibodies of known specificity are mixed, usually on a slide, with virus-infected cell culture material or with the patient's sample that contains the unknown viral antigen. In some latex testing, especially if the material is a fecal sample, the sample must be prepared by extraction, centrifugation, or filtration before testing. The prepared material is mixed with the coated latex. If the viral antigen in the sample is recognized by the known antibody coating the latex particles, the antibodies bind, resulting in agglutination of the particles. Latex agglutination

TABLE 5–6 COMPARISON OF THE SENSITIVITIES AND SPECIFICITIES OF VARIOUS ENZYME IMMUNOASSAY (EIA) METHODS FOR HERPES SIMPLEX ANTIGEN DETECTION

METHOD (MANUFACTURER)/ DESCRIPTION	SENSITIVITY (%)*	SPECIFICITY (%)*	NO. SAMPLES TESTED	REFERENCE
Fairleigh Dickinson ELISA/manual microwell EIA	63	95	148	13
Herpchek (Du Pont)/manual microwell EIA	93	92	346	14
	85	96	377	15
	84	98	473	15
	72	100	80†	15
	84	97	168†	15
	99	100	422	16
	59	99	119	16
Ortho ELISA/manual microwell EIA	35	100	186	17
SureCell (Kodak)/packet EIA	76	99	440	18
	70	99	365	18
	73	100	25	U
VIDAS (Vitek)/automated EIA	92	89	356	14

*Sensitivity and specificity compared with virus isolation.
†Genital specimens only.
ELISA = enzyme-linked immunosorbent assay; U = unpublished data from the Indiana University Virology Laboratory.

testing requires only 2 to 20 minutes to perform, and results of several latex test methods compare favorably with more technically difficult methods.

Latex agglutination products are marketed for detection of rotavirus in stool samples. Rotavirus latex test sensitivity was reported at 69 to 79% compared with enzyme immunoassay [19]. In a second study, latex testing showed greater sensitivity than the enzyme immunoassay [20]. A newer rotavirus antigen latex agglutination test (Meritec rotavirus latex detection procedure, Meridian Diagnostics, Inc.) identified as positive 39 of 41 fecal samples that had been previously shown by electron microscopy to have rotavirus.

CYTOMEGALOVIRUS ANTIGENEMIA ASSAY

CMV is not one of the viruses that has routinely been identified in clinical samples by rapid antigen detection methods. Both immunofluorescence and enzyme immunoassay methods have been only minimally successful in detecting CMV antigen in clinical samples. However, a new assay has been developed and is available commercially. This assay detects CMV lower matrix early structural protein (pp65) in peripheral blood leukocytes. The method combines a technique for separating peripheral blood leukocytes from erythrocytes and a staining method for identifying CMV antigen within the leukocytes. Separated leukocytes are placed on a microscope slide and stained with a preparation containing two monoclonal antibodies directed against the CMV antigen. After incubation and rinsing, horseradish peroxidase–labeled antimouse antibodies are added, followed by a substrate solution. Then the cells are examined by light microscopy for dark or red-brown nuclear staining. The entire procedure requires 5 hours to complete.

Because this technique is a new one, few reports have described the CMV antigenemia assay. However, in one comparison of the antigenemia assay, CMV shell vials, and conventional viral culture, the antigenemia assay identified more positives than shell vial cultures and more positives than conventional cell cultures [21]. The antigenemia assay is, however, labor intensive and expensive and must be performed with strict adherence to the guidelines provided by the manufacturer of the testing system.

REFERENCES

1. Leland DS. Concepts of clinical diagnostic virology. In Lennette EH (ed), Laboratory Diagnosis of Viral Infections, 2nd ed. New York: Marcel Dekker, 1992, pp 3–43.
2. Dominguez EA, Taber LH, Couch RB. Comparison of rapid diagnostic techniques for respiratory syncytial and influenza A virus respiratory infections in young children. J Clin Microbiol 1993;31:2286–2290.
3. Halstead DC, Todd S, Fritch G. Evaluation of five methods for respiratory syncytial virus detection. J Clin Microbiol 1990;28:1021–1025.
4. Kok T, Barancek K, Burrell CJ. Evaluation of the Becton Dickinson Directigen Test for respiratory syncytial virus in nasopharyngeal aspirates. J Clin Microbiol 1990;28:1458–1459.
5. Rothbarth PH, Hermus M-C, Schrijnemakers P. Reliability of two new test kits for rapid diagnosis of respiratory syncytial virus infection. J Clin Microbiol 1991;29:824–826.
6. Johnston SLG, Siegel CS. Evaluation of direct immunofluorescence, enzyme immunoassay, centrifugation culture, and conventional culture for the detection of respiratory syncytial virus. J Clin Microbiol 1990;28:2394–2397.
7. Thomas EE, Book LE. Comparison of two rapid methods for detection of respiratory syncytial virus (RSV) (TestPack RSV and Ortho RSV ELISA) with direct immunofluorescence and virus isolation for the diagnosis of pediatric RSV infection. J Clin Microbiol 1991;29:632–635.
8. Miller H, Milk R, Diaz-Mitoma F. Comparison of the VIDAS RSV assay and the Abbott Testpack RSV with direct immunofluorescence for detection of respiratory syncytial virus in nasopharyngeal aspirates. J Clin Microbiol 1993;31:1336–1338.
9. Wren CG, Bate BJ, Masters HB, Lauer BA. Detection of respiratory syncytial virus antigen in nasal washings by Abbott TestPack enzyme immunoassay. J Clin Microbiol 1990;28:1395–1397.
10. Leonardi GP, Leib H, Birkhead GS, et al. Comparison of rapid detection methods for influenza A virus and their value in health-care management of institutionalized geriatric patients. J Clin Microbiol 1994;32:70–74.
11. Johnston SLG, Bloy H. Evaluation of a rapid enzyme immunoassay for detection of influenza A virus. J Clin Microbiol 1993;31:142–143.
12. Döller G, Schuy W, Tjhen KY, et al. Direct detection of influenza virus antigen in nasopharyngeal specimens by direct enzyme immunoassay in comparison with quantitating virus shedding. J Clin Microbiol 1992;30:866–869.
13. Needham C, Hurlbert P. Evaluation of an enzyme-linked immunoassay employing a covalently bound capture antibody for direct detection of herpes simplex virus. J Clin Microbiol 1992;30:531–532.
14. Johnston SLG, Hamilton S, Bindra P, et al. Evaluation of an automated immunodiagnostic assay system for direct detection of herpes simplex virus antigen in clinical specimens. J Clin Microbiol 1992;30:1042–1044.
15. Ogburn JR, Hoffpauir JT, Cole E, et al. Evaluation of new transport medium for detection of herpes simplex by culture and direct enzyme-linked immunosorbent assay. J Clin Microbiol 1994;32:3082–3084.
16. Verano L, Michalski FJ. Herpes simplex virus antigen direct detection in standard virus transport medium by DuPont Herpchek enzyme-linked immunosorbent assay. J Clin Microbiol 1990;28:2555–2558.
17. Gonik B, Seibel M, Berkowitz A, et al. Comparison of two enzyme-linked immunosorbent assays for detection of herpes simplex virus antigen. J Clin Microbiol 1991;29:436–438.
18. Kodak Clinical Products. Kodak SureCell Herpes (HSV) Test Kit. Product Information. Kodak Clinical Products, 1992.
19. Sambourg MA, Goudeau A, Courant C, et al. Direct appraisal of latex agglutination testing, a convenient alternative to enzyme immunoassay for the detection of rotavirus in childhood gastroenteritis, by comparison of two enzyme immunoassays and two latex tests. J Clin Microbiol 1985;21:622–625.
20. Pai CH, Shahrabad MS, Ince B. Rapid diagnosis of rotavirus gastroenteritis by a commercial latex agglutination test. J Clin Microbiol 1985;22:846–850.
21. Erice A, Holm MA, Gill PC, et al. Cytomegalovirus (CMV) antigenemia assay is more sensitive than shell vial cultures for rapid detection of CMV in polymorphonuclear blood leukocytes. J Clin Microbiol 1992;30:2822–2825.

REVIEW QUESTIONS

1. All of the following are advantages of viral antigen detection over other approaches for viral disease diagnosis **except**
   a. Quick and easy to perform; use standard equipment
   b. Virus does not need to be viable
   c. Antigen may be shed longer than infectious virus
   d. More sensitive than virus isolation

2. Immunofluorescence is one popular viral antigen detection method. In collecting samples and preparing smears for these tests
   a. The sample should be smeared on a glass microscope slide to cover the entire surface of the glass
   b. For optimal sensitivity, the patient's sample should include mucus, watery secretions, blood, and pus
   c. The sample should not be placed in liquid transport medium because this dilutes the sample
   d. Intact infected cells concentrated in small test areas on Teflon-coated slides are optimal

3. In immunofluorescence testing for detection of viral antigens
   a. The antigen smear fixed on the slide is a cell preparation infected with virus of known type
   b. The antibodies used in testing are usually high-quality monoclonal antibodies of known specificity
   c. The staining protocols for both direct and indirect immunofluorescence staining are lengthy and time consuming
   d. Any fluorescence, regardless of intensity or distribution, is considered positive when results are interpreted

4. The sensitivity of viral antigen detection by immunofluorescence compared with virus isolation varies from virus to virus. Which of the following statements is accurate concerning the relative sensitivity?
   a. Immunofluorescence for respiratory syncytial virus (RSV) detects 90% or more of RSV that would be isolated in cell culture.
   b. Immunofluorescence has uniform sensitivity in detecting antigens of all of the various respiratory viruses.
   c. Herpes simplex virus types 1 and 2 antigen detection sensitivity is 95% or higher by immunofluorescence.
   d. Immunofluorescence is the method of choice for detection of enterovirus antigens.

5. Enzyme immunoassays (EIAs) are available for detection of many viral antigens. Which of the following statements describes the level of performance and advantages or disadvantages of EIA in detecting various viruses?
   a. EIA is not useful for rotavirus antigen detection.
   b. Hepatitis B virus antigens cannot be detected by EIA because they are too small.
   c. Respiratory syncytial virus antigen detection by EIA has shown good sensitivity and specificity.
   d. EIAs in general are useful in testing small numbers of samples but are not useful for handling large batches of tests.

6. In latex agglutination testing for viral antigen detection
   a. The procedure is lengthy, usually requiring an overnight incubation
   b. The test features latex particles coated with antiviral antibodies
   c. Viral antigens in the sample are acted on by enzyme-labeled antibodies
   d. A positive (antigen present) assay result appears as a smooth suspension of latex particles

7. The cytomegalovirus (CMV) antigenemia assays are a recent addition to the list of viral antigen detection methods. These assays are performed and interpreted as follows:
   a. The test sample is urine from the infected individuals
   b. The assay involves simply mixing anticoagulated whole blood with labeled antiviral antibodies and is completed after a 2-minute mixing of cells and stain
   c. A positive result appears as red-brown staining of infected lymphocytes
   d. Viral antigen is free in suspension and is captured by antiviral antibodies attached to a solid phase

$\mathcal{S}$erodiagnosis of Viral Infections

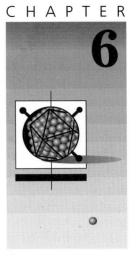

OBJECTIVES

At the completion of this unit of study, the student will be able to do the following:

1. Explain the basis of viral diagnosis through serology, and list three general circumstances in which serology rather than virus isolation or viral antigen detection is the test of choice.

2. Describe quantitative and qualitative testing, and give examples of how each type of determination may be helpful in viral disease diagnosis.

3. Using rubella virus infection as an example, and, assuming that assays detect primarily immunoglobulin (Ig) G, provide answers to the following for serodiagnosis of acquired and congenital infections and for determination of immune status:
   How many serum samples should be tested?
   When should these samples be collected?
   Should the test be in a quantitative or qualitative format?
   How are the results of testing interpreted?

4. Describe test modifications and pretreatments used to make assays specific for IgM, and explain how IgG and rheumatoid factor may interfere in IgM-specific assays.

5. Give examples of clinical situations in which IgM-specific assays may be of use and discuss the problems, both technical and biological, that must be considered in interpreting the results of IgM-specific assays.

6. Be able to diagram at least three methodologies used routinely in viral antibody detection.

7. List at least five viruses whose diagnosis at present relies on the serological approach.

8. Describe the proper collection and storage of blood samples that will be tested for viral antibodies.

9. When presented with sample results of quantitative serological test, be able to differentiate significant from nonsignificant differences in titer, and use the proper format in reporting or following up results when all dilutions of a quantitative assay yield positive or negative results.

HOW AND WHY ARE VIRAL INFECTIONS DIAGNOSED THROUGH SEROLOGY?

The basic principles of serodiagnosis of viral infection are the same as those used in serological confirmation of other infectious diseases. Experience with most microorganisms, including viruses, induces the formation of specific antibody. This specific antibody, when identified in the serum, provides proof that an individual has been exposed to or infected by a given agent. Identification of such antibody may be vital in viral diagnosis, especially in the following circumstances: (1) when the infecting organism is difficult to isolate or to identify, (2) when proper clinical specimens for culturing or antigen assays are difficult to obtain (i.e., a brain biopsy), (3) when specimens for virus isolation were collected too late in the disease, or (4) when a virus has been isolated, but its role in the present disease process is uncertain. Examples of this include echovirus, which has no defined role as a pathogen but may be important in some cases, and cytomegalovirus, which may be shed by immunocompromised patients even when the cytomegalovirus is not significant in the present infection. In each of these situations, the serological approach provides an alternate or ancillary route for making the diagnosis. Antibodies in the serum may be conveniently identified, and the required test sample, serum from a peripheral blood sample, is easy to collect.

For diagnosis of viral infections, serology is used often because viral isolation is generally viewed as "difficult," and virus isolation services or viral antigen detection assays are simply not always readily available. As laboratories expand their viral diagnostic services, the serological approach will become less popular, especially for those viruses that can be isolated in traditional cell cultures or can be accurately detected with viral antigen detection methods. However, serological diagnosis will continue to be important in defining the role of certain viruses in the disease process and in diagnosing viral infections caused by viruses that cannot be isolated in traditional cell culture systems, for example, hepatitis B virus. Serology is also useful in determining a patient's immune status, that is, whether the individual has been infected by or immunized against a certain virus and has antibodies against the virus. Antibody detection is the only avenue for confirming previous infections and exposures because the infecting agent is no longer present; only the antibodies remain to serve as proof that the infection or exposure occurred.

In general, serology serves as an indirect method for diagnosing viral infections. In serodiagnosis, viral antibodies produced in various clinical syndromes are identified and quantitated. This is in contrast to the more direct methods of viral disease diagnosis that require isolation or observation of the infecting virus or its antigens. Most serological procedures use a known antigen that will react with specific antibody to produce a visible reaction. The principles of many immunoserological testing methods are discussed in Chapter 2.

Traditional serological assays detect primarily immunoglobulin G (IgG). IgG is the "memory" immunoglobulin that is produced in highest quantities during infections and persists lifelong after most viral infections. IgG is also the predominant immunoglobulin in serum, representing approximately 76% compared with 16% for IgA, 8% for IgM, and less than 1% for IgD and IgE [1]. Because of the enormous excess of IgG, it is the immunoglobulin that is usually detected. IgM, which is produced first but in lower quantities in infections and declines to undetectable levels early on, may be detected along with IgG in traditional methods that measure total antibody, but IgG and IgM are not differentiated in these methods. IgA may or may not be detected. IgA onset, level, and duration are less predictable than IgM or IgG [2], and IgD and IgE, whose role in viral infections has not been elucidated and whose quantity is minimal, probably are not detected.

QUANTITATIVE SEROLOGICAL DETERMINATIONS

The serological approach may involve either a qualitative or a quantitative serological determination. **Quantitative determinations** are performed in clinical situations in which the amount of antibody, not simply its presence or absence, is important. The need in some cases for quantitative determination of the antibody level is based on the traditional antibody response to infection. On acquiring a primary infection, the body produces IgM specific for the infecting agent. This usually appears within several days after onset of symptoms, peaks within 7 to 10 days, and then declines to undetectable levels or disappears within 1 to 2 months. Within several days after IgM production is initiated, IgG of the same specificity appears. This immunoglobulin reaches higher levels than IgM and, after most viral infections, persists lifelong in reduced quantities. Because IgG persists, it is difficult to determine whether IgG detected in serological assays is associated with current or very recent infection or whether it is "old" IgG resulting from infections or exposures from many months or years ago. Comparing IgG levels in samples collected at the appropriate intervals allows differentiation of old IgG, which should stay at a steady level, and IgG produced in current or very recent infections, which should increase in amount.

Quantitative serological determinations are also required in evaluating congenital infections in neonates. Congenitally *(in utero)* infected fetuses, despite their immature immune systems, are capable of producing antibodies. Initially, these are IgM class antibodies, but at birth or shortly thereafter, IgG production begins. Therefore, identification of antibodies in the infant's serum should be helpful in determining whether or not the infant has been infected. However, this determination is complicated by the fact that maternal IgG crosses the placenta into the infant's serum before birth. In fact, most of the IgG in an infant's serum is maternal in origin, and serological tests cannot differentiate maternal from infant IgG. By comparing antibody levels in sequential serum samples collected from an infant at birth and at intervals during the next 4 to 6 months, maternal antibodies and antibodies produced by the infant can be differentiated. Maternal antibodies will steadily decline. However, infant IgG antibodies associated with congenital infection will increase or persist at elevated levels.

For traditional quantitative determinations, the serum is diluted in a series of twofold (doubling) dilutions. Once these dilutions are prepared, the given test procedure is performed on each dilution. The highest dilution of serum that produces a reaction is the end point or "titer" of the reaction, and this titer is reported to the physician. When antibody titers of two samples are compared, a twofold (one tube or one twofold dilution) difference is not considered to be significant. A twofold difference in any serological determination may be due simply to random variations such as lot-to-lot variation in reagents or minor differences in serological technique. A fourfold (two tube or two twofold dilutions) or greater difference is thought to be significant. A difference of this magnitude should not occur as a result of simple random laboratory variables. A difference in titer of fourfold or greater is usually seen in two samples collected at appropriate intervals during an acquired infection.

Some of the newer serological testing methods, although quantitative, are performed on a single dilution of serum. Although only one dilution is tested, the results are evaluated by a readout device such as a spectrophotometer that provides a numerical, quantitative result. These technologies are based on the concept that antigens and antibodies react quantitatively to produce results that reflect the magnitude of the reaction. Although the numerical reactivity scores for some antibody assays have been correlated with traditional serological titers, the relationship is not linear between the two, and conversion of the scores to titers is not encouraged. Routinely, the patient's numerical value and a cutoff value that must be met or exceeded for the test to be considered positive are reported. By evaluating the magnitude of difference between the patient's value and the cutoff value, the physician has a quantitative determination of the patient's antibody level. Some manufacturers of these assay systems provide guidelines that allow comparison of two values to determine whether the magnitude of difference in antibody level is significant or insignificant. Reporting conventions are discussed later under Technical Hints.

QUALITATIVE SEROLOGICAL DETERMINATIONS

Qualitative determinations are used diagnostically in clinical situations in which the knowledge that a particular antibody is present (or absent) is useful in medical decision making, and the quantity or level of the antibody is not important. Qualitative test results are usually reported as "positive" or "negative." Qualitative testing is often used to evaluate an individual's "**immune status**" in regard to viruses such as measles, mumps, and rubella, which confer lifelong immunity. An example of immune status testing follows.

In some states, serum from all females is tested for rubella virus antibodies as part of required premarital testing. A "positive" (antibody present) result indicates that the female has been previously exposed to the virus, either through vaccination or infection, and that she should be immune to future rubella infections. This is important because rubella infection in nonimmune pregnant females may cause damage to the fetus. If the result of a premarital rubella antibody test is "negative" (no antibody detected), the female has not had experience with the rubella virus and is not immune to future rubella infection. Women who have negative rubella antibody test results should be immunized.

Qualitative determinations are also useful for diagnosis of infections caused by viruses such as human immunodeficiency virus, type 1 (HIV-1). Antibodies to HIV-1 should not be present in uninfected individuals, so a negative test is helpful in ruling out HIV-1 infection. The presence of HIV-1 antibodies, regardless of antibody level, indicates HIV-1 infection and, in symptomatic individuals, provides supportive evidence in the diagnosis of AIDS. A positive qualitative test result indicates that the individual has been infected with HIV-1 but does not confirm active disease and certainly does not indicate protection against AIDS.

Although qualitative testing is often used to determine immune status, a positive qualitative test indicating the presence of viral antibodies does not necessarily ensure that a patient is protected from further disease complications when certain viruses are involved. The viruses of the *Herpesviridae* family, including cytomegalovirus, Epstein-Barr virus, herpes simplex virus, and varicella-zoster virus, persist in the body in a latent state after infection. Although the body produces antibodies against these viruses and the antibodies remain at detectable levels throughout life, these viruses are fully capable of reactivating to cause disease if the host is stressed or weakened. In these situations, a positive qualitative test indicates that the individual has been infected previously by the virus but does not ensure that reactivation will be prevented.

Qualitative determinations are not helpful in determining previous exposure or immune status for viruses that do not confer lifelong group-specific immunity. Most of the respiratory viruses, including the influenzas, the parainfluenzas, respiratory syncytial virus, and adenovirus, will induce type-specific antibody production during infection. Although these antibodies may remain long term after infection, the host is not protected against future infection by viruses of the same group but of other subtypes.

PROTOCOLS FOR SEROLOGICAL EVALUATION OF ACQUIRED AND CONGENITAL INFECTIONS AND IMMUNE STATUS—EXAMPLE: RUBELLA

The proper specimen collection sequence and guidelines for interpretation of both quantitative and qualitative results are described for three clinical situations: acquired infection, congenital infection, and immune status determinations. The virus rubella is used as an example because it is important clinically in all three clinical circumstances. For both acquired infection and congenital infection, quantitative evaluation of antibody levels is important in making the diagnosis, whereas qualitative determinations are suitable for immune status assessment.

Rubella (German measles) is usually a mild disease and was common in children and young adults in the United States before the implementation of rubella immunizations for all children. Rubella infection typically produces mild symptoms for 3 days, including low-grade fever, headache, mild conjunctivitis, lymphadenopathy, and rash [3]. Complications of rubella infection in children are rare. Rubella infection in nonimmune pregnant women during the first trimester of pregnancy may cause anomalies in the fetus, including heart lesions, ocular complications, ear malfunctions, hepatosplenomegaly, meningoencephalitis, and lesions of the long bones [3]. Although virus isolation may be helpful in the diagnosis of rubella infections, especially in congenital rubella, the rubella virus is one of the more difficult viruses to isolate. Therefore, serological methods for diagnosis of rubella infections remain an economical and practical diagnostic service.

A description of the protocols for serological evaluation of acquired and congenital infection and for determination of immune status for rubella follow. **These guidelines apply for traditional serological tests that detect primarily IgG.**

ACQUIRED INFECTION. In confirming rubella infection in patients with clinical signs of rubella infection, the serological diagnosis is based on a fourfold or greater rise in antibody titer. Quantitative testing on two serum specimens is required. The first sample (acute) must be collected as soon as possible after onset, and the second (convalescent) is collected 14 days later. The following interpretations are used:

1. If there is a fourfold or greater increase in antibody level (or a significant difference on the basis of other quantitative comparison criteria) between the acute and convalescent sample, present acquired infection is confirmed.
2. If no significant difference in antibody level is observed and there is antibody present in the acute specimen, past rubella infection is indicated. This diagnosis can be made only when date of onset and date of acute specimen collection are within 2 or 3 weeks of each other. If the acute specimen is collected several months after onset, newly produced IgG may have already increased fourfold or more but will now be at a steady level. No diagnosis can be made when the date of onset and acute specimen collection are too far apart.
3. If no antibody is detected in either specimen, the patient is negative for present or past rubella infection.

CONGENITAL RUBELLA VIRUS INFECTIONS IN INFANTS. This testing may be requested for infants who are born with obvious congenital defects or for apparently normal infants born of mothers who had rubella during pregnancy. To evaluate and confirm congenital rubella infection, a quantitative rubella antibody assay must be performed on the infant's serum collected at birth and at intervals during the first 6 months of life. Antibody present in the infant's serum may be antibody produced by the infant in response to intrauterine infection or may be maternal antibody. Maternal antibody will normally be lost at 5 to 6 months; therefore, persistence of (or increase in) antibody level up to and after 6 months indicates intrauterine infection. Sequential serum specimens should be collected from the infant; one is collected soon after birth, and the others are collected at intervals during the next 5 to 6 months. The following interpretations may be used:

1. If antibody is detected in the initial specimen and persists at the same level or higher in the 5- to 6-month specimens, congenital rubella is confirmed.
2. If antibody is detected in the initial specimen but the level declines to low or undetectable levels in the 5- to 6-month specimens, congenital rubella is ruled out.

IMMUNE STATUS. The presence of rubella antibodies indicates past rubella infection or immunization. Individuals with rubella antibodies are considered to be immune to further rubella infection. Determination of immune status is desirable in the following cases:

1. **In all women of childbearing age.** Such testing is designed to identify women of childbearing age who may be susceptible to rubella infection. Susceptible women are usually immunized to make them immune to rubella. Then rubella infection will not be a danger during pregnancy.
2. **In men who will work with pregnant women.** Male health-care professionals and any other males who deal with large numbers of pregnant women may serve as sources of accidental rubella infection for these women. Those men who are not immune should be vaccinated; then they will be immune and no longer serve as possible sources of rubella transmission to female patients [4].

3. **In pregnant women exposed to rubella.** Determination of immune status of such women may be a critical factor in deciding completion or termination of pregnancy. Women with immunity need not fear fetal damage as a result of exposure to rubella. In nonimmune women exposed to rubella during pregnancy, fetal damage may be considerable.

To determine whether a person is immune to rubella, qualitative testing on only one serum specimen is required:

1. In healthy men and women, the specimen may be collected at any time. The following interpretations are used:
   a. If antibody is present in the serum (at the standard dilution for the method utilized), past infection or immunization is indicated. The result is reported as "positive," "antibody detected," or "immune."
   b. If antibody is not detected, there is no evidence of past infection or immunization. The result is reported as "negative," "antibody not detected," "not immune," or "susceptible."
2. In pregnant women exposed to rubella, the specimen must be collected within 10 days of exposure. Both exposure date and collection date must be known if the results are to be of value. The 10-day limit is imposed because rubella antibodies are usually produced in a new infection within 10 days of exposure. To ensure that antibodies measured are "old," preexisting antibodies rather than newly produced antibodies, the sample must be collected within 10 days of exposure. The following interpretations can be used:
   a. If antibody is present (at standard dilutions used in testing) in a serum specimen collected within 10 days after exposure, the individual is immune due to past infection or immunization, and the fetus is not considered to be at risk.
   b. If antibody is present in a serum specimen collected more than 10 days after exposure (or relationship to exposure is unknown), results are inconclusive and immune status before exposure cannot be determined.
   c. If no antibody is detected, there is no evidence of immunity resulting from past infection or immunization. A second specimen should be collected in 2 to 3 weeks and tested to determine whether antibodies appear. If antibodies appear, the pregnant woman has been infected by the virus. If antibodies do not appear, there was no infection.

IMMUNOGLOBULIN M–SPECIFIC SEROLOGICAL TESTING

Some of the classic serological methods have been modified to allow them to detect IgM alone rather than IgG or total antibody. Such methods can be used to differentiate recent from past infections because IgM ordinarily is present only early in the course of most infections. A positive IgM result usually indicates present or very recent infection. Testing of acute and convalescent samples is not required as it is with methods detecting primarily IgG.

In the evaluation of congenital infections, detection of IgM in the serum of an infant confirms that the infant is infected. IgM does not cross the placenta and cannot be maternal in origin. If testing detects IgM in the infant's serum, infection of the infant is confirmed.

IgM-specific testing is not useful for immune status determinations. IgM is transient and should be present only in current or very recent infection. Antibodies identified in immune status determinations are "memory antibodies" of the IgG type rather than those that are involved with current or recent infections.

Several of the serological methods can be modified to make them specific for detection of IgM. Each of these methods involves the use of "conjugates" composed of antihuman globulin or antihuman IgG, which are usually labeled with a fluorescent dye or with an enzyme. By replacing this conjugate with antihuman IgM, testing can be directed toward detection of IgM rather than of IgG or total antibody.

Use of IgM-specific conjugates is important in modifying traditional serological tests for use in IgM detection. However, this modification alone is not sufficient for IgM detection. IgM is present in serum in small quantities compared with IgG and is, therefore, more difficult to detect. IgG has been shown to interfere in IgM detection, as follows:

1. **If both IgG and IgM directed against the same antigen are present in a test sample,** the smaller and more numerous IgG molecules may bind to the antigen and block the larger, less numerous IgM molecules from binding (Fig. 6–1). If this happens, a test result may be **falsely negative** because of the IgG interference.

2. **If a test sample contains rheumatoid factor as well as IgG that is specific for the antigen in the test system,** there is a potential for **false-positive** results in IgM specific testing. (Reminder: Rheumatoid factors are antibodies, predominantly of the IgM class, and they bind to IgG, any IgG!). In IgM-specific testing of serum containing both rheumatoid factor and specific IgG, when the test serum is exposed to the test antigen, the specific IgG may bind to the antigen (Fig. 6–2). Then the rheumatoid factor in the test serum will bind to the bound IgG. When the IgM-specific conjugate is added, it will bind to the IgM rheumatoid factors. This produces a false-positive result for the test.

When IgG is removed from the sample, the interference just described in items 1 and 2 is eliminated. When IgG is absent, the larger IgM molecules have access to antigen binding sites, and false-negative results are eliminated. When IgG is removed, false-positive results caused by rheumatoid factor are also eliminated. Because no IgG is present to bind to the test antigen, the rheumatoid factor (which binds to IgG) can no longer bind.

Because IgG is known to cause interference in IgM-specific testing, many of the IgM-specific procedures now include an additional separation step at the beginning of the procedure. In this step, IgG is separated from the IgM. There are many approaches for separating IgG and IgM. Three of these methods are described next.

1. **Ion exchange column separation:** The test serum is added to a separation column packed with a resin. The immunoglobulin molecules will pass into the column and will migrate according to their size and charge. Elution buffers are added to elute the IgM molecules from the column. This eluate is used for the IgM-specific serological test.

2. **Anti-IgG:** The test serum is treated with antibodies against IgG. These antibodies will bind the IgG in the sample so that it is unable to react in the IgM-specific assay.

3. **IgM capture:** An initial step can be added at the beginning of enzyme immunoassay procedures. In this step, the "**capture**" step, anti-IgM antibodies attached to a solid phase bind or "capture" any IgM in the test serum. The assay is completed by adding reagents that will determine the specificity of the captured IgM (Fig. 6–3).

Although demonstration of specific IgM may be very helpful in diagnosis, these test results, like all laboratory values, cannot be accepted as 100% sensitive or specific. Certain biological and technical problems complicate the interpretation of IgM testing results.

Technical Factors

1. IgM testing is difficult to standardize because control sera must be of human origin and must contain the specific IgM. Because IgM is transient in infection, control sera must be harvested from individuals who are actively infected and producing IgM. Such sera are expensive and often difficult to obtain commercially.

2. Serum pretreatments for separation of IgG and IgM dilute the serum sample. This may cause false-negative results in sera with very low levels of IgM.

3. Pretreatments are not 100% effective, so IgG may interfere in some IgM tests, even after pretreatment.

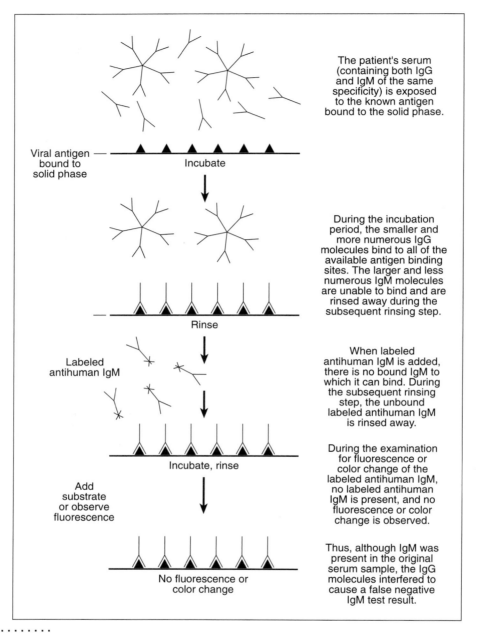

The patient's serum (containing both IgG and IgM of the same specificity) is exposed to the known antigen bound to the solid phase.

Viral antigen bound to solid phase

Incubate

During the incubation period, the smaller and more numerous IgG molecules bind to all of the available antigen binding sites. The larger and less numerous IgM molecules are unable to bind and are rinsed away during the subsequent rinsing step.

Rinse

Labeled antihuman IgM

When labeled antihuman IgM is added, there is no bound IgM to which it can bind. During the subsequent rinsing step, the unbound labeled antihuman IgM is rinsed away.

Incubate, rinse

Add substrate or observe fluorescence

During the examination for fluorescence or color change of the labeled antihuman IgM, no labeled antihuman IgM is present, and no fluorescence or color change is observed.

No fluorescence or color change

Thus, although IgM was present in the original serum sample, the IgG molecules interfered to cause a false negative IgM test result.

FIGURE 6–1 FALSE-NEGATIVE IMMUNOGLOBULIN M (IgM) TEST RESULT CAUSED BY IgG INTERFERENCE. In testing for IgM alone, when IgM is present in serum along with IgG of the same specificity, the IgG may interfere, producing a false-negative result. The mechanism of this interference is shown.

Biological Factors

1. IgM production in some individuals, such as children with congenital rubella or immunocompromised patients with chronic cytomegalovirus infections, may persist indefinitely after infection. In such cases, a positive IgM test does not indicate current or recent infection [5].

2. Some cross-reactivity exists between IgM antibodies and closely related viruses [5].

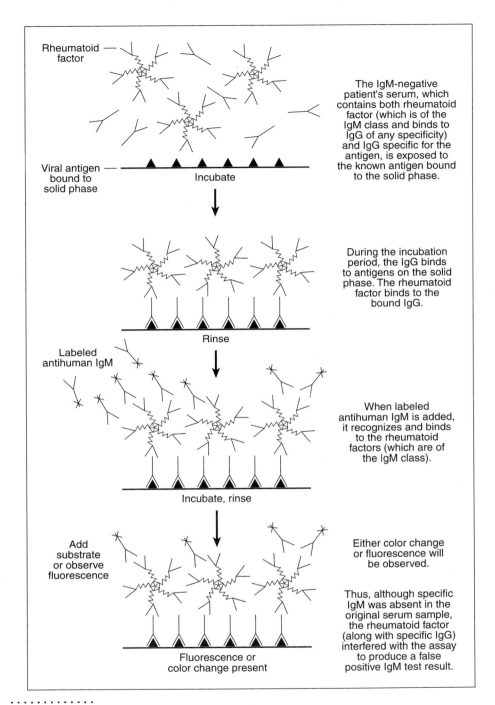

Rheumatoid factor

Viral antigen bound to solid phase

Incubate

The IgM-negative patient's serum, which contains both rheumatoid factor (which is of the IgM class and binds to IgG of any specificity) and IgG specific for the antigen, is exposed to the known antigen bound to the solid phase.

Rinse

During the incubation period, the IgG binds to antigens on the solid phase. The rheumatoid factor binds to the bound IgG.

Labeled antihuman IgM

Incubate, rinse

When labeled antihuman IgM is added, it recognizes and binds to the rheumatoid factors (which are of the IgM class).

Add substrate or observe fluorescence

Either color change or fluorescence will be observed.

Fluorescence or color change present

Thus, although specific IgM was absent in the original serum sample, the rheumatoid factor (along with specific IgG) interfered with the assay to produce a false positive IgM test result.

FIGURE 6–2   FALSE-POSITIVE IMMUNOGLOBULIN M (IgM) TEST RESULT CAUSED BY RHEUMATOID FACTOR INTERFERENCE. In testing for IgM alone, when IgG and rheumatoid factor are present in serum and IgM is absent, a false-positive result may occur. The mechanism of this interference is diagrammed.

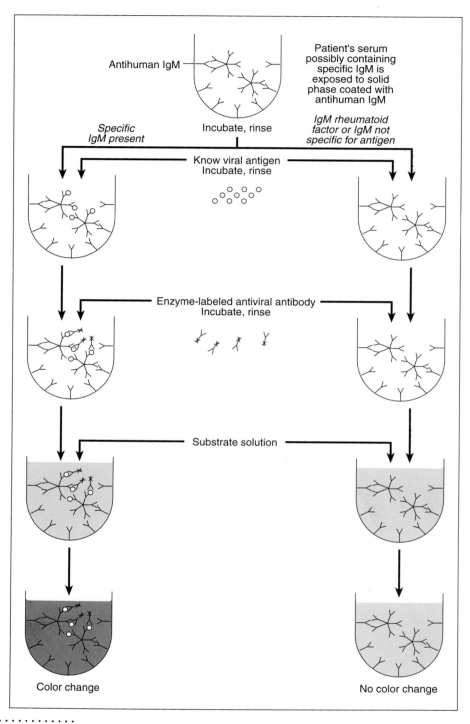

FIGURE 6–3 IMMUNOGLOBULIN M (IgM) CAPTURE ENZYME IMMUNOASSAY.
Patient's serum possibly containing IgM is exposed to antihuman IgM attached to a solid phase. Any IgM in the serum is "captured" or bound by the antihuman IgM. Subsequent steps in the assay (addition of known viral antigen, enzyme-labeled antiviral antibodies, and substrate) are performed to determine the specificity of the captured IgM. Captured IgM of the proper specificity will produce a final result of color change. Captured IgM of other specificity, including rheumatoid factor, will not produce an end result of color change.

3. Polyclonal IgM production has been reported in acute infectious mononucleosis. When stimulated by the Epstein-Barr virus, IgM class antibodies are produced by clones already committed to production of antibodies not related to Epstein-Barr virus [5].

AVAILABILITY AND APPLICATION OF VARIOUS VIRAL SEROLOGICAL ASSAYS

The assortment of commercially available diagnostic test kits designed to detect the various viral antibodies is enormous. Because each viral antibody can be detected by many different serological test mechanisms, the decision to select one method over the other may be difficult. General guidelines concerning the applicability and availability of various viral serological assay products are presented next. No procedures are presented in this text. Most commercially available viral antibody detection kits and systems are distributed with specific testing protocols. These protocols should be followed without modification to ensure accurate test results.

Passive agglutination tests, which involve mixing the patient's serum with particles that are coated with viral antigens, are probably the quickest and least technically complicated tests available at this writing. The test mechanism for passive agglutination is discussed in Chapter 2. The most popular passive agglutination methods involve antigen-coated latex particles that are mixed on a slide with the patient's serum. Rubella, cytomegalovirus, and varicella antibodies can be identified by latex agglutination. In comparison studies, the latex agglutination methods have been shown to produce results that are comparable in sensitivity and specificity to those of other methods for detection of antibodies [6,7]. The latex agglutination tests are reported to detect both IgG and IgM class antibodies. These tests are convenient to perform and are well suited to low-volume testing. Some passive hemagglutination tests involve the use of erythrocytes that are coated with antigens. Often the mixing of patient's serum with coated particles is performed in a microwell plate, and the plate is incubated for several hours or overnight before results are evaluated.

Indirect immunofluorescence is a popular and versatile serological approach for detecting viral antibodies. The indirect immunofluorescence method is discussed in Chapter 2. Dilutions of the patient's serum are added to smears of virus-infected cells fixed on a microscope slide. After incubation and rinsing, a preparation of fluorescein-labeled antispecies globulin is added to the smear. The smear is examined with a fluorescence microscope for the presence of fluorescing viral inclusions. The indirect immunofluorescence approach usually requires 2 to 3 hours for the staining of smears and a technologist with some expertise to examine the stained smear. At this writing, indirect immunofluorescence testing systems are available for detecting several types of antibodies against Epstein-Barr virus, measles, mumps, respiratory syncytial virus, cytomegalovirus, and herpes simplex virus. The indirect immunofluorescence procedures are well standardized and produce high-quality results when a trained technologist is the evaluator.

More expertise is required for performance and evaluation of indirect immunofluorescence assays than for passive agglutination methods. In immunofluorescence, the virologist must observe the pattern of fluorescence as well as the intensity. For the various viruses, patterns of staining are known (see Chapter 5). As virologists observe the results of indirect immunofluorescence tests for identification of viral antibodies, they must ensure that any fluorescence that is observed is distributed appropriately for the virus in question. The viruses of the *Herpesviridae* family (cytomegalovirus, Epstein-Barr virus, herpes simplex virus, and varicella) are known to induce Fc-binding receptors in the cytoplasm of the cells they infect. When indirect immunofluorescence is used for detection of antibodies against any of the *Herpesviridae* viruses, the virologist must examine the resulting fluorescence carefully. If fluorescence is visible in the cytoplasm rather than in the nucleus of the cells, nonspecific binding of antibodies by virus-induced cytoplasmic receptors is suspected. True fluorescence resulting from anti-*Herpesviridae* antibodies would be seen in the nucleus or in the nucleus and cytoplasm of virus-infected cells where viral inclusions are located. This Fc binding complicates the interpretation of indirect immunofluorescence test results involving *Herpesviridae* family viruses.

Another type of interference may be observed when immunofluorescence is used for identification of viral antibodies. If the patient's serum contains autoimmune antibodies, especially antinuclear antibodies, the antibodies may bind to nuclear or other nonviral antigens in the virus-infected substrate cells. This binding usually produces fluorescence in all cells in the substrate preparation. For this reason, most substrate smears for viral antibody immunofluorescence tests are prepared from mixtures of virus-infected and uninfected cells or from infected-cell populations in which only approximately 10 to 30% of the cells express viral antigens. Therefore, uniform fluorescence of all cells due to binding of autoimmune antibodies can be differentiated from fluorescence produced by viral antibodies because virus-specific fluorescence will be restricted to the less frequent virus-infected cells.

Enzyme immunoassays of various configurations are available commercially for detection of many viral antibodies. Various solid-phase enzyme immunoassay systems are discussed in Chapter 2. The systems include a solid phase such as a bead or the wall of a test tube or microwell that is coated with viral antigen. The patient's serum is exposed to the solid phase, and after incubation and rinsing, a preparation of enzyme-labeled antihuman globulin is added. After incubation and rinsing, a substrate solution is added. The color change of the substrate is measured by a spectrophotometric reader. Manual enzyme immunoassay systems with testing performed in microwell plates are available for detecting antibodies against cytomegalovirus; herpes simplex virus; hepatitis A, B, and C; HIV; Epstein-Barr virus; measles; rubella; varicella-zoster; and perhaps others. The manual microwell enzyme immunoassays usually require minimal expertise from the technologist and are completed in 3 to 4 hours.

The test pack configuration has been developed for enzyme immunoassay measurements of several viral antibodies. Cytomegalovirus antibodies can be measured in a "cube" test pack. The procedure requires only 20 minutes to perform, and the method has been reported to provide results that are comparable to those of the other more sophisticated and cumbersome enzyme immunoassay methods [8].

Several manufacturers have developed automated enzyme immunoassay systems. Such systems can perform a variety of viral antibody detection immunoassays, most commonly cytomegalovirus IgG and IgM, Epstein-Barr virus viral capsid antibody IgG and IgM, herpes simplex virus types 1 and 2 IgG and IgM, measles IgG, rubella IgG and IgM, and varicella IgG. This list is expanding rapidly as the technology is refined. The basic principle of these procedures is the same as for the comparable manual enzyme immunoassays, except that in the automated system, an instrument dilutes, transfers, mixes, rinses, and evaluates results for all of the assays. Routinely, the technologist "builds" a microplate by assembling microwells coated with the antigen that will be used in the test system. This microwell plate is positioned on the instrument along with tubes containing undiluted serum samples that will be assayed for the presence of antibodies. The steps of the immunoassay then commence: (1) The serum samples are diluted in sample diluent and added to the antigen-coated microwells; (2) antibodies, if present in the serum samples, bind to the antigen in the wells and subsequent washing removes unreacted serum components; (3) enzyme-labeled antihuman immunoglobulin (conjugate) is then added, which binds to the antibody that has bound to the antigen, and unreacted excess conjugate is washed away; and (4) the enzyme substrate is then added. The substrate is acted on by the bound enzyme, thus changing the color of the reaction mixture. The reaction is then stopped, and the intensity of the color, which is proportional to antibody concentration in the sample, is measured photometrically.

After the technologist positions tubes of undiluted patients' samples and the required reagents (diluent, conjugate, substrate) in the rack and constructs a microtiter plate of antigen wells of the type needed for the assay, the instrument is activated and its microcomputer directs the instrument through the appropriate timed cycles of diluting, reagent addition, and rinsing. When the entire test protocol is completed, the microcomputer signals the technologist. The technologist then transfers the microtiter plate to a spectrophotometric plate reader that measures the color of each microtiter well. The plate reader processes this information to calculate the final values and interpret the results for each sample.

With these instruments a single immunoassay (e.g., rubella IgG) can be performed on all of the samples, or two or more compatible assays (e.g., rubella IgG and cytomegalovirus IgG) can be performed simultaneously on all of the samples. With some systems, three to eight compatible separate assays may be performed on limited numbers of samples in the same run of testing.

Many other types of serological assays are used in viral antibody testing. Hemagglutination inhibition, neutralization, and complement fixation are three that are versatile and produce high-quality results. Each of these methods is described in Chapter 2. All are time consuming and require specialized reagents and technical expertise. **Hemagglutination inhibition** is useful in identifying IgG and IgM (together) produced against viruses that have the capacity to hemagglutinate. This includes the influenza and parainfluenza viruses, rubella, measles, and mumps. These antibodies rise early and persist for long periods. This method allows differentiation of antibodies against the various subtypes of influenza viruses such as influenza A/Victoria, A/Texas, and A/Hong Kong, differentiations that cannot be made with other serological assays. The assay is complicated by the presence of nonspecific inhibitors and natural agglutinins that must be removed from patients' sera before testing. Although this method was used originally to detect antibodies to many hemagglutinating viruses, it is now available primarily in research and reference settings because of the cumbersome nature of the assays.

Virus neutralization is the most specific antibody assay, depending on antibodies to bind to the known live virus, inactivate it, and render it incapable of proliferating. Biologically, neutralizing antibodies are the most important in response to infection and in establishing immunity. In the neutralization test system (discussed in Chapter 2), quantitation of the live virus is required before use in testing, and the test proper must incubate for 4 to 7 days before results are evaluated. Although all types of viral antibodies can be measured through neutralization, the method has been replaced by the less cumbersome and more standard assays. Neutralization testing is still the method of choice for evaluation of enterovirus antibodies, which include coxsackievirus, echovirus, and poliovirus antibodies.

Complement fixation testing is available at some larger laboratories where it is usually retained because it is so versatile. This system can be used to measure IgG and IgM (together) against many viral, bacterial, and fungal agents. At present, complement fixation is often used for adenovirus, influenza A and B, and parainfluenza 1, 2, and 3 antibody detection. Complement fixation is used sometimes for enterovirus antibody detection, but this is not recommended. Complement fixation in general is less sensitive than many other methods. Antibodies measured in the complement fixation system tend to decline to undetectable levels after infection, which makes the complement fixation test unacceptable for immune status determinations.

At this writing, the serological approach is still the only method widely available to aid in diagnosis of infections associated with each of the following viruses: HIV-1; Epstein-Barr virus; the classic encephalitis viruses; hepatitis A,B, and C; and parvovirus. The serological response for each of these viruses is described in Chapters 8 and 9. Although rubella virus proliferates in standard cell cultures, its isolation is a challenge; therefore, its diagnosis is often approached serologically. Rubella serodiagnosis is discussed extensively in this chapter. Some viral infections, notably rotavirus, are not routinely approached serologically. Antibody response in rotavirus is neither strong nor predictable. Rotavirus diagnosis relies on detection of viral antigen in stool samples, usually by enzyme immunoassay or passive agglutination.

TECHNICAL HINTS FOR SEROLOGICAL TESTING

1. In many serological procedures, specimens must be "heat inactivated" before testing. Heat inactivation destroys complement and other enzymes or lipoproteins that may be active in the serum and interfere with the desired serological reaction, especially in tests performed by the

complement fixation method. For other testing methods, heat inactivation of the sample is not required and, in many cases, may be prohibited. Be sure to consult the manufacturer's guidelines or the procedure manual to determine whether heat inactivation is necessary. Such heating does not destroy most antibodies. Heat inactivation is accomplished by incubating serum samples in a water bath at 56°C for 30 minutes.

2. Serum that is hemolyzed (has red discoloration) or contaminated should not be accepted for serological testing. Hemolysis products may interfere with or obscure serological reactions, and bacterial or fungal contaminants may produce substances that inactivate test reagents.

3. In quantitative testing involving twofold serial dilutions, each dilution tube is one doubling dilution different from the next. The dilutions may begin at any given point. Some examples of serial twofold dilutions follow:
   a. 1:10, 1:20, 1:40, 1:80, 1:160
   b. 1:85, 1:170, 1:340, 1:680
   c. 1:1, 1:2, 1:4, 1:8, 1:16

4. In quantitative testing, if all dilutions of a sample have failed to show a reaction, the final report is given in terms of the lowest dilution tested. For example, in a procedure in which dilutions 1:10 to 1:1280 were tested, if none of the dilutions reacted, the final report would be "<1:10;" the term "negative" is not used. If all of the dilutions, including the 1:1280, showed reactivity, the sample should be diluted further and retested to obtain an end point. A report of greater than or equal to 1:1280 is not usually acceptable; a definite end point is desirable.

5. In reporting of quantitative results from systems that provide results in the form of a numerical value rather than as a dilution end point, several methods may be used:
   a. The actual absorbance reading (or appropriate numerical score) for the test sample may be reported. Then the absorbance value or score that represents the "cutoff value" for the test method—the value that must be met or exceeded in order for the test to be considered positive—will be presented. If the sample value falls below the cutoff value, the result is considered "negative" or "antibody not detected." If the sample value meets or exceeds the cutoff value, the result is considered "positive" or "antibody detected." By comparing the magnitude of the sample value to that of the cutoff value, the physician can estimate the level of antibody. If the sample value far exceeds the cutoff value, the sample has a high level of antibody. If the sample value falls very near the cutoff value, the sample has a low level of antibody. Because actual absorbance readings are presented, the numbers are largely meaningless unless the cutoff value is reported.
   b. Another method for reporting the results involves dividing the absorbance reading of the test sample by the cutoff value to calculate a quotient termed the **index value.** Because the index value represents a comparison of the test sample value and the cutoff value, all values can be interpreted by the same criteria: an index value of less than 1.0 indicates a negative test (antibody not detected) and an index value of greater than or equal to 1.0 indicates a positive test (antibody detected). The magnitude of the index value correlates with quantity of antibody. For example, if two samples are tested for the same antibody, a sample with an index value of 8.6 has more of the antibody than a sample with an index value of 2.3. Consult the manufacturer's instructions for guidelines to use in differentiating significant from insignificant differences in index values. One manufacturer suggests that a quotient of greater than or equal to 2.0 between two index values indicates a significant difference in antibody level for some types of antibodies (Diamedix rubella IgG enzyme immunoassay, Diamedix Inc., Miami, FL). However, the necessary quotient for significance varies according to antibody type. Many manufacturers do not indicate parameters for evaluating magnitude of difference.

6. In all quantitative serological determinations, if two results are to be compared for antibody level, the two samples must be tested in parallel in the same run of testing. Comparing antibody levels determined days or weeks apart may allow insignificant random variations in testing to appear as significant differences.

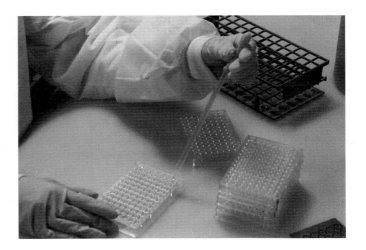

FIGURE 6–4 THE MICROTITRATION SYSTEM. This miniaturized system designed for preparation of twofold serial dilutions features microwell plates, micropipettes that deliver a single specified volume, and microdilutors (either hand held or automated). This system requires lower volumes of reagents and patient's samples and speeds accurate preparation of serial dilutions.

7. Quantitative serological testing involving twofold serial dilutions is facilitated by microtitration technology (Fig. 6–4). This system consists of microwell plates—either U-shaped bottom or V-shaped bottom, disposable or nondisposable micropipettes that deliver either 0.025 ml or 0.05 ml per drop, microdiluters (either hand held or in an automated format) of either 0.025 ml or 0.05 ml that are used to dilute the sample, and blotter paper (either 0.025 ml or 0.05 ml) for use in monitoring the accuracy of the microdiluters. The microtitration equipment is important in serology laboratories that perform assays in microtitration plates or routinely prepare serial twofold dilutions, portions of which can be transferred for testing in another system such as glass microscope slides bearing smears for use in indirect immunofluorescence techniques. The microtitration system allows for use of less serum and smaller volumes of costly reagents and provides a quick, accurate, and efficient system for preparing serial twofold dilutions.

8. In qualitative assays, undiluted serum or a single dilution of serum is tested. The result obtained is either "positive" or "negative"; no attempt is made to determine or report the amount of antibody present.

9. Testing of cerebrospinal fluid (CSF) for viral antibodies is sometimes requested when central nervous system involvement is suspected. Assaying of CSF or of other body fluids presents a problem in the laboratory because most serological assays are designed for testing of serum. The test systems have been developed, standardized, validated, and approved only for testing of serum, and the evaluation of other types of fluids in these systems will likely produce results that cannot be interpreted. Testing of body fluids other than serum with methods designed specifically for serum antibody determinations should be discouraged for this reason. If other body fluids are to be tested, the assay should be validated in the laboratory by testing of the appropriate types of body fluid from both infected and uninfected patients.

   A serum sample from the patient should always be tested in parallel with the body fluid. For CSF, an attempt should be made to determine whether the CSF contains antibodies produced within the central nervous system or is contaminated with serum antibodies that have crossed the blood-brain barrier. This differentiation involves evaluating the serum albumin level and the specific antibody level in both serum and CSF. This evaluation and the guidelines for interpretation are described elsewhere [2].

SPECIMEN COLLECTION AND STORAGE

Blood specimens for most serological assays must be collected in tubes without anticoagulant. The serum should be promptly separated from the clot and refrigerated at 2 to 8°C if the testing will be performed within 24 hours. Freeze the serum if testing will not be performed within 24 hours. A few assays can be performed on plasma from blood anticoagulated with EDTA or acid citrate dextrose; heparin is usually not acceptable. Be sure to consult manufacturer's instructions before using plasma in any serological assay. Plasma should be separated and stored as directed previously for serum.

The timing of blood collection will vary according to the clinical situation under investigation. Serodiagnosis of acquired and congenital infections requires that antibody levels in two or more sera be evaluated. Appropriate time intervals for these situations are discussed earlier in this chapter and may vary slightly from virus to virus. Immune status determinations or qualitative screening for antibodies involves testing of only a single sample collected at random.

SERUM BANK

If sample quantity and laboratory freezer space permit, it is helpful to freeze and store a portion of each serum sample that has been tested for viral antibodies. Samples may be maintained for 6 months to 1 year or longer. Such specimen storage allows physicians to order assays in retrospect as the patient's progress or lack of progress is evaluated. This system also facilitates the parallel testing recommended for acute and convalescent sera. When sera are stored in the laboratory, the frozen acute sample can be retrieved from storage and tested in parallel with the convalescent sample when it arrives.

A convenient storage system can be implemented using 2-ml cryovials. Approximately 1000 tubes can be stored per cubic foot of freezer space by using $5\frac{1}{8} \times 5\frac{1}{2} \times 2\frac{5}{8}$-in. cardboard or plastic storage boxes, which are divided into 81 compartments for cryovials. Number the boxes consecutively and identify each specimen's position by row and position number.

R E F E R E N C E S

1. Hyde RM, Patnode RA. Antibodies. In Immunology. Reston, VA: Reston Publishing Company, 1978, pp 33–45.
2. Cremer NE. Antibodies in serodiagnosis of viral infections. In Lennette EH (ed), Laboratory Diagnosis of Viral Infections, 2nd ed. New York: Marcel Dekker, 1992; pp 69–88.
3. Horstmann DM. Rubella. In Evans AS (ed), Viral Infections of Humans, Epidemiology and Control. New York: Plenum, 1976, pp 409–427.
4. U.S. Department of Health, Education, and Welfare. Exposure of patients to rubella by medical personnel—California. MMWR 1978; 27:123.
5. Herrmann KL. IgM determinations. In Spector S, Lancz GJ (eds), Clinical Virology Manual. New York: Elsevier, 1986:219–227.
6. Leland DS, Barth KA, Cunningham EB, et al. Evaluation of four methods for cytomegalovirus antibody detection tests for use by a bone marrow transplantation service. J Clin Microbiol 1989; 27:176–178.
7. Steinberg SP, Gershon AA. Measurement of antibodies to varicella-zoster virus by using a latex agglutination test. J Clin Microbiol 1991; 29:1527–1529.
8. Gleaves CA, Wendt SF, Dobbs DR, Meyers JD. Evaluation of the CMV-CUBE assay for detection of cytomegalovirus serologic status on marrow transplant patients and marrow donors. J Clin Microbiol 1990; 28:841–842.

R E V I E W Q U E S T I O N S

1. Serodiagnosis of viral infections is described as an indirect diagnostic method because
   a. A two-stage procedure involving antihuman globulin is used in many of the immunoserological procedures
   b. Infecting viruses are isolated indirectly from serum rather than directly from the site of infection
   c. Diagnosis relies on detection of viral antibodies in serum rather than on isolation or observation of the infecting agent
   d. Antibodies identified in serum are not type specific enough to identify the infecting virus definitively, so such diagnosis only "indirectly" implicates the causative agent

2. Serodiagnosis rather than isolation of the virus or identification of viral antigens is preferred in each of the following situations **except**
   a. When a virology laboratory is available and the infecting virus is easy to isolate and identify
   b. When proper samples for culturing or antigen detection are difficult to obtain
   c. When culture and antigen detection specimens were collected too late in the infection
   d. When the significance of a viral isolate needs to be clarified

3. In enzyme immunoassays in which the "answer" is read spectrophotometrically, an index value may be calculated on each sample and reported to the physician. Which of the following phrases accurately describes the index value?
   a. The index value is a ratio of the absorbance values of acute and convalescent samples from a patient; values of greater than or equal to 4 indicate a significant difference in titer.
   b. The index value is a ratio representing the spectrophotometric readout of the patient's sample divided by that of the calibrator (or cutoff value) sample; values of greater than or equal to 1 indicate a positive (antibody present) result.
   c. The index ratio is calculated by multiplying a sample's absorbance value by the dilution factor.
   d. The index ratio is simply a sample's absorbance reading from the spectrophotometer.

4. Before performance of many serological procedures, serum specimens must be heat inactivated. This heating
   a. Precipitates any hemolysis products that are present
   b. Destroys most antibodies
   c. Destroys complement and other enzymes
   d. Is accomplished by incubating samples at 37°C for 15 minutes

5. In a quantitative serological test, the results shown below were obtained. How should this result be reported (+ = antibody detected, 0 = no antibody detected)?

	SERUM DILUTION					
	1: 10	1: 20	1: 40	1: 80	1: 160	1: 320
Test result	+	+	+	+	+	+

   a. Report "negative" for antibody.
   b. Report "positive" for antibody.
   c. Repeat the test because this pattern is impossible.
   d. Perform testing on additional dilutions until an end point is reached.

6. An 8-year-old boy was tested to determine whether the rash he experienced recently was due to rubella. One serum sample was collected 4 days after the rash appeared, and a second sample was collected 14 days later. Results of a traditional rubella antibody test (which detects primarily IgG) were as follows: sample 1 = <1:10 and sample 2 = 1:160. What do these results indicate about the cause of the rash?
   a. The results are inconclusive.
   b. Several additional samples collected in a 6-month period should be tested.
   c. The rash was due to rubella infection.
   d. The boy was immune to rubella before the rash.

7. To determine the rubella immune status of a normal, healthy individual (using a traditional rubella antibody test that detects primarily IgG), the following serum specimens are required:
   a. One random sample
   b. Two samples collected 2 weeks apart
   c. Several samples collected during a 6-month period
   d. One sample collected within 10 days of exposure

8. A pregnant woman was tested for rubella antibodies (using a traditional rubella antibody test that detects primarily IgG) because she thought she had been exposed. Her sample was collected within 10 days of exposure, and her rubella titer was 1:32. What do these results indicate?
   a. She was immune before exposure.
   b. She has active rubella presently.
   c. A second sample is required to evaluate results.
   d. She has not been exposed to or immunized against rubella.

9. An infant was tested for rubella antibodies (using a traditional rubella antibody test that detects primarily IgG) at birth and at age 6 months. His results were as follows: at birth = 1:160 and at 6 months = <1:10. What do these results indicate?
   a. He did not have congenital rubella.
   b. He was exposed to rubella shortly after he was born.
   c. He is probably immunodeficient.
   d. Data are insufficient to make a diagnosis.

10. Consider the following rubella antibody testing results from tests for rubella IgM and IgG:

PATIENT	AT INFANT'S BIRTH		3 MO AFTER BIRTH		6 MO AFTER BIRTH	
	IgG	IgM	IgG	IgM	IgG	IgM
Mother	1:128	1:10	1:64	<1:10	1:64	<1:10
Infant	1:128	1:40	1:256	1:20	1:512	1:10

What do these results suggest?
   a. The infant probably has a congenitally acquired rubella infection.
   b. The infant was born with something in his serum that gave false-positive results in the rubella IgM test.
   c. The infant was infected by rubella at age 3 months.
   d. The infant's high rubella titer at 6 months is due to maternal antibody.

11. Which of the following phrases describes the first step in the IgM capture enzyme immunoassay method?
   a. Patient's IgM binds to antigen that is bound to the solid phase.
   b. Patient's IgM is bound by anti-IgM that is bound to the solid phase.
   c. IgM that is bound to a solid phase "captures" test antigen.
   d. Enzyme-conjugated IgM reacts with a substrate to produce a color change.

12. True or false? A serum sample collected from an 8-year-old girl with a rash showed a rubella antibody titer of 1:40. This result proves that the rash is due to rubella infection.

13. True or false? In IgM-specific testing, untreated sera containing rheumatoid factors are likely to yield false-negative results because the rheumatoid factors bind to the test antigen and block the specific IgM from reaching the binding sites.

14. True or false? IgG interference in IgM-specific assays can be eliminated (or significantly reduced) by treating the serum with antibodies against IgG; these antibodies bind to IgG in the serum.

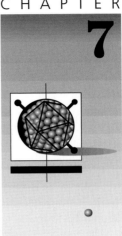

Diagnostic Laboratory Equipment, Quality Control/ Assurance, and Safety

EQUIPMENT AND MAINTENANCE
  Laminar Airflow Hood (Biological Safety Cabinet)
  Centrifuge
  Rotating Racks (Roller Drums)
  Incubator
  Standard Light Microscope
  Fluorescence Microscope
  Inverted Microscope
  −70°C Freezer
  Liquid Nitrogen Freezer
  Small Equipment
    Railroad Track Test Tube Holder
    Needle for Manipulating Shell Vial Coverslips
    Scrapers
    Repipettors
    Teflon-Coated Slides
    Tissue Grinders

QUALITY CONTROL AND QUALITY ASSURANCE
  Routine Quality Control
  Quality Assurance Program

SAFETY TIPS
  Personal Protective Equipment
  Engineering Controls

OBJECTIVES

At the completion of this unit of study, the student will be able to do the following:

1. Describe the following pieces of equipment and explain how they are used in the virology laboratory: laminar airflow hood, centrifuge, rotating racks (roller drums), incubator, standard light microscope, fluorescence microscope, inverted microscope, −70°C freezer, liquid nitrogen freezer, railroad track, scrapers, repipettors, Teflon-coated slides, and tissue grinders.

2. Trace the flow of air through the laminar airflow hood (biological safety cabinet, class II), and describe features of this piece of equipment.

3. List features that are necessary or desirable for a desktop centrifuge for use in routine clinical virology.

4. List advantages of the inverted microscope in clinical virology laboratory practice.

5. Explain how the quality of cell cultures is monitored in the virology laboratory.

6. Describe splash shields and face shields, and give the advantages of each in providing protection.

7. Discuss various aspects of evaluating specimen quality.

8. Define "engineering controls," and give examples of how this concept is applied in safety programs in the virology laboratory.

EQUIPMENT AND MAINTENANCE

The equipment required in the diagnostic virology laboratory includes many of the components routinely used in other areas of the diagnostic microbiology laboratory and varies depending on the level and sophistication of virology services provided. Viral serology and viral antigen detection assays involve pipetting devices, slides or appropriate sample containers, and instruments, either manual or automated, for mixing and transferring reagents. Most of the procedures are well standardized, and equipment and reagents are specified and provided by or available from the manufacturer of the various test kits. The success of these assays may depend on use of the appropriate instrumentation, and instructions from each system's manufacturer should be followed conscientiously.

The equipment used in virus isolation is much less standardized and may involve a few pieces of apparatus designed specifically for use in viral and cell culturing. Several pieces of equipment that are essential for virus isolation or other virology laboratory functions are described next. This list is not comprehensive and serves to highlight equipment used extensively in virology laboratories.

Laminar Airflow Hood (Biological Safety Cabinet)

Biological safety cabinets (hoods) have long been used in all areas of microbiology to prevent exposure of the microbiologist to infectious microorganisms, to prevent contamination of the materials being manipulated within the cabinet, and to protect the environment. Hoods have two major components: (1) a cabinet that holds the samples and provides a working area for the technologist and (2) an air-handling system that directs the flow of air. Most hoods also disinfect the air moving through and subsequently out of the hood. These are **not** chemical fume hoods, and they do not remove volatile nonparticulates.

Hoods identified as class II (laminar flow) are appropriate for clinical virology (Fig. 7–1). In class II laminar flow hoods, a unidirectional flow of air is created by a blower fan (Fig. 7–2). Air from the laboratory enters the cabinet through the front opening and, along with vertical airflow, passes downward through the front air intake grill. The blower fan forces the air out of the lower airspace. It travels to the upper airspace via a conduit along the back of the hood. Some of the air leaves through the top of the hood after passing through an exhaust high-efficiency particulate air (HEPA) filter. HEPA filters are composed of emulsified submicron glass fibers separated by crimped aluminum in a fire-resistant frame [1]. These filters effectively trap 99.97% of microscopic particles [2] and are very efficient with particles that are the size of viruses [1]. The portion of the air that does not leave the cabinet is forced downward through a different set of HEPA filter and enters the work area. This air is now clean and filtered. The clean air descends and, near the center of the work surface, splits. Half of it then passes downward through the front air grills, creating a protective air curtain across the front opening [3]. The other half of the air passes downward through the rear air exhaust grill into the lower space and simply continues to recirculate. Many class II hoods are now bench-top models with the blower fan located above the lower set of HEPA filters. Most hoods are also equipped with ultraviolet lights that can be turned on to sterilize the surface of the work space within the hood when it is not in use.

For all class II cabinets, appropriate rate and direction of airflow and excellent condition of the HEPA filters are imperative for optimal function. These criteria must be evaluated by a reputable hood inspector. Each hood should be certified after installation but before first use, at least annually thereafter, when HEPA filters are changed, when maintenance or repairs are necessary, and when the cabinets are relocated [3]. It is the responsibility of the laboratory

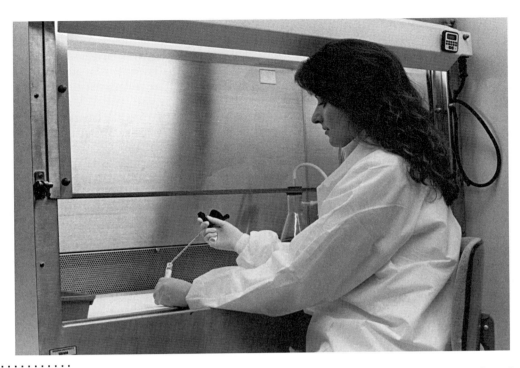

....
FIGURE 7–1 CLASS II BIOLOGICAL SAFETY CABINET. This cabinet provides a work area for safe handling of infectious materials. The work area is surrounded by a unidirectional flow of air that prevents contamination of materials within the cabinet and protects the environment from contamination from inside the cabinet.

....
FIGURE 7–2 AIRFLOW IN CLASS II BIOLOGICAL SAFETY CABINET. A unidirectional flow of air, created by a blower, enters the cabinet, passes downward through the front air intake grill, travels through the lower space, and moves upward along the back of the cabinet into the upper air space. After passing through an exhaust high-efficiency particulate air (HEPA) filter, some air leaves the hood. The remainder travels downward through HEPA filters and into the work area, where it splits, half providing a protective air curtain across the front opening and half passing downward through the rear air exhaust grill.

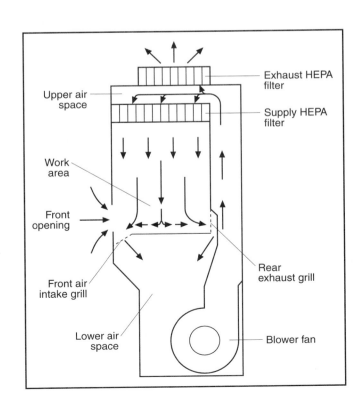

personnel to summon the inspector at the appropriate time. The inspector must evaluate hood functions such as the airflow velocity across the work space, the airflow across the access opening, the integrity of the HEPA filters, and the airflow smoke pattern (which ensures that the airflow along the entire perimeter of the work access opening is inward). Also inspected are lighting intensity, temperature increase, vibration, and noise, which are factors that do not involve contamination but do affect the safety and comfort of the operator [3].

In addition to ensuring that the hood is inspected at the appropriate time, the laboratorian must be sure to use the hood according to established guidelines (Table 7–1). If virus isolation services are offered along with general microbiology, which includes culturing of bacteria, fungi, mycobacteriology, or mycoplasma, it is best to dedicate a hood for processing of virus samples rather than sharing one hood for the various microbiology services. This will help eliminate the possibility of contaminating cell cultures with organisms from other cultures. Likewise, within the larger diagnostic virology laboratory, it is wise to designate one hood for specimen processing and another for feeding of cell cultures or passing or preparing of cell cultures. Hoods function optimally when they are located in a closed room. The use of fans in the area is discouraged because fans may disrupt the airflow in the hood.

Within the hood in the virology laboratory, it is convenient to have discard containers for sharp and nonsharp wastes, containers of sterile pipettes, and an electrical pipetting device. An aspiration (vacuum) device or system (Fig. 7–3) installed within the hood will also be useful in aspirating fluid from cultures and shell vials. The waste fluid from the aspirator must be discarded daily, and, periodically, the rubber tubing on the flasks should be replaced. The work space in the floor of the hood should be covered with absorbent paper, which is changed daily when the hood is cleaned and disinfected.

Centrifuge

Standard desktop centrifuges are suitable for daily routine tasks in the virology laboratory. High-speed or ultra-centrifuges are not required. Swinging bucket (horizontal head) centrifuges equipped with several sizes of specimen carriers are the best to accommodate the various tubes, vials, and microplates that require centrifugation. Specimen carriers should be equipped with safety covers to prevent formation of aerosols. Programmable centrifuges are convenient in that they allow push-button activation of various programs with specified combinations of centrifugation times, speeds, and temperatures required for various activities.

TABLE 7–1   GUIDELINES FOR USE OF CLASS II LAMINAR AIRFLOW HOODS

"DO'S" FOR HOOD USE
Turn on the hood 15 to 20 minutes before work begins.
Plan and organize the task to be completed in the hood so that all materials that will be needed can be placed in the hood, and the work can be completed without passing materials in or out through the air barrier.
Keep discard receptacles in the rear of the work area.
Conduct manipulations in the center of the work area, not over the intake grill.
When the work is complete, let the motor run for 15 additional minutes to allow removal of infectious particles.
At least daily, decontaminate the interior work surfaces of the hood by wiping them with a disinfectant solution; do not use bleach on stainless steel surfaces.

"DON'TS" FOR HOOD USE
Do not place supplies or pipette discard containers outside the hood on the floor or on carts.
Do not block the front intake or rear exhaust grills with paper or equipment.
Do not rapidly insert or withdraw arms.
Do not tape notes and so on to the front window; this may obstruct vision or decrease light intensity.

Modified from Kruse RH, Puckett WH, Richardson JH. Biological safety cabinetry. Clin Microbiol Rev 1991; 4:207–241.

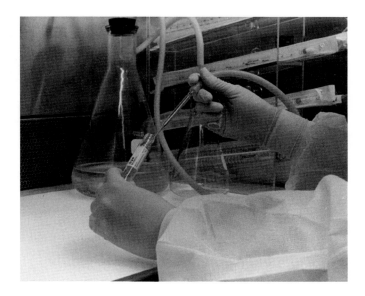

FIGURE 7–3 ASPIRATION SYSTEM FOR BIOLOGICAL SAFETY CABINET. Installed in the biological safety cabinet, a simple aspiration system with a large waste reservoir is helpful in aspirating fluid from cultures and shell vials.

For example, clinical samples in transport medium are spun at room temperature for 10 minutes at 1500*g* while shell vials are spun at 33 to 35°C for 1 hour at 700*g*. Although heating and cooling by the centrifuge are not required, this feature is useful in virology procedures such as shell vial inoculation in which it is recommended that vials be spun at 33 to 35°C.

Centrifuges require calibration checks periodically to ensure that they revolve at the desired number of revolutions per minute. Tachometers are available for performing this function. Another maintenance function involves monitoring and replacing commutator (motor) brushes. Commutator brushes are devices composed of a graphite head mounted on a spring. These function in delivery of power within the centrifuge motor. As the instrument is used, the graphite wears away, and the brush fails to function. Consult the instructions from the centrifuge manufacturer to determine where the commutator brushes are located and whether the technologist should be monitoring the condition of the brushes.

Rotating Racks (Roller Drums)

Rotating racks that hold standard 16-mm cell culture tubes are important to the clinical virologist. The function of rotating racks is described, and the rack is pictured in Chapter 3. Most roller drums hold 164 standard viral cell culture tubes and rotate these tubes at a rate between 0.2 and 2 revolutions per minute. These instruments require little maintenance even though they operate continuously for prolonged periods of months to years within the warm environment of an incubator. The laboratory maintenance program for roller drums must include instrument lubrication and the changing of commutator (motor) brushes, which, as described for the centrifuge, are the spring-loaded graphite devices that function in the delivery of electrical power. A procedure for instrument lubrication and for replacing of commutator brushes is included in the Appendix.

Incubator

An ambient air incubator (a carbon dioxide incubator is not needed) should be dedicated to virus isolation. It should have sufficient space to house roller drums, inoculated and uninoculated cell culture tubes, inoculated and uninoculated shell vial cultures, and antigen detection tests requiring incubation. This may be a free-standing floor model incubator with internal power sources and adjustable shelves or, in large laboratories, a large, walk-in incubator. Temperature must be maintained at 35 to 37°C.

Standard Light Microscope

Standard light microscopes equipped with 10 × objectives are sufficient for examination of cell culture tubes. The only special feature that is needed is an adjustable stage; this allows the stage to be lowered to accommodate a "railroad track" test tube holder and the cell culture tube. Some of the newer microscope models feature ergonomic design to ensure the comfort of the user (Fig. 7–4). This is important in the virology laboratory where virologists may spend long hours at the microscope examining cell culture tubes. In laboratories that frequently host student technologists, medical students, or house staff, a second head on at least one microscope allows for more effective and convenient teaching.

Fluorescence Microscope

A fluorescence microscope is a virtual necessity for most clinical diagnostic virology laboratories because so many of the routine procedures involve immunofluorescence. The fluorescence microscope does not need specialized features; the standard equipment will suffice for most virology-related tasks. An epifluorescence condenser is appropriate, and 20 or 25 × and 40 × dry objectives will be useful.

Inverted Microscope

Inverted microscopes have their optical system installed in positions that are opposite those of the standard microscope. The objectives are below the microscope stage, and the condenser is above the stage (Fig. 7–5). The advantage of this arrangement is that the objective is under the stage to focus on cells that may be contained in vessels that are filled with fluid and have configurations that cannot be accommodated on the standard light microscope. This arrangement is especially helpful in examining cells grown in cell culture flasks, shell vial cultures, and microwell plates, which are difficult to examine with most standard microscopes. Therefore, an

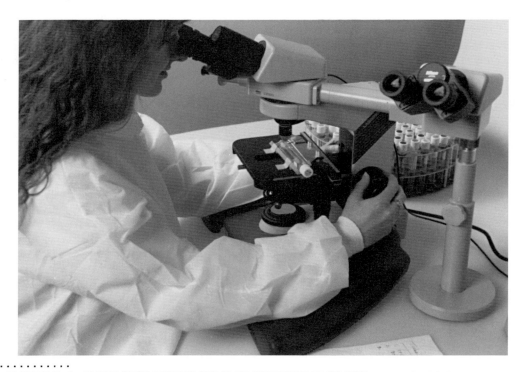

. . . .
FIGURE 7–4   LIGHT MICROSCOPE WITH ERGONOMIC FEATURES. A standard light microscope with ergonomic features such as armrests provides more comfort for virologists who may spend long hours examining cell cultures.

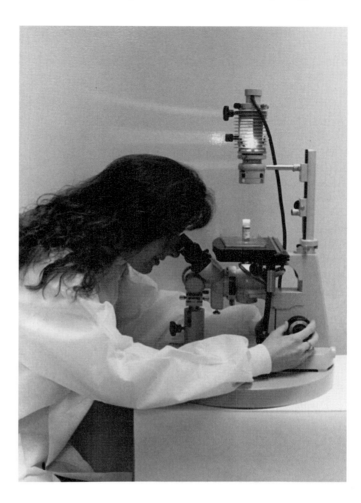

FIGURE 7–5 INVERTED MI-CROSCOPE. This inverted microscope design, with objectives beneath the stage and condenser above, accommodates cell culture flasks, shell vial cultures, and cultures in microwells, configurations that are difficult to examine with standard light microscopes.

inverted microscope is not a necessity for many routine clinical virology laboratory functions, but it is a welcome addition if it can be procured. The inverted microscope is useful with some of the newer technologies such as the enzyme-linked virus inducible system (ELVIS) described in Chapter 10. In this system, cells growing in microwell plates or in shell vials must be examined for color development. Although some of the color change reactions are strong enough to be observed macroscopically, the inverted microscope is an important tool to use with weak or questionable reactions. Inverted microscopes can be purchased for both standard light microscopy and for immunofluorescence work.

−70°C Freezer

It is convenient to have a −70°C freezer located within the virology laboratory or nearby. Because viruses do not tolerate storage at −20°C, viral culture specimens that must be frozen before inoculation into cell cultures or excess processed specimen material that will be stored after culture inoculation should be frozen at −70°C or colder. The temperature of the freezer must be checked daily, and it must be defrosted or otherwise cleared of frost periodically. Either a −70°C freezer or a liquid nitrogen freezer is required for storing stock viruses.

Liquid Nitrogen Freezer

A liquid nitrogen freezer is not essential for routine clinical virology, but it provides the optimal storage conditions for long-term storage of stock viruses and cells. The configuration of the freezer will be determined according to the needs and available space of the individual laboratory. A 15-ft^3 chest-type freezer is ideal. The unit is maintained by a 50-gallon liquid nitrogen tank. The tank should last 10 days before replacement is required. If less nitrogen freezer storage is required and laboratory space is limited, portable nitrogen Dewar freezers (Fig. 7–6) are available. These are usually mounted on wheels and easily slide beneath the laboratory work bench for convenient storage. These Dewar freezers are filled from a central liquid nitrogen tank, which may be located in a nearby laboratory area and shared by others. Dewar freezers will maintain their low temperatures for a period of 1 to 2 weeks. Materials that may require liquid nitrogen storage are stock viruses, stored portions of processed clinical specimens, and preserved cells that will be used to initiate cell cultures. Routine maintenance for the liquid nitrogen freezer includes monitoring of the nitrogen supply in the storage tank.

Small Equipment

RAILROAD TRACK TEST TUBE HOLDER. This device is taped in place on the stage of the microscope and functions in holding the cell culture tube in place and at an angle while the cells are being examined. These holders are pictured and described in Chapter 3. They are inexpensive, require no maintenance, and are available from several commercial sources.

NEEDLE FOR MANIPULATING SHELL VIAL COVERSLIPS. The coverslip that supports the cell culture monolayer in the bottom of the shell vial must be removed from the vial and mounted on a microscope slide during the process of evaluating shell vial culture results.

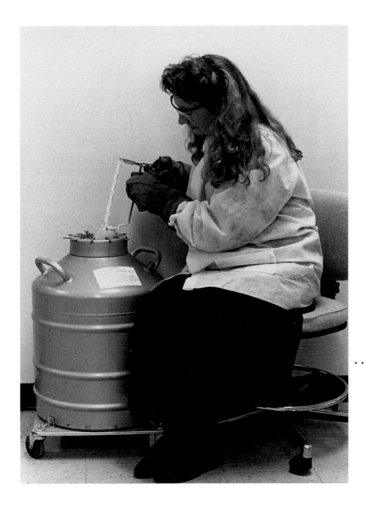

FIGURE 7–6 NITROGEN DE-WAR FREEZER. These small nitrogen freezers, with a "storage tank" configuration, are usually mounted on wheels and fit beneath standard laboratory benches. They provide the low temperatures of liquid nitrogen, yet do not take up as much space as a standard nitrogen freezer.

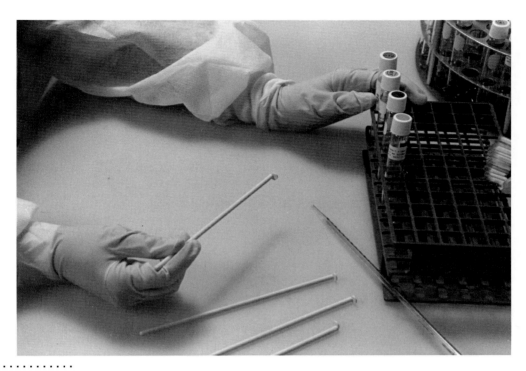

. . . .
FIGURE 7–7 CELL SCRAPER. Simple cell scraper devices can be used to dislodge adherent cells from the walls of their culture vessels.

Several devices can be prepared in-house for this purpose. One of these consists of an 18-gauge needle mounted on a tuberculin syringe. The bevel of the needle is bent with a hemostat to form a tiny hook that will slip under the edge of the coverslip to lift it up from the bottom of the vial. This device is pictured in Chapter 4. A standard microbiological wire probe can also be used for this purpose.

SCRAPERS. When cells are to be dislodged from the wall of a cell culture tube or flask during smear preparation or cell passaging, devices ranging from a plastic disposable serological pipette to a special cell scraper may be used. Scraping with a pipette will dislodge cells from the culture vessel, although the integrity of many of the cells may be disrupted and the removal may not be thorough. Specialized scraping devices will provide a better quality product with less effort from the virologist. One device, officially termed a "rubber policeman" and consisting of an elongated, flattened rubber tip attached to a glass rod, is very effective. These can be washed, sterilized, and reused repeatedly. Another device, commercially available as a "cell scraper," is a one-piece plastic apparatus with flat, circular head attached to a long plastic rod. These are disposable but can be reused after disinfecting, cleaning, and sterilizing. One type of cell scraper is pictured in Figure 7–7.

REPIPETTORS. In Chapter 3 the use of repipettors in feeding cell cultures was described. Repipettors are dispensing devices that include a calibrated plunger-type dispensing pump mounted on a reservoir that holds the fluid that will be dispensed (Fig. 7–8). Repipettors are available in many sizes, and each can be adjusted to dispense fluid in volumes within the range for the particular size of the device. In purchasing a repipettor for use in dispensing cell culture media or other fluids in the virology laboratory, be sure to select repipettors with parts that can be autoclaved. Sterility will be critical if the repipettor is to be useful in dispensing cell culture media into cell culture tubes. Repipettors can also be used in the virology laboratory for dispensing fixatives (use a glass repipettor for this) or buffers such as phosphate-buffered saline into shell vials during the staining process.

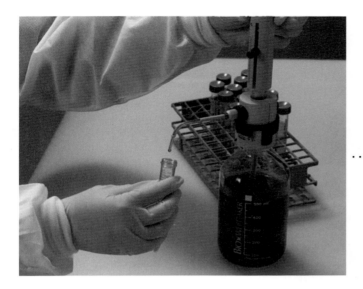

. . . .
FIGURE 7–8 REPIPETTOR.
These plunger-topped devices allow convenient delivery of a
measured volume of fluid simply
by depressing the plunger. Repipettors can be used in the virology laboratory for dispensing of
sterile cell culture media, phosphate-buffered saline, fixatives,
and other solutions.

TEFLON-COATED SLIDES

Although plain, frosted-end glass slides are acceptable for use for all virologic techniques, Teflon-coated slides featuring designated specimen test wells simplify all staining procedures. The raised Teflon coating that encircles each indented test area holds reagents on the test site. This eliminates the requirement for encircling smears with paint or marker and efficiently keeps expensive reagents confined to the desired area. Teflon-coated slides are pictured and discussed in Chapter 5. Although these slides are more expensive than the plain, frosted-end slides, they save time and expensive reagents. They are available from several manufacturers in a variety of colors and well configurations.

TISSUE GRINDERS

After large pieces of tissue have been minced with a scalpel, the minced pieces must be further dissociated by grinding with a manual tissue grinder. Both reusable and disposable grinders are available commercially. These consist of a cylindrical specimen container and a rough-surfaced plunger that fits snugly into the specimen container and is moved up and down and rotated to grind the tissue. The reusable grinders are washed and sterilized between uses. If the plunger has a glass shaft, the shaft should be protected during the washing and sterilizing steps to keep the shaft from chipping, cracking, or breaking. The fragile nature of the shaft is the greatest disadvantage of the reusable grinders. The disposable grinders are discarded after one use, which may prove costly. Grinders are available from several manufacturers.

QUALITY CONTROL AND QUALITY ASSURANCE

Quality control refers to the day-to-day operations that are a vital part of each procedure and laboratory operation and are designed to prove that each reagent, piece of equipment, or assay is functioning as it should to produce the desired result. The quality control program confirms that results are of high quality, prevents as many errors as possible, and detects errors that occur. Routine quality control is an important part of the quality assurance program, which is the overall total of related activities, including quality control, that monitor the process and practice of the laboratory and how the results are used in patient care.

Routine Quality Control

The routine quality control activities in the diagnostic virology laboratory are the same as those in most clinical laboratories, involving preparing and maintaining procedure manuals, selecting test methods, ensuring reagent quality, monitoring equipment and instrument function, and keeping records. The list of these activities is lengthy, and most are specified and defined by a variety of accrediting and inspecting agencies. One simple rule is universal in its application in quality control monitoring:

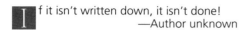 f it isn't written down, it isn't done!
—Author unknown

The following items do not constitute a comprehensive quality control program, and suggestions are not designed to supersede or redefine mandatory regulations. Some of the items listed are important in many types of laboratories, whereas others are unique to clinical virology. The information presented is intended to provide ideas concerning how various components of a quality control program can be implemented in the virology laboratory.

1. *Read and record the temperatures of all freezers, refrigerators, water baths, and incubators daily.* If any temperatures do not fall within acceptable ranges (which must be posted), take appropriate corrective action and recheck the temperature again in a reasonable time period. Be sure all activities are carefully documented. If corrective action does not remedy the problem, consult the supervisor, and take the instrument out of service, if necessary.

2. *For each assay, including antigen and antibody detection as well as molecular diagnostic techniques, ensure that both known positive and known negative controls are included in each run of testing or are tested in the first daily run of tests for any assays that are performed more than once each day.* Be sure that all results of control samples are documented. Results of patients' samples may be reported only when the control samples yield the expected results. If the control samples fail to yield the expected results, do not report results of patient's samples. When there are control failures, consult the supervisor, and take appropriate remedial action. The steps in a sample remedial action policy are shown in Table 7–2. Remedial action may involve repeating all testing using the same reagents, repeating all testing using different reagents, or referring specimens to a reference laboratory until the problems in the testing system can be resolved.

When controls do not yield the expected results, all patient samples tested between the time of the last successful run and the failed run must be tested. For example, samples from six patients

TABLE 7–2   STEPS FOR REMEDIAL ACTION WHEN CONTROL SAMPLES HAVE FAILED TO YIELD THE EXPECTED RESULTS*

REMEDIAL ACTION PROTOCOL
1. If the source of error is not obvious, repeat all testing using the same reagents from the same kit or lot as in the initial unsuccessful run. If the source of error is obvious, replace the faulty reagent and so on with a new lot of the product, and repeat all testing.
2. If the problem persists after repeating the procedure, repeat all testing using reagents or controls, or both, from a different lot of reagents.
3. Analyze any persistent problems to identify the source of the malfunction. Make sure the unsatisfactory reagents are discarded and any faulty equipment is repaired or taken out of service.
4. Complete any additional corrective action recommended by the supervisor or the director.
5. If problems cannot be resolved, refer samples to a reference laboratory for testing. This will keep laboratory dificulties from disrupting patient care. Continue to work to resolve the problems in the laboratory.
6. When the problem is resolved and the procedure yields acceptable results on all controls, evaluate any patients' results reported since the last successful quality control run; repeat testing may be required.
7. Document any remedial action, and keep these records in a location that will ensure that anyone who encounters similar problems has easy access to the information.

*For each procedure in which known positive and negative control samples or any additional control systems are included in testing, results of all control samples must be evaluated and recorded before evaluation of results from test samples. If all controls have yielded results that fall within the limits defined for the particular procedure, the results from patients' samples may be evaluated and reported. If any controls have not yielded results that fall within the limits defined for the particular procedure, do not evaluate or report results of patients' samples. Review the results with the supervisor or director, and implement remedial action.

were tested on Tuesday morning in a direct immunofluorescence test for respiratory syncytial virus (RSV) antigens; all controls yielded the expected results. On Tuesday afternoon, four additional samples were tested by the same method using the same reagents for RSV antigen detection. No controls were included because the daily controls had been tested in the morning run, and they had produced the expected results that morning. On Wednesday morning, seven samples were tested for RSV antigens, and the positive control showed no fluorescence. This was *not* an acceptable result, so the results for the seven patients were not reported. In follow-up to this failure, the seven samples from Wednesday morning (the failed run) must be retested, and the results of the four samples from Tuesday afternoon (samples tested since the last successful run on Tuesday morning) must be reviewed and evaluated; retesting may be appropriate.

At this writing, the regulations concerning testing of control samples are under review by accrediting agencies. It is likely that testing of both positive and negative controls soon will be required in each run. When controls are included with each run, situations such as the one described previously will not be encountered.

3. *Evaluate and control the quality of commercially purchased or in-house prepared cell cultures.* Keep detailed records concerning each batch or lot of cell cultures. Indicate the manufacturer, type of cell, lot number, date received in the laboratory, date put into service, and any comments concerning shipping, quality control assessments, and so on. Many of the manufacturers of commercially prepared cell cultures are now providing quality control information along with their cell culture tubes. This information indicates which types of testing have been done by the manufacturer and the results of this testing. These records should be maintained along with the in-house quality control data on the cell cultures and can be an important part of the quality control program. If the laboratory uses a sufficient number of commercially purchased cell culture tubes and more than one distributor is available, it is wise to purchase cultures from more than one manufacturer. This ensures a supply of cell cultures when one manufacturer has production problems or there are shipping delays and so on.

Immediately on receipt of commercially purchased cell cultures (traditional tube cultures, flask cultures, or shell vial cultures) or just before initiation of use of cell cultures prepared in house, select several tubes from each lot and observe them grossly and under the microscope. Be sure that there are no obvious signs of contamination or toxicity and that monolayers are healthy and confluent. If cells do not appear healthy, incubate them and observe them again later to determine whether problems may have been related to shipping or to slow growth and will resolve. Change culture medium at this time if the pH is not appropriate. If problems with commercially prepared cultures do not resolve, contact the manufacturer, and do not use the cultures for clinical testing. Keep careful written records about each lot of cell cultures [4].

If cultures appear healthy and ready for use, select at least one uninoculated culture from each lot. This uninoculated culture should be held for the full length of the maximum incubation period that will be used for any of the inoculated cultures from the lot [5]. For example, for fibroblast tubes that are held 30 days for cytomegalovirus isolation, hold the uninoculated tube for the entire 30 days. The uninoculated control tubes serve as negative reading standards for technologists, who may sometimes have difficulty differentiating nonspecific cellular degeneration from virus-induced changes. The uninoculated tubes are especially helpful with primary monkey kidney cultures, which may sometimes be infected with indigenous monkey viruses. If the uninoculated control tubes begin to show a cytopathogenic effect (CPE), the virologist knows that the cell cultures, rather than the clinical samples inoculated into the cell culture tube, are responsible for the CPE.

For newly arrived cell cultures that are ready for use, select one additional tube of each lot and inoculate it to serve as a positive control tube. Use a stock solution of an appropriate virus that has been previously titered, diluted, aliquoted, and stored frozen. Observe the inoculated tube daily, and record the observations on a quality control data sheet. Define acceptable limits for the time and intensity of CPE expected for each cell line. If the time and appearance of CPE are as expected, continue with use of the cell cultures (which will probably already be in use for clinical testing). If the control tubes do not yield the expected result, select yet another tube from the same lot and repeat the process. For repeated failure, discontinue use of the cultures from that lot. Be sure to report any failures to the manufacturer, or, if the failure involved cultures prepared in house, carefully evaluate the culture preparation procedure to identify and correct sources of errors. For clinical samples that were inoculated into cell cultures from the unsatisfactory lot, use stored, frozen, processed sample material to inoculate tubes from another lot of the same tissue, a lot that does yield acceptable control results.

For inoculation of all types of cell cultures except primary monkey kidney cultures (primarily used for cultivation of respiratory viruses) and fibroblast shell vial cultures (primarily used for cultivation of cytomegalovirus), use herpes simplex virus type 1 to inoculate the positive control tubes. For primary monkey kidney cultures, use a stock hemadsorbing virus (we recommend parainfluenza 2), and for fibroblast shell vial cultures, use cytomegalovirus. For standard cell culture tubes, observe tubes daily and record observations. Use the guidelines just provided to evaluate results. For fibroblast shell vial cultures inoculated with cytomegalovirus, incubate for the time interval used in the laboratory for clinical testing involving the vials, and, at the appropriate time interval, stain the coverslip just as would be done for a clinical specimen. The positive control should yield positive results at this time. If it does not, repeat the procedure with another vial. If the failure is repeated, follow the directions just provided for cell culture tubes.

For cost-effective quality control of cell cultures and virus isolation procedures, some of the quality control tubes can serve dual purposes. For example, primary monkey kidney cell cultures that are inoculated with parainfluenza 2 can be placed in a stationary slant rack in the refrigerator as soon as they show the desired CPE. These refrigerated infected tubes can be used as positive controls for evaluating guinea pig erythrocytes received each week for use in hemadsorption testing. One positive control tube is tested with each new lot of erythrocytes before the erythrocytes are put into service for routine testing. The uninoculated cell culture tubes that are held from each lot of primary monkey kidney cell cultures can be used as negative controls for new lots of erythrocytes. These negative control tubes can be rinsed free from erythrocytes at the completion of hemadsorption testing and reincubated as negative control tubes.

When excess fibroblast shell vials are available, the vials can be inoculated with cytomegalovirus instead of discarding them. After a suitable incubation period, one vial is fixed in methanol and stained with cytomegalovirus monoclonal antibodies; if this vial yields satisfactory results, all of the inoculated vials can be fixed in methanol and then allowed to dry completely. On completion of drying, the vials can be recapped and stored at $-20°C$. One of these vials can be used with each run of shell vial staining to serve as a positive control.

Other inoculated positive control tubes or unused, uninoculated tubes can be used for preparing control smears for use in immunofluorescence testing. A procedure for preparing control smears is included in the Appendix.

Quality Assurance Program

Quality assurance is a broad concept applied in the analysis of processes to find the cause of deficiencies, to improve the process, and to anticipate and prevent problems, all in hopes of making permanent improvement. Quality assurance involves more than intralaboratory quality control of testing and reagents. The quality assurance process involves all aspects of the testing process from specimen collection and transport to reporting and interpreting test results. Often evaluation and improvement of quality through the quality assurance program involves not only laboratory personnel but also physicians, hospital staff, and others involved in patient care. Several aspects of a diagnostic virology laboratory quality assurance program are now addressed.

Again, this is not a comprehensive list, presenting examples rather than mandates for addressing quality assurance.

SPECIMEN QUALITY. The importance of the quality of the patient's sample in providing meaningful diagnostic virology laboratory services is explained in Chapter 3. Appropriate types of specimens for use in virus detection in various clinical syndromes are listed, and specimen collection guidelines are presented. A good-quality specimen that facilitates rapid and accurate viral diagnosis is of medical and financial benefit to all: the patient, the payer, the physician, and the laboratory [6].

Certain aspects of specimen quality are easily evaluated. One of these aspects is simply ensuring that the correct type of sample is submitted for the test or virus suspected. Occasionally, the wrong type of sample may be submitted. For example, if the specimen received is a stool sample and the test requested is for RSV antigen, the mismatch is obvious and the physician or ward can be notified of the confusion. The sample will likely be replaced with an appropriate respiratory sample or the proper assay identified. In this case it is likely that rotavirus antigen rather than RSV antigen testing was desired. Similar mix-ups occur daily, and each should be followed up by notifying the appropriate individuals. This notification process should be completed before the specimen is discarded!

For all samples, if the paperwork (or computer request information) that accompanies the sample is complete, the time of collection of the sample should be noted. This time can be compared with the time of delivery of the sample to the laboratory, and the elapsed time can be appraised as acceptable or unacceptable for the type of sample. For example, leukocytes in an anticoagulated peripheral blood sample collected 96 hours before receipt in the laboratory may fail to separate properly when processed; this sample probably will not yield useful information. In this case, the appropriate individuals should be notified that the sample is unsuitable for testing. Not only is the time required for transport of the sample important, but the transport temperature is often very important as well. Specimens for virus isolation should be kept refrigerated or on wet ice and should not be frozen. If the sample is not handled as required, it should not be accepted for testing.

Other aspects of specimen quality are less easily determined. Although the number of intact cells present in a sample can be evaluated in immunofluorescence testing for viral antigens, this is not the case for samples that are submitted for virus isolation or for enzyme immunoassay testing for detection of viral antigen. Manipulations of specimens for the latter assays do not involve microscopic examination for counting of cells. Even if such counting was done, it would be inappropriate to reject these specimens based solely on low cell count. For both of the types of assays mentioned, extracellular virus present in fluids may well be detected.

To avoid or decrease problems involving specimen collection and transport, the laboratory must effectively communicate the information to the collectors. The following activities have been recommended [6]: (1) Provide physicians and hospital staff with a handbook of information concerning collection techniques; (2) provide specimen selection and collection information in hospital computers if this is available in the data system; (3) provide diagrams or "cartoons" of how to collect samples; (4) provide written recollection guidelines with all notifications of unacceptable samples; (5) utilize laboratory or infectious disease personnel to serve on physician education teams; and (6) prepare collection videotapes for physician education.

COMMUNICATION OF RESULTS. Regardless of the quality of the work being done in the laboratory, the application of this information in patient care and effective patient management relies on effective and efficient communication of test results from the laboratory to those who need to know the result in order to make decisions. Telephoning of results or computer-communicated "stat" reports of viral antigen testing are very helpful and are probably the virologists' greatest contribution to patient management. Likewise, immediate notification to the physician when a positive viral culture is discovered is very helpful. A positive culture result that is not reported until the end of the 2-week culture period is not likely to be useful in patient management.

SAFETY TIPS

In the virology laboratory as in all areas of the laboratory, safety is of paramount importance. Guidelines for safe performance of tasks in the clinical virology laboratory are the same as those for all laboratory areas and must conform to the regulations of the various accrediting agencies that certify the facility. Programs for controlling exposure to blood-borne pathogens and chemical hazards and for safe practices involving electrical hazards, fire, and other hazards are essential. Several safety hints are now provided. This is not a comprehensive safety program, only suggestions for safe operation of the diagnostic virology facility.

Personal Protective Equipment

In addition to the laboratory coat and gloves that are mandated by various inspecting agencies, the virologist's eyes and face should be protected when splash is imminent. This is a built-in protection in biological safety hoods, which have glass windows that separate the work area from the user. By restricting specimen manipulations to the safety hood, the virologist's face is protected, and no additional face protection is required.

Antibody assays involving serum are often performed on open benches rather than in the safety hood. For these activities, face protection must be provided during the time that the samples are being manipulated and the chance of splash is great. There are many options for providing the necessary protection. Splash shields can be mounted on flexible arms that are attached to bench-top cabinetry or to flat bench-top platforms. These allow a protective Plexiglas shield to be positioned between the worker and the work surface to prevent splashes from reaching the face or eyes of the technologist (Fig. 7–9). In cramped surroundings or when portability of the shield is important, a simple disposable face shield can be used (Fig. 7–10). Face shields feature a transparent plastic shield that is attached at the technologist's forehead by an elastic band and

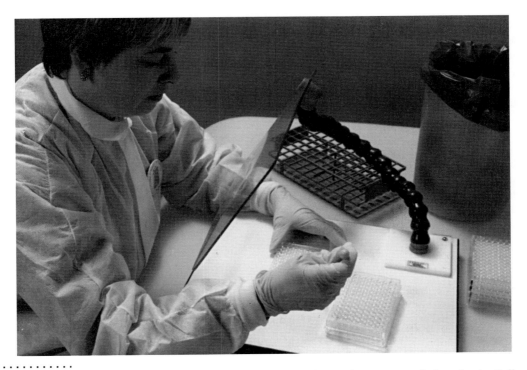

FIGURE 7–9 SPLASH SHIELD. Bench-top splash shields can be used to prevent splashes of potentially infectious or caustic liquids from reaching the face or eyes of the technologist.

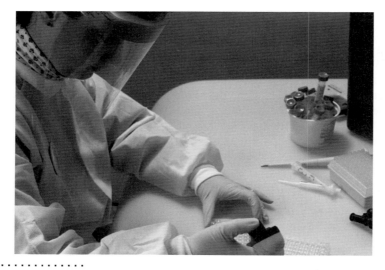

FIGURE 7–10 FACE SHIELDS. Face shields can be worn to protect the eyes and face from splashes of liquids handled in the laboratory. These are lightweight and fit comfortably over regular glasses. They do not occupy bench space and are highly portable.

extends below the chin. These are lightweight and comfortable to wear and protect eyes and face from splashes.

Engineering Controls

One important aspect of safety in the laboratory involves taking advantage of new or improved equipment and devices that are engineered for safe laboratory practice. In other words, identify sources of danger and find alternate methods and devices so that the dangerous items or practices can be eliminated. Such modifications and substitutions are called *engineering controls*. Although this sounds complicated, many engineering controls are actually very simple. For example, one of the best ways to protect virologists from accidental needle sticks and cuts from broken glass pipettes and tubes is to eliminate the use of these supplies in routine tasks. Rather than using a syringe to withdraw and transfer antibiotics from their vials into cell culture media bottles, open the antibiotic vial, and use a sterile plastic serologic pipette to draw up and dispense the antibiotic. Likewise, rather than using glass sterile, disposable serological pipettes, use plastic serological pipettes; instead of using glass centrifuge tubes, use plastic tubes. Inexpensive disposable glassware often has tiny flaws that result in excess fragility. Simply by replacing the glass items with plastic, many accidents can be eliminated.

REFERENCES

1. First MV. Testing of Class II Biological Safety Cabinets. Boston, MA: Harvard School of Public Health, 1980.
2. Gilbert H, Palmer JH. High efficiency filter units. Washington, DC: U.S. Atomic Energy Commission, Office of Technical Services, Department of Commerce, 1961.
3. Kruse RH, Puckett WH, Richardson JH. Biological safety cabinetry. Clin Microbiol Rev 1991; 4:207–241.
4. Clarke LM, McPhee JM, Cummings RV. Isolation of viruses in conventional tube culture: selection and inoculation of cell cultures. In Isenberg HD (ed), Clinical Microbiology Procedures Handbook. Washington, DC: American Society for Microbiology, 1992; pp 8.5.1–8.5.13.
5. Aarnaes S, Daidone BJ. Observation and maintenance of inoculated cell cultures. In Isenberg HD (ed), Clinical Microbiology Procedures Handbook. Washington, DC: American Society for Microbiology, 1992, pp 8.7.1–8.7.16.
6. Warford A. Monitoring and improving the quality of specimens. Pan American Group for Rapid Viral Diagnosis Newsletter 1994; 20:1–4.

REVIEW QUESTIONS

1. A "railroad track" test tube holder functions as follows:
   a. Holds tubes in a vertical position during cell culture inoculation
   b. Holds tubes horizontally and at an angle on the stage of the microscope
   c. Holds tubes at a 45-degree angle during centrifugation in a swinging-bucket centrifuge
   d. Holds tubes horizontally in stationary racks used for cell culture incubation

2. A main reason that a −70°C freezer is useful in the virology laboratory is
   a. The components of cell culture media are fragile and require storage at −70°C
   b. Antiviral antibodies in serum are unstable except at −70°C
   c. −70°C is the temperature used for hemadsorption testing
   d. Viruses do not tolerate −20°C storage (regular freezer temperature) and should be stored at −70°C if they must be frozen

3. Which of the following describes the function or purpose of the laminar airflow hood?
   a. The cabinet prevents exposure of the virologist to infectious microorganisms, protects the environment, and prevents contamination of the experiment being conducted in the cabinet.
   b. Air is processed to remove volatile nonparticulates.
   c. High-efficiency particulate air filters filter out viruses from samples and from the air and concentrate them in an area where the virologist can access them for use in inoculating cell cultures.
   d. Airflow vents may be blocked without affecting hood function as long as the blockage is due to required equipment or papers.

4. A desktop centrifuge for routine use in the clinical virology laboratory should have the following features:
   a. Must have ultra-centrifuge capacity to generate 30,000 to 100,000 × g force
   b. Must have the capacity to cool to −20°C during centrifugation
   c. Needs a nonadjustable revolution per minute setting because all routine virology laboratory functions require the same gravity force
   d. Should be a standard swinging-bucket centrifuge equipped with several sets of sample carriers of various sizes

5. A program for monitoring the quality of cell cultures involves all the following **except**
   a. Maintaining careful records of manufacturer, cell type, lot number, and dates received and put into service
   b. On receiving cultures from manufacturer, observing uninoculated cultures, both grossly and microscopically, for evidence of contamination or toxicity
   c. Inoculating cells into eggs or animals to ensure freedom from otherwise noncultur- able viruses and rickettsia
   d. Incubating of uninoculated cultures from each lot to monitor cell quality through- out the incubation period

6. Although it is not possible to monitor all aspects of specimen quality, the following activities are recommended **except**
   a. Ensuring that the assay and virus suspected are appropriate for the type of sample submitted
   b. Evaluating collection time and date and delivery time and date
   c. Providing physicians and hospital staff with specimen collection guidelines
   d. Performing a cell count on all samples submitted for all assays; reject those with fewer than 20 cells per high-power field

7. Various splash and face shields are available for eye and face protection. These should be configured and used as follows:
   a. Face shield should be worn at all times while the virologist works at the laminar flow hood
   b. A shield of some sort should be used whenever chance of splash in imminent
   c. A desktop shield features a unidirectional airflow that draws aerosols downward and away from the technologist
   d. Face shields cover only the mouth and must be worn along with safety glasses
8. The inverted microscope is useful in the virology laboratory because
   a. It magnifies at a higher power than the standard light microscope
   b. It has ergonomic features that make it much more comfortable to use than a standard light microscope
   c. The inverted configuration accommodates cell culture vessels of shapes and sizes that cannot be conveniently examined with a standard light microscope
   d. The inverted microscope has the condenser below the stage and the objectives above it
9. *Engineering controls* is a term used to describe
   a. Eliminating unsafe equipment and activities by providing improved equipment or by modifying processes to eliminate the unsafe practice
   b. Hiring a clinical engineer to monitor daily laboratory activities
   c. Using specially engineered cell lines in virus isolation
   d. Designing better control samples through advanced technologies such as molecular cloning
10. True or false? A repipettor is a device consisting of a plunger top mounted on a storage vessel. When the plunger is depressed, a measured volume of fluid is expelled.
11. True or false? A Teflon-coated microscope slide features test areas coated with transparent Teflon. This holds cells on the glass and eliminates the need for fixation.

DNA Viruses

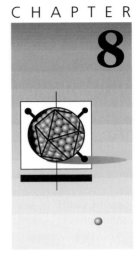

ADENOVIRIDAE
  Adenovirus

HEPADNAVIRIDAE
  Hepatitis B Virus

HERPESVIRIDAE
  Cytomegalovirus
  Epstein-Barr Virus
  Herpes Simplex Virus Types 1 and 2
  Varicella-Zoster Virus

PAPOVAVIRIDAE
  Papillomavirus, Polyomavirus

PARVOVIRIDAE
  Human Parvovirus B19

POXVIRIDAE
  Variola, Molluscum Contagiosum, Others

O B J E C T I V E S

After completion of this unit of study, the student will be able to do the following for each virus described:

1. Give the classification by family.

2. List disease syndromes with which each virus is commonly associated.

3. Identify the approaches (virus isolation, viral antigen detection, serodiagnosis) that are useful in laboratory diagnosis of infection.

4. Indicate whether viral antigen detection methods are available and useful clinically, and list and describe specific methodologies used for this purpose.

5. Indicate which types of clinical samples should be collected and submitted for diagnosis.

FAMILY: *ADENOVIRIDAE*   VIRUS: ADENOVIRUS

Disease Association: Upper and lower respiratory tract infections, ocular infections, gastroenteritis, cystitis, serious complications in transplant recipients.

Laboratory Diagnosis:

Virus isolation: Standard cell cultures of human neonatal kidney cells or A-549 for most serotypes; cytopathogenic effect of grapelike clusters in 5 to 8 days. Most enteric adenoviruses (types 40 and 41) are nonculturable in standard cell lines.

Viral antigen detection: Immunofluorescence for identification of adenovirus group (typing must be done by neutralization).

Serodiagnosis: Complement fixation for determining seroconversion and monitoring changes in antibody level.

Box continued on following page

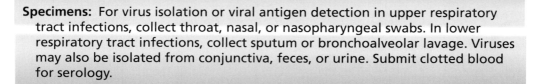

Specimens: For virus isolation or viral antigen detection in upper respiratory tract infections, collect throat, nasal, or nasopharyngeal swabs. In lower respiratory tract infections, collect sputum or bronchoalveolar lavage. Viruses may also be isolated from conjunctiva, feces, or urine. Submit clotted blood for serology.

Adenovirus infections are spread from human to human through the fecal-oral route and by aerosols. Forty-seven serotypes of human adenoviruses have been described. Adenoviruses produce 2 to 10% of all respiratory tract infections, with symptoms ranging from mild cough and pharyngitis to acute respiratory disease and pneumonia. Ocular infections include conjunctivitis in conjunction with respiratory disease and in the form of epidemic kerato-conjunctivitis characterized by conjunctivitis, which lasts 2 weeks and is typically followed by corneal keratitis that can persist for months. Adenoviral gastroenteritis is usually seen only in children younger than 2 years, whereas adenoviral cystitis is seen in boys aged 6 to 15 years. Adenovirus follows only cytomegalovirus and herpes simplex virus in frequency of involvement in serious infections in transplant recipients; bone marrow transplant recipients are especially susceptible. In seriously infected transplant recipients the virus may be isolated from many sites, including the respiratory tract, urine, and various infected internal organs (liver, lung, kidney).

Clinical samples should be collected from the site of infection and submitted to the laboratory for virus isolation and for viral antigen detection by immunofluorescence. Throat and nasal swabs, conjunctival swabs, stools, and urine may be appropriate specimens. Although the enteric adenoviruses (types 40 and 41) cannot be isolated in standard cell cultures, most adenoviruses proliferate, usually in 5 to 7 days, in human neonatal kidney cells and in 5 to 8 days in A549 cells; some types may produce a cytopathogenic effect (CPE) in primary monkey kidney cells and in diploid fibroblasts. Typical CPE is grapelike clusters. Viral isolates are usually tested by immunofluorescence to confirm that they are adenoviruses. The immunofluorescence tests detect adenovirus group (family) antigens. Although it is known that certain serotypes tend to be isolated from particular sites, typing of adenovirus isolates is rarely helpful in diagnosis and clinical management of adenovirus infections. Typing may be very useful in epidemiological studies, and, when typing is required, the procedure must be performed using the neutralization technique in which the isolated adenovirus is mixed with adenovirus antibodies of various specificities and then tested for viability. This service is not available in most diagnostic laboratories but may be offered by state health laboratories or in research facilities.

Although either direct and indirect immunofluorescence methods may be applied for nonenteric adenovirus antigen detection in clinical specimens, neither of the immunofluorescence techniques is highly sensitive for adenovirus infections. Routinely, immunofluorescence testing for viral antigen in respiratory samples detects only 55 to 60% of respiratory adenovirus infections (see discussion of immunofluorescence versus virus isolation presented in Chapter 5).

Serological testing is routinely approached by the complement fixation method. A conversion from antibody negative to antibody positive or a fourfold increase in antibody level is evidence of current adenovirus infection. Adenovirus antibodies are serotype specific and long lasting [1]. However, immune status determinations by complement fixation are not useful in predicting immunity or susceptibility to future infections. In complement fixation, group antibodies rather than type-specific antibodies are measured, using an adenovirus group (family) antigen that detects antibodies of all serotypes. Hemagglutination inhibition or neutralization is required for antibody serotyping.

FAMILY: *HEPADNAVIRIDAE*   VIRUS: HEPATITIS B VIRUS

Disease Association: Is the agent of classic "serum" hepatitis.
Laboratory Diagnosis:
   Virus isolation: Cannot be isolated in standard cell cultures.
   Viral antigen detection: Several hepatitis B–related antigens can be detected in serum by enzyme immunoassay.
   Serodiagnosis: Several hepatitis B–related antibodies can be detected by enzyme immunoassay.
   Other: Molecular diagnostics may be used to detect viral nucleic acids.
Specimens: Submit clotted blood for use in antigen and antibody detection assays.

Hepatitis B virus is found worldwide and is the primary cause of hepatitis associated with exposure to blood and body fluids; it is often called "serum" hepatitis. Infection occurs after transfusions of infected blood or contact with infected body fluids such as semen and saliva. HBV is the most important blood-borne pathogen for laboratory workers, producing numerous infections each year in this population. Symptoms appear within 6 weeks to 6 months after infections and include hepatosplenomegaly and jaundice. HBV infection may result in a variety of syndromes: subclinical infection; acute hepatitis with resolution of illness; fulminant hepatitis or subacute hepatic necrosis with possible death within 3 months; chronic active hepatitis frequently resulting in cirrhosis; chronic persistent hepatitis; or a silent carrier state with minimal (or absent) liver damage. Primary hepatocellular carcinoma is known to be associated with HBV infections. Of the large number of individuals who acquire chronic HBV infections, all continue to shed the virus. However, some chronic cases simply persist with benign consequences, whereas chronic active infections may involve severe liver necrosis and may result in the development of primary hepatocellular carcinoma.

Several morphological forms of HBV antigen can be found in the serum of HBV-infected patients. One of these is the infectious 42-nm spherical Dane particle (also called Australia antigen). Dane particle is the name given to the viral nucleic acid, protein coat, and envelope. Other forms of the antigen include spherical and filamentous incomplete particles consisting of HBV surface antigen; these are devoid of nucleic acid. These normally occur in 100- to 1000-fold excess over mature virions.

The virus does not proliferate in standard cell cultures. However, HBV antigens can be identified in the peripheral blood of infected individuals. Identification of HBV surface antigen (HBsAg) is the hallmark of current or recent infection. The viral core-related e antigen (HBeAg) is also detectable in the early stages of infection. During the incubation period, HBsAg is the first marker to appear. Soon after, HBeAg can also be detected, and this indicates that the patient is infective.

HBV has a complicated serological profile (Fig. 8–1). The first antibody produced is antibody against the HBV core (anti-HBc), which appears during acute infection and persists for years. Both IgM anti-HBc and total (IgG plus IgM) anti-HBc are measured in the laboratory. The next antibody to appear is antibody against the HBV core–related (e) antigen (anti-HBe), which is followed months or years later by the development of antibody against the HBV surface antigen (anti-HBs). The presence of anti-HBs signals the late stages of disease and the development of immunity.

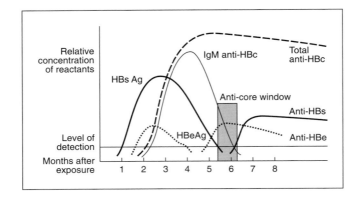

FIGURE 8–1 HEPATITIS B VIRUS (HBV) ANTIBODY-ANTIGEN PROFILE. Various antibodies and antigens associated with HBV infection can be detected in the serum of infected individuals. These appear in this order: surface antigen (HBsAg), core-related e antigen (HBeAg), IgM anticore antibody (IgM anti-HBc) and total (IgG and IgM) anticore antibody (total anti-HBc), antibody to core-related e antigen (anti-HBe), and surface antibody (anti-HBs). After HBsAg declines to undetectable levels and before anti-HBs is detectable, total and IgM anti-HBc may be the only serological markers that are reliably positive. This time period is called the anticore window.

Of interest serologically is a period in the course of most HBV infections when HBsAg forms immune complexes with anti-HBs produced as part of the recovery process. This immune complexing of antigen and antibody may render both the HBsAg and the anti-HBs undetectable. During this time, the only serological markers that are reliably positive are the total and IgM anti-HBc. This time period is often called the "anticore window."

HBsAg is the diagnostic marker for chronic HBV infections; this may last for 6 months to several years after initial infection. HBeAg may also be present. Anti-HBc is usually present in high titer. If anti-HBe appears along with a decrease in HBeAg, chronic persistent hepatitis is indicated. If high titers of HBeAg persist and anti-HBe fails to appear, chronic active infection is indicated, and the patient is likely to experience serious liver disease. The serological profiles seen in the various types of HBV disease are shown in Table 8–1.

TABLE 8–1 HBV SEROLOGICAL PROFILES*

	SEROLOGICAL MARKERS					
STAGE OF INFECTION	HBsAg	HBeAg	IgM Anti-HBc	Total Anti-HBc	Anti-HBe	Anti-HBs
Acute Infection						
Incubation period	+	+	0	0	0	0
Acute	+	+	+	+	0	0
Early convalescent	+	0	+	+	+	0
Convalescent	0	0	+	+	+	0
Late convalescent	0	0	0	+	+	+
Past infection	0	0	0	+	+/0	+
Chronic infection (active, persistent, carrier)	+*	+/0†	+/0	+	+/0†	0
HBsAg Immunization	0	0	0	0	0	+

*HBsAg-negative chronic infection may occur.
†Liver disease in chronic infection is seen more frequently in the presence of HBeAg than of anti-HBe.
HBV = hepatitis B virus; HBsAg = HBV surface antigen; HBeAg = HBV e antigen; Anti-HBc = antibody to HBV core; Anti-HBs = antibody to HBV surface antigen; + = present; 0 = absent; +/0 = may be present or absent.
Modified from Escobar MR. Viral hepatitis. In Spector S, Lancz GJ (eds), Clinical Virology Manual, 2nd ed. New York: Elsevier, 1992; pp. 397–423.

HBV assays, both antigen and antibody, were originally developed as radioimmunoassay techniques. Now most of these have been converted to enzyme immunoassays to eliminate the hazard of working with radioactive reagents in the laboratory. Many HBV antibody and antigen enzyme immunoassay systems, both manual and automated, are now available commercially and are reported to produce high-quality results.

FAMILY: *HERPESVIRIDAE*   VIRUS: CYTOMEGALOVIRUS

Disease Association: In immunocompetent individuals, most infections are sub-clinical or insignificant, although a mononucleosis-like syndrome is seen in teenagers and young adults, and primary infections in seronegative pregnant females may produce congenital infections, which result in a variety of symptoms. The virus establishes latency, and, in immunocompromised individuals, especially bone marrow transplant recipients, serious and often fatal pneumonia is seen.

Laboratory Diagnosis:

Virus isolation: Standard cell cultures of diploid fibroblasts; CPE of foci of small, rounded cells in 10 to 30 days. Shell vial cultures used often.

Viral antigen detection: Not routinely productive, although newer antigen-emia assays have been reported to be useful.

Serodiagnosis: Many methods (passive latex agglutination, enzyme immu-noassay, indirect immunofluorescence) are used for determining antibody status, detecting seroconversion, and monitoring changes in antibody level.

Specimens: Urine and peripheral blood are the two samples that yield virus most frequently in culture. In infected immunocompromised patients, bronchoalveolar lavage as well as lung and other appropriate biopsy samples are most useful. Anticoagulated peripheral blood is used for antigenemia assays. Submit clotted blood for serology.

Cytomegalovirus (CMV) was named as such because it produces massive enlargement of affected cells *in vivo*. CMV infections are spread from human to human through contaminated blood and body fluids such as urine, saliva, semen, breast milk, and cervical secretions. Most CMV infections in immunocompetent but otherwise healthy individuals are subclinical or insignificant, although a mononucleosis-like syndrome has been reported that includes sore throat, fatigue, and lymphadenopathy. CMV-related mononucleosis can be differentiated from classic Epstein-Barr virus (EBV) infectious mononucleosis through serological evaluations. This evaluation should begin with testing for heterophile antibodies. These antibodies are described in the section of this text that deals with EBV. Heterophile antibodies are found in 80 to 90% of EBV mononucleosis cases, whereas CMV mononucleosis is not associated with heterophile antibody production. A negative heterophile antibody test may be helpful in confirming CMV mononucleosis. However, differentiation of heterophile-negative EBV mononucleosis, seen in 10 to 20% of EBV mononucleosis cases, and CMV mononucleosis must rely on quantitative serological testing for both EBV-related antibodies and for CMV antibodies. IgM production, seroconversion, or fourfold increases in antibody level should be seen for CMV antibodies if that virus is causing the mononucleosis. EBV serological testing is described in the EBV section of this chapter, and CMV serology is described next.

The most important CMV infection in otherwise healthy individuals involves pregnant CMV seronegative women who have a primary CMV infection during pregnancy. In approximately

15% of these cases, the fetus will have a congenital infection that results in hepatospleno-megaly, chorioretinitis, deafness, microcephaly, or mental retardation [2]. If the virus can be isolated from the neonate or if CMV IgM can be identified in the infant's serum, the diagnosis of congenital CMV is supported. CMV is one of the viruses included in the TORCH complex of congenital infections: *t*oxoplasma; *o*ther, usually syphilis; *r*ubella, *c*ytomegalovirus; and *h*erpes simplex.

CMV, like all of the members of the *Herpesviridae* family, establishes latency within the host after initial infection. CMV is believed to reside in the mononuclear cells of the immune system. The virus can be reactivated when the host is stressed. Although infections resulting from reactivation in seropositive individuals are usually not as severe as primary infections, such reactivation infections may be devastating in immunocompromised individuals. This is usually observed during disease-related processes or therapy, including cancer chemotherapy and organ transplant–related therapy.

In immunocompromised individuals, especially those with T-cell deficits (organ transplant recipients, AIDS patients), CMV may cause serious infections in both CMV-seronegative and seropositive individuals; the infection may be due to reactivation of the individual's own latent CMV or to infection by a heterologous strain of the virus. The infections are often severe, usually beginning with a pneumonia and ending with multisystem infection. Pneu-monitis, retinitis, hepatitis, pancreatitis, meningoencephalitis, and gastrointestinal infections have been reported. Serious CMV infections currently can be treated with ganciclovir, which is routinely effective in diminishing the severity of the symptoms; however, the infection may relapse when therapy is withdrawn. The antiviral foscarnet may be used to treat CMV retinitis.

For virus isolation, peripheral blood, urine, throat swabs, or appropriate samples from other infected sites (bronchoalveolar lavage, lung biopsy, stomach biopsy) should be submitted. The virus proliferates slowly, usually requiring 10 to 30 days to produce CPE in standard cell cultures of fibroblast cells such as MRC-5 lung fibroblasts or MRHF human foreskin fibroblasts. The CPE consists of foci of rounded cells. Because the CPE is characteristic and because confirmatory testing on viral isolates often fails to confirm CMV even with bona fide CMV isolates, confirmatory testing is usually not performed, and the identification relies on the appearance of the typical CPE. If the CPE is not typical, the infected cells can be transferred to a shell vial fibroblast culture, and the shell vial can be incubated and then stained for CMV early antigens. See Chapter 4 for information about shell vial cultures.

A modified system involving culturing of CMV in fibroblasts grown in shell vials (described in detail in Chapter 4) has been shown to be effective in detecting CMV in many types of clinical samples after an incubation period of only 24 to 48 hours [3]. This system may be nearly as effective as 30-day cell cultures in detecting CMV in urine samples and provides CMV identification in 80 to 90% of samples from other sources such as peripheral blood and bronchoalveolar lavage samples. This system is not as effective with throat swab samples, identifying only 50% of the CMV-positive samples. The shell vial system is very important in the laboratory diagnosis of CMV infection, providing confirmation of CMV infection within 24 to 48 hours rather than in 10 to 30 days as with traditional cell cultures.

Because CMV is known to establish latency and to emerge during periods of stress, the interpretation of the diagnostic significance of a positive CMV culture is complicated. CMV is routinely shed in the urine of seropositive individuals after renal transplants, although this shedding is usually asymptomatic. Likewise, CMV may be isolated from the respiratory tract of asymptomatic immunocompromised individuals. Unless the virus can be shown to be involved in the actual disease process, the isolation of CMV may not be helpful in patient management. It is currently believed that isolation of CMV from peripheral blood may be a much better indication of the involvement of the organisms in the disease process. Isolation of large quantities of the virus from carefully collected samples from lung, liver, spleen, and so on in symptomatic individuals, detection of CMV IgM, and observation of cytomegalic "owl's eye" inclusions in histological sections of tissue may be required to confirm that the virus is involved in the actual disease process.

One viral antigen detection test that has been recommended for use in detecting CMV antigen in clinical samples is a new CMV antigenemia assay that is performed on anticoagulated peripheral blood. This assay (described in detail in Chapter 5) involves staining blood leukocytes for detection of a CMV protein pp65. The assay is time consuming but has been reported to be as sensitive as shell vials in detecting CMV antigen in peripheral blood.

CMV serodiagnosis is complicated by the fact that CMV establishes latency. Therefore, although a patient has CMV antibodies, he or she is not "immune" to CMV infection. Infections occur in seropositive individuals as a result of reactivation of their own CMV or to infection with a new strain of the virus. CMV immune status testing is important in determining whether the patient has CMV antibodies because infections from reactivation or reinfection with a new strain are usually not as severe as those seen in primary infections. In therapy of CMV-seronegative immunocompromised individuals and in newborns, CMV seronegative blood and blood products may be used in therapy to avoid exposing the patients to CMV.

CMV antibody levels may increase in primary as well as in reactivation disease, and quantitative testing may be helpful in disease diagnosis. CMV IgM detection is probably more helpful, and this testing is widely available. Many commercial products are available for CMV antibody determinations. The passive latex agglutination methods are of high quality and are very convenient to perform; they detect both IgG and IgM and do not differentiate between the two. Indirect immunofluorescence assays are used, but they may be more difficult to interpret because of the nonspecific binding of antibodies to Fc receptors present in the cytoplasm of CMV-infected cells used in testing. Immunofluorescence assays are usually specific for either IgG or IgM. Enzyme immunoassays for CMV IgG or IgM detection are widely available, and many of these are in formats that allow for automation of the assay. These usually provide high-quality results in these assays; at this writing, the IgG assays are more standardized than the IgM assays.

FAMILY: *HERPESVIRIDAE*   VIRUS: EPSTEIN-BARR VIRUS

Disease Association: Produces classic EBV infectious mononucleosis in otherwise healthy adolescents and young adults. Subclinical infections are common in children. The virus establishes latency after primary infection and may reactivate when the host is stressed. Immunocompromised patients may experience reactivation disease.

Laboratory Diagnosis:
Virus isolation: Cannot be isolated in standard cell cultures.
Viral antigen detection: Not available.
Serodiagnosis: Classic EBV infectious mononucleosis is usually associated with heterophile antibodies. Heterophile-negative cases occur. Several methods (enzyme immunoassay, indirect immunofluorescence) are used to detect and identify a variety of EBV-related antibodies for determining antibody status and in detecting seroconversion and monitoring changes in antibody level.

Specimens: Submit clotted blood for serology.

EBV is distributed worldwide and is associated with a variety of infections. The virus is transmitted by oral secretions and also through blood transfusions. EBV may infect individuals of all ages to produce subclinical infections or mild cold or flulike illness, but it is more well known as the agent of classic infectious mononucleosis (IM). This infection occurs most frequently in teenagers and young adults and presents routinely with a low-grade fever, sore throat, lymphadenopathy, and fatigue. There is no specific treatment, and patients usually improve in 3 to 6 weeks with rest and restricted activity.

Once infected with EBV, humans harbor the virus lifelong, with reactivation disease possible on stress. Bone marrow transplant recipients and other EBV-seropositive individuals who are immunocompromised may demonstrate EBV symptoms. The virus has also been implicated as the agent of malignancies, including Burkitt's lymphoma and nasopharyngeal carcinoma. Neither of these is common in the United States, although both have been reported. Burkitt's lymphoma is most common in parts of South America and Africa, and nasopharyngeal carcinoma is most common in eastern China. EBV has been implicated in other malignancies such as lymphoma and leukemia, although the etiological link has not been conclusively demonstrated.

Because EBV does not proliferate in standard cell cultures and methods for detection of EBV antigens in clinical specimens are not available, laboratory confirmation of EBV infection relies on serological detection of antibodies. The approach for serological confirmation will vary depending on the type of infection.

Laboratory diagnosis of EBV IM usually begins with serological testing for heterophile antibodies. **Heterophile antibodies** are antibodies that react with antigens that are different from and phylogenetically unrelated to the antigens responsible for their production. The heterophile antibodies of IM are capable of reacting with sheep erythrocytes. Although IM heterophile antibodies are not the only heterophile antibodies that have been identified in humans, they are the most common type, and serological assays that detect these antibodies and differentiate them from other non-IM heterophile antibodies are widely available. Differentiation of heterophile antibodies usually involves absorption of two portions of the test serum, one portion with kidney extract (either guinea pig or horse kidney) and one with beef erythrocyte extract, before reacting the serum with erythrocytes (either sheep or horse erythrocytes). The reactivity of the two absorbed sera is compared to confirm the identification of IM heterophile antibodies. IM heterophile antibodies will not be absorbed (or will be absorbed only minimally) by kidney antigens, so that kidney-absorbed serum will agglutinate erythrocytes. The IM heterophile antibodies will be absorbed by beef erythrocyte extract, so that beef extract–absorbed serum will not agglutinate erythrocytes. Table 8–2 compares the reactivity of several types of heterophile antibodies in absorbed serum.

Heterophile antibodies are produced in 80 to 90% of EBV IM cases, which indicates that 10 to 20% of infected individuals will be negative when tested for heterophile antibodies. The diagnosis of heterophile-negative IM relies on detection of antibodies directed against components of EBV itself. At this writing, testing for at least four types of EBV-related antibodies is widely available; these include antibodies, both IgG and IgM, against viral capsid antigens (VCA) and antibodies against EBV early antigens (EA) and Epstein-Barr nuclear antigens (EBNA). The sequence of appearance-disappearance of the four types of antibodies in classic IM is shown in Figure 8–2. VCA IgM is first to appear and becomes undetectable within 4 weeks. VCA IgG also appears very early in infection, and, although it may decline, it persists at detectable levels for life. Antibodies against EBV EA, which are sometimes

TABLE 8–2 REACTIVITY OF HETEROPHILE ANTIBODIES IN ABSORBED SERUM

TYPE OF HETEROPHILE ANTIBODY	AGGLUTINATION OF ERYTHROCYTES AFTER ABSORPTION WITH ANTIGEN SHOWN	
	Guinea Pig Kidney	Beef Stroma
Infectious mononucleosis	+	0
Forssman	0	+
Serum sickness	0	0

+ = positive for agglutination; 0 = negative for agglutination.

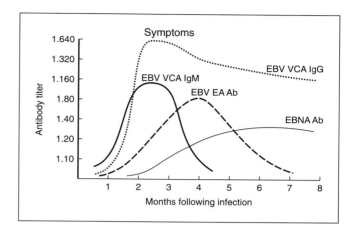

FIGURE 8–2 EPSTEIN-BARR VIRUS (EBV) ANTIBODY RESPONSE. At least four types of antibodies can be monitored in EBV infection. They appear in this order: immunoglobulin M (IgM) against viral capsid antigen (EBV VCA IgM), IgG against viral capsid antigen (EBV VCA IgG), antibody against early antigens (EBV EA Ab), and antibodies against nuclear antigens (EBNA Ab).

differentiated into diffuse and restricted types, also appear during the acute phase of the infection; these are usually no longer detectable within 3 months after onset of disease, although persistence of EA antibodies has been demonstrated. Antibodies against EBNA are the slowest to appear; they are rarely present during the acute phase of the illness but increase during convalescence and are maintained in most individuals for life. In acute EBV IM, VCA IgM should be detectable, and EBNA antibodies should be absent. In other EBV-related infections, the pattern of reactivity of the four types of EBV antibodies differs, and the interpretation of atypical patterns is extremely difficult. Table 8–3 shows typical antibody response patterns in the various EBV-related diseases.

VCA antibodies are measured routinely by indirect immunofluorescence and by enzyme immunoassay. In indirect immunofluorescence, EBV producer cells (that allow production of viral capsid antigens) are fixed on the microscope slides. Testing can be modified to differentiate IgG and IgM antibodies. Likewise, in enzyme immunoassay testing for VCA antibodies, the capsid antigens are affixed to a solid phase, and the patient's antibodies bind to the antigens; the patient's antibodies can be differentiated as to their class, either IgG or IgM. The VCA IgG tests are usually performed in a quantitative format because these antibodies persist lifelong after infection so that their mere presence does not confirm current infection; increases in VCA IgG level must be demonstrated to confirm current EBV infection. VCA IgM testing may be done either qualitatively or quantitatively; with VCA IgM, the fact that the antibody is present is helpful in making the diagnosis.

EBV EA antibodies are also usually tested by indirect immunofluorescence or enzyme immunoassay. For detection of these antibodies by immunofluorescence, the EBV-infected cells on the microscope slide are treated to make them express early antigens. The same antigens are used in enzyme immunoassay. The detection of EA antibodies is routinely performed in a

TABLE 8–3   EBV ANTIBODY PROFILES IN EBV-RELATED SYNDROMES

| EBV-RELATED SYNDROME | EBV-RELATED ANTIBODIES PRESENT-ABSENT | | | | |
| | EBV VCA IgM | EBV VCA IgG | EBV EA | | EBNA |
			Diffuse	Restricted	
No past or present EBV	0	0	0	0	0
Past infection	0	+	0	0	+
Reactivation	+/0	+	+/0	+/0	+
Burkitt's lymphoma	0	+	0	+	+
Nasopharyngeal carcinoma	0	+	+	0	+

EBV = Epstein-Barr virus; EA = early antigen; VCA = viral capsid antigen, + = present, 0 = absent, +/0 = may be present or absent.

qualitative format because presence of EA antibodies usually indicates current infection. EA antibodies seldom persist for long periods after infection. Although these antibodies may be differentiated in immunofluorescence testing into diffuse and restricted patterns, this testing is not well standardized and is usually available at reference and research facilities only.

EBNA antibodies are detected in anticomplement immunofluorescence methods. Such testing involves EBV-infected cells that express only EBNA. These cells are fixed on the microscope slide. Because the amount of EBNA expression is low, the sensitive anticomplement immunofluorescence method is used in EBNA antibody detection (Fig. 8–3). Patient's serum is added; after incubation and rinsing, complement is added. If antigen-antibody complexes were formed in the first step, complement (the C3 component) will bind to the complexes. After incubation and rinsing, a preparation of fluorescein-labeled anticomplement antibodies is added, which will bind to bound complement. This methodology is sensitive and specific and is the reference method for detecting EBNA antibodies. Other types of assays for EBNA detection are not widely available at this writing. The anticomplement immunofluorescence test for EBNA is usually performed in a qualitative format. Presence of EBNA antibodies is consistent with past EBV infection.

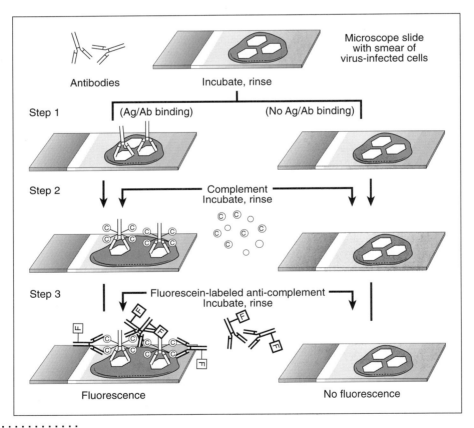

FIGURE 8–3 ANTICOMPLEMENT IMMUNOFLUORESCENCE. In step one, antibodies are exposed to virus-infected cells fixed on a microscope slide. In step two, complement is added and binds to antigen-antibody (Ag/Ab) complexes formed in step one. In step three, fluorescein-labeled anticomplement is added and binds to complement that bound in step two, and fluorescence is seen. If antibodies do not bind in step one, complement cannot bind in step two, fluorescein-labeled anticomplement cannot bind in step three, and no fluorescence is seen.

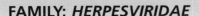

FAMILY: *HERPESVIRIDAE*

VIRUS: HERPES SIMPLEX VIRUS TYPES 1 AND 2

Disease Association: Produces recurrent lesions in oral and genital areas. The virus establishes latency after primary infection and may reactivate when the host is stressed. Congenital infections may occur in infants born to mothers who have genital herpes.

Laboratory Diagnosis:

Virus isolation: Standard cell cultures of rabbit kidney, mink lung, human neonatal kidney, and others; CPE of enlarged, rounded cells in 1 to 4 days.

Viral antigen detection: Immunofluorescence or enzyme immunoassay.

Serodiagnosis: Many methods (enzyme immunoassay, indirect immunofluorescence) are used for determining antibody status, detecting seroconversion, and monitoring changes in antibody level.

Specimens: For virus isolation and antigen detection, submit swabs from lesions or other infected sites. Submit clotted blood for serology.

Herpes simplex virus (HSV) infections are spread from human to human through direct contact. There are two major types of HSV: HSV type 1 (HSV-1) and HSV type 2 (HSV-2). Both oral and genital infections are common; HSV-1 is more common in oral infections (cold sores, fever blisters), and HSV-2 is more common in genital infections. Genital herpes is one of the most common sexually transmitted diseases. HSV lesions tend to recur whenever the host is stressed. Lesions are painful and usually last for 10 to 14 days. Lesions will heal without treatment, but their duration can be shortened through treatment with the antiviral agent acyclovir, both topical and oral. Although these lesions are unsightly and inconvenient, they are not usually life threatening; occasionally, meningitis or encephalitis may develop as a result of severe HSV infection. In immunocompromised individuals, reactivation of HSV occurs with great frequency unless acyclovir is administered prophylactically. This is now a routine part of the posttransplantation protocol for most HSV-seropositive transplant recipients.

Congenital HSV infection occurs both *in utero* and during delivery in women with genital HSV. Congenital infections are frequent and severe unless the mother receives prophylactic acyclovir near the time of delivery. HSV is one of the agents included in the TORCH complex of congenital infections. It is most severe in women who experience primary infection during pregnancy. A cesarean delivery will be performed on any woman who has active HSV lesions at the time of delivery. Congenitally infected infants may have gross lesions or may be largely asymptomatic at birth, abruptly developing severe symptoms within 48 to 72 hours after delivery.

HSV proliferates rapidly and vigorously in traditional cell cultures, producing CPE ranging from enlargement and rounding of infected cells to complete destruction of the cell monolayer, often within 24 to 48 hours after inoculation. HSV proliferates in many types of cells, including rabbit kidney, mink lung, human neonatal kidney, A549, various diploid fibroblast lines, and primary monkey kidney. Confirmation of the identity of the isolated virus can be performed by direct immunofluorescence. Depending on the antibodies used for testing, this identification may simply confirm that the virus is HSV or may be used to differentiate HSV-1 and HSV-2. Enzyme immunoassay may also be used for culture confirmation, but this method routinely confirms HSV and does differentiate HSV-1 and HSV-2.

Because HSV is such a frequent isolate and such a rapid grower, modified cell culture systems are often used. These systems are designed specifically for HSV detection and are especially useful in laboratories that limit their virus isolation services. These systems are described in Chapter 4 and include shell vials and herpes isolators. Most of the modified systems depend on an immunological staining method (immunofluorescence or immunoperoxidase) rather than CPE production to identify HSV antigens in the cell monolayer. Most of these systems identify HSV but do not differentiate HSV-1 and HSV-2.

HSV antigens are detectable in clinical materials by several techniques, including direct immunofluorescence and enzyme immunoassay. These methods are rapid, producing results within 1 to 3 hours after the patient's sample is received in the laboratory. HSV antigen detection methods are described, and comparisons of sensitivity and specificity of these methods relative to virus isolation are presented in Chapter 5.

HSV antibodies can be detected by many methods, including enzyme immunoassay and immunofluorescence. A conversion from antibody negative to antibody positive or a fourfold or greater change in antibody titer is consistent with current infection. Many enzyme immunoassay products for HSV antibody determinations use two different antigens in an attempt to differentiate HSV-1 and HSV-2 antibodies. Because of the extensive cross-reactions of HSV-1 and HSV-2 antibodies, this differentiation is difficult. HSV-1 invariably reacts more strongly than HSV-2, and calculations of ratios representing relative reactivity must be made to offset this stronger reactivity. There are also methods available for detection of HSV IgM.

Evaluation of HSV "immune status" is complicated by the fact that HSV establishes latency. Therefore, presence of HSV antibodies indicates prior experience with the virus but does not signal immunity to subsequent infections. Recurrent infections are common because of reactivation of latent HSV.

FAMILY: *HERPESVIRIDAE* **VIRUS: VARICELLA-ZOSTER**

Disease Association: Is the agent of chickenpox and of shingles.
Laboratory Diagnosis:
  Virus Isolation: Standard cell cultures of human neonatal kidney; CPE of small, rounded cells in 6 to 8 days.
  Viral antigen detection: Immunofluorescence.
  Serodiagnosis: Many methods (passive latex agglutination, enzyme immunoassay, indirect immunofluorescence) are used for determining immune status, detecting seroconversion, and monitoring changes in antibody level.
Specimens: For virus isolation and viral antigen detection, scrapings or swab samples collected from lesions should be submitted. Submit clotted blood for serology.

Varicella-zoster (VZ), also called varicella or herpes zoster, is the etiological agent of the classic childhood disease chickenpox. This is one of the few childhood viral illnesses for which a vaccine is not used widely, so chickenpox persists, whereas rubella, measles, and mumps have been largely eliminated. Chickenpox is seen most frequently in young children. It is highly transmissible, so exposure of nonimmune individuals usually results in typical disease. The infection is characterized by vesicular lesions with indented centers; lesions may be many or few. Fever and other symptoms are also variable in their incidence and severity; some children experience few if any symptoms and only one or two lesions, whereas others may have fever and extreme discomfort because of extensive lesions. Most chickenpox cases last 7 to 10 days, with lesions crusting over by day 10. Complications are rare in immunocompetent children, but chickenpox in adults may be more severe. Chickenpox can be a life-threatening infection in immunocompromised individuals. Chickenpox is usually not treated, except in severe infections; these are treated with high doses of the antiviral acyclovir. A vaccine, used in the past on a limited basis with individuals who are at high risk of severe disease, has been approved for use with all children.

Varicella is not frequently associated with congenital infections. However, the infant may be affected when seronegative mothers experience primary varicella infections at or near the time of the infant's birth.

Once individuals have experienced chickenpox, antibodies are produced that persist lifelong, eliminating susceptibility to further chickenpox. However, the virus persists indefinitely within the body, being sequestered in nerve cells, and may re-emerge to produce another clinical syndrome: shingles. Shingles is different clinically from chickenpox but is simply a reactivation disease that occurs when the host is stressed. In shingles, large, painful, vesicular lesions are produced on the skin that overlies the pathway of a nerve. Lesions are restricted to the specific area and produce a burning sensation that is so severe that it may be debilitating. Shingles is a frequent complication in both pediatric and adult transplant recipients, cancer patients, and others who are immunocompromised.

VZ will proliferate in standard cell cultures of human neonatal kidney and may produce CPE in human diploid fibroblasts. CPE appears in 6 to 8 days and consists of small, rounded cells. The isolated virus can be identified by direct immunofluorescence. Direct immunofluorescence can also be used to detect VZ antigen in clinical samples. Cells from moist lesions must be collected for this assay.

Serological detection of VZ antibodies can be performed by immunofluorescence, enzyme immunoassay, and latex agglutination. Most of these assays detect VZ IgG, although latex agglutination detects IgM as well as IgG. All of these methods produce high-quality results. Presence of antibody indicates prior experience with the virus and immunity to chickenpox; however, any seropositive individual is at risk for shingles on immunosuppression. A seroconversion from antibody negative to positive or a fourfold change in titer can be used to confirm current infection. Most typical VZ infections are not confirmed serologically; only those cases in which lesions or other clinical signs and symptoms are atypical are evaluated serologically. The primary usefulness of serological evaluation of VZ antibodies is to determine immunity to chickenpox. This evaluation is required routinely for many health-care personnel, especially those who will work with immunocompromised children. It is important to evaluate the immune status of these individuals before the start of employment so that, if a chickenpox outbreak or exposure occurs, the immune status of the individual will have already been established and proper infection control measures can be implemented to protect the employee as well as the patients.

FAMILY: *PAPOVAVIRIDAE*　　　　VIRUSES: PAPILLOMAVIRUS, POLYOMAVIRUS

Disease Association: Associated with various warts and dermatological anomalies.

Laboratory Diagnosis:
  Virus isolation: Cannot be isolated in standard cell cultures.
  Viral antigen detection: Not widely available.
  Serodiagnosis: Not available.
  Other: Diagnosis usually rests with clinical evaluation and histological confirmation. Molecular diagnostic techniques may be necessary to identify viral nucleic acids.

Specimens: Contact reference or research laboratory to determine acceptable samples.

The *Papovaviridae* family name is based on an acronym: *pa*pillomavirus; *po*lyomavirus; and *va*cuolating virus (from monkeys). Thus, the name *Papovaviridae* indicates the groupings of viruses included within the family. Both the papillomaviruses and the polyomaviruses infect humans and are distributed worldwide. The papillomaviruses spread via direct close contact. They infect epithelial cells and produce localized disease of skin and mucous membranes. They are not disseminated systemically. About 35 serotypes of papillomaviruses infect the skin, producing various types of warts, including plantar warts and laryngeal papillomas; about 20 serotypes infect the genital tract, where they produce warts and have been shown to be related to cervical cancer.

The polyomaviruses enter through the respiratory tract or the gastrointestinal tract, where they multiply and are then distributed to other internal organ systems. The name "polyoma" (meaning agent of many tumors) virus was assigned to this group because members of this group are oncogenic in laboratory animals. However, there is no consistent association of these viruses with human malignancies. Two human polyomaviruses, BK virus and JC virus, have been identified. JC virus causes progressive multifocal leukoencephalopathy, which is a progressive fatal neurological disease. BK virus infection in healthy individuals is usually subclinical, although cystitis is seen occasionally; the BK virus has been isolated from the urine of infected patients. Both BK and JC viruses are known to infect a high proportion of the world population and seroprevalence of both types of antibodies is between 75 and 100% in adults in the United States. Both viruses remain latent in the kidneys and may produce disease on reactivation, especially in immunocompromised patients.

Because the papillomaviruses and polyomaviruses are not reliably isolated in cell cultures and require specialized reagents for staining of viral antigens within paraffinized tissue, laboratory confirmation of infection is not provided by most clinical virology laboratories. Serological evaluations are not helpful. Specialized testing for these viruses is available at reference facilities only. Nucleic acid probes may be used to detect viral nucleic acids in tissue.

FAMILY: *PARVOVIRIDAE*   VIRUS: HUMAN PARVOVIRUS B19

Disease Association: Has been implicated as the agent of fifth disease in children, in aplastic crisis in patients with hematological disorders, and in fetal hydrops.

Laboratory Diagnosis:
  Virus isolation: Cannot be isolated in standard cell cultures.
  Viral antigen detection: Not available.
  Serodiagnosis: Antibody testing is available in reference laboratories. Molecular techniques may be used.
  Other: Molecular diagnostic techniques may be used to detect parvovirus B19 DNA.

Specimens: Submit clotted blood for serology.

Viruses in the family *Parvoviridae* were associated primarily with infections in animals until the early 1980s, when parvovirus B19 was identified as the agent of several human infections. Human parvovirus infections are diverse in their clinical associations and include erythema infectiosum (fifth disease), aplastic crisis, fetal hydrops, and others. The virus is thought to be transmitted through infected respiratory secretions. Erythema infectiosum was named fifth disease because it was the fifth illness described with a somewhat similar rash; the first four diseases were rubella, measles, scarlet fever, and Filatov-Dukes disease (now considered a mild atypical form of scarlet fever)[4]. Fifth disease is seen in children and is characterized by high fever and a rash on the cheeks that is described as "slapped cheek" rash. The rash and fever disappear, and no complications are experienced. Aplastic crisis resulting from parvovirus B19 is experienced by immunocompromised individuals and is especially severe in those with hematological anomalies such as hereditary spherocytosis, sickle-cell disease, thalassemia, and blood loss. The virus appears to infect the erythrocytes to cause anemia in these individuals. Most recover within 7 to 10 days. Fetal hydrops is seen in some pregnant women who experience primary parvovirus B19 infection. The complications are often severe, resulting in death of the fetus.

Parvovirus B19 cannot be isolated in standard cell cultures, and there are no tests available for antigen detection. Serological detection, especially of IgM antibodies, is required to establish a diagnosis of current or recent parvovirus infection. A positive IgG result alone is not sufficient to establish a diagnosis because more than 50% of the adult population in the United States is seropositive for parvovirus antibodies. Several reference laboratories offer serological testing for parvovirus B19 antibodies, and an enzyme immunoassay for this purpose has become available commercially. Larger reference laboratories and the Centers for Disease Control have used nucleic acid technology to identify parvovirus B19 DNA in infected tissue.

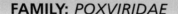

FAMILY: *POXVIRIDAE*   **VIRUSES: VARIOLA, MOLLUSCUM CONTAGIOSUM, OTHERS**

Disease Association: Variola virus produces classic smallpox. This virus is now reported by the World Health Association to be eradicated worldwide. Molluscum contagiosum produces skin or genital lesions.
Laboratory Diagnosis: No testing available in routine clinical laboratories.

Variola virus (smallpox virus) was eradicated worldwide by 1980. This infection was transmitted from individual to individual by direct contact or contact with clothing, bedding, or utensils. The infection began with fever, headache, and pain in the limbs, followed in 3 to 4 days by a rash that developed pustules within 5 or 6 days. Variola major, the clinically severe form of the disease, resulted in 15 to 40% mortality, whereas variola minor, a less severe variant, was less often fatal. Through a conscientious vaccination program, smallpox was virtually eliminated in the United States before 1950 [5].

The only remaining viruses of the *Poxviridae* family that produce disease in humans are vaccinia virus and molluscum contagiosum. Vaccinia virus, which is believed to be an attenuated cowpox or horsepox strain, is the strain that is used in the smallpox vaccination. Although smallpox vaccinations have been discontinued in many countries, complications resulting from the vaccination still are seen in populations being vaccinated. These complications include an allergic rash, progressive vaccinia, and postvaccinial encephalitis.

Molluscum contagiosum has two manifestations. One occurs in children and is characterized by lesions on the face, trunk, and limbs. The other form of infection occurs in young adults and is characterized by lesions in the genital area that are transmitted by sexual contact.

Because the poxvirus diseases are usually diagnosed clinically, most laboratories do not offer poxvirus diagnostic services. Arrangements for diagnostic testing can be made through the Centers for Disease Control.

R E F E R E N C E S

1. Ellner PD, Neu HC. Overview of upper respiratory tract infections. In Understanding Infectious Disease. St. Louis, MO: Mosby Year Book, 1992, pp 27–34
2. Stagno S, Pass RF, Cloud G, et al. Cytomegalovirus: incidence, transmission to fetus, and clinical outcome. JAMA 1986; 256:1904

3. Leland DS, Hansing RL, French MLV. Clinical experience with cytomegalovirus isolation using both conventional cell cultures and rapid shell vial techniques. J Clin Microbiol 1989; 27:1159-1162

4. Nelson WE, Vaughan VC, McKay RJ Jr, Behrman RE (eds). Erythema infectiosum (fifth disease). In Textbook of Pediatrics. Philadelphia: WB Saunders, 1976, p 867

5. Noble J. Smallpox. In Gorbach SL, Bartlett JG, Blacklow NR (eds), Infectious diseases. Philadelphia: WB Saunders, 1992, pp 1112–1113

REVIEW QUESTIONS

1. Which of the following viruses are closely related and members of the same family?
   a. Cytomegalovirus and varicella-zoster virus
   b. Papillomavirus and parvovirus
   c. Hepatitis B virus and herpes simplex virus
   d. Adenovirus and Epstein-Barr virus

2. You are working with a sample from a lip lesion. Herpes simplex virus (HSV) is suspected. What information is accurate concerning availability and timeliness of HSV laboratory testing?
   a. HSV grows slowly in cell culture, so do not expect a positive result before 7 to 10 days.
   b. Tests for HSV antigen detection are not widely available, so virus isolation is the test of choice.
   c. The lesion sample can be tested for HSV antigen and inoculated into cell cultures. Antigens test are widely available and HSV grows quickly in culture.
   d. A serum sample, rather than the lip lesion sample, should be collected and tested for HSV antibodies. If antibodies are present, the patient is immune to HSV and the lip lesion cannot be a result of HSV infection.

3. Cytomegalovirus (CMV) is associated with all of the following clinical syndromes **except**
   a. Congenital infection in infants whose mothers experienced primary CMV infections during pregnancy
   b. An infectious mononucleosis–like syndrome in adolescents and young adults
   c. Serious, often fatal, pneumonia in immunocompromised individuals, especially bone marrow transplant recipients
   d. Painful genital lesions in individuals with multiple sex partners

4. You are a virologist working in the clinical virology laboratory and have just received a throat swab sample in transport medium with Epstein-Barr virus (EBV) marked as the viral suspect. You should
   a. Process the sample as usual and inoculate standard cell cultures, including primary monkey kidney and various fibroblast lines
   b. Spin the transport medium and stain the cell pellet with fluorescein-isothiocyanate-labeled anti-EBV viral capsid antigen (VCA) antibodies
   c. Call the physician to communicate that EBV does not proliferate in standard cell cultures; perhaps suggest that clotted blood be submitted for EBV antibody testing
   d. Spin the transport medium and use the supernatant in an enzyme immunoassay for detection of anti-EBV VCA antibodies

5. In a patient with conjunctivitis or keratoconjunctivitis, which of the following viruses would be the most likely suspect?
   a. Papillomavirus
   b. Adenovirus
   c. Variola virus
   d. Epstein-Barr virus

6. A physician contacts the laboratory to ask about tests available for detection of hepatitis B (HBV)–related antigens. Which tests are available and which specimens are appropriate?
   a. Submit clotted blood so that the serum can be tested by enzyme immunoassay for HBV antigens
   b. Submit infected liver tissue for immunofluorescence staining for HBV antigens
   c. Submit anticoagulated peripheral blood for inoculation of viral cultures so that the infected cultured cells can be tested for HBV antigen
   d. Submit a scraping from the skin for testing by latex agglutination for HBV antigens

7. Erythema infectiosum (fifth disease) is the name given to the clinical syndrome associated with which of the following viruses?
   a. Hepatitis B virus
   b. Varicella
   c. Molluscum contagiosum
   d. Human parvovirus B19

8. A battery of serological tests is available for identifying various Epstein-Barr virus (EBV) antibodies. Which of the following statements describes these tests?
   a. They are often performed by direct agglutination by mixing erythrocytes with patient's serum.
   b. They usually detect IgG and IgM against the viral capsid, antibodies against EBV early antigens, and antibodies against EBV nuclear antigens.
   c. They are positive only in current EBV infection.
   d. They involve heterophile antibodies.

9. Varicella virus is associated with all of the following clinical syndromes **except**
   a. Smallpox
   b. Chickenpox
   c. Shingles
   d. Congenital infection when seronegative mothers experience primary varicella infection at or near the time of the infant's birth

10. A physician suspects that her patient has papilloma virus and wants laboratory confirmation of the infection. Which laboratory assays will provide this confirmation?
    a. Virus isolation in standard cell cultures
    b. Viral antigen detection by enzyme immunoassay
    c. Molecular probe detection of viral nucleic acids
    d. Detection of antibodies against papilloma virus

11. All of the following statements are true about variola virus **except**
    a. It is the agent of smallpox
    b. Some forms of the infection result in high mortality
    c. It is occasionally seen at present in the United States in southern Arizona
    d. It is closely related to molluscum contagiosum and vaccinia virus

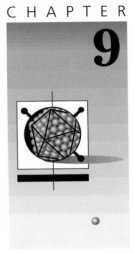

RNA Viruses

O B J E C T I V E S
. . . .

After completion of this unit of study, the student will be able to do the following for each virus described:

1. Give the classification by family.
2. List disease syndromes with which each virus is commonly associated.
3. Identify the approaches (virus isolation, viral antigen detection, serodiagnosis) that are useful in laboratory diagnosis of infection.
4. Indicate whether viral antigen detection methods are available and useful clinically, and list specific methodologies used for this purpose.
5. Indicate which types of clinical samples should be collected and submitted for diagnosis.

FAMILY: *ARENAVIRIDAE* VIRUSES: LASSA FEVER VIRUS, LYMPHOCYTIC CHORIOMENINGITIS VIRUS, OTHERS

Disease Association: Hemorrhagic fevers found in Africa (Lassa virus), aseptic meningitic (lymphocytic choriomeningitis virus).
Laboratory Diagnosis: Not available in routine clinical virology facilities. Make special arrangements with reference or research laboratory

All Arenaviruses are associated with rodents (mice, hamsters, guinea pigs) or bats, and humans are infected by inhalation of aerosols or dust, by direct contact with the animal, or by animal bite. Lassa fever is a hemorrhagic fever virus found in West Africa. It is one of the most dangerous infections known to humans. It produces high fever, hemorrhage, and shock, resulting in 15 to 50% mortality. Lassa fever can be treated with ribavirin.

Lymphocytic choriomeningitis virus (LCM) may be found worldwide and is associated with the house mouse. LCM produces an influenza-like disease that may progress to aseptic meningitis but is rarely fatal. Many other Arenaviruses exist, but they are not associated with naturally occurring human disease. Most are arthropod-borne serious systemic diseases and fevers.

FAMILY: BUNYAVIRIDAE VIRUSES: CALIFORNIA ENCEPHALITIS VIRUS, OTHERS

Disease Association: California encephalitis, a mosquito-borne encephalitis found in the midwestern United States.
Laboratory Diagnosis
Virus isolation: Cannot be isolated in standard cell cultures.
Viral antigen detection: Not available.
Serodiagnosis: Antibodies can be detected by hemagglutination inhibition and complement fixation testing; usually not available except in endemic areas during the summer months or at reference laboratories and state health facilities.
Specimens: Submit clotted blood for serology.

California encephalitis (CE) virus, more specifically named La Crosse virus, is in the *Bunyaviridae* family, which includes nearly 300 other viruses. All of these are arthropod borne, most produce hemorrhagic fevers (Rift Valley fever, Crimean-Congo hemorrhagic fever), and most are not found in the United States. Although CE was first isolated in California, it is found in Wisconsin, Minnesota, Iowa, Michigan, Ohio, Indiana, Illinois, New York, and other neighboring states. CE is transmitted by mosquitos, and infections are most common during the summer months when mosquitos are present. CE may produce severe disease, especially in children, but permanent impairment and death are not common. CE virus will not proliferate in standard cell cultures, and tests for detection of viral antigens are not available. The diagnosis relies on serological testing of paired sera. Such serological testing is usually available at state health laboratories and reference centers and is not offered at most clinical facilities.

FAMILY: *ORTHOMYXOVIRIDAE*   VIRUS: INFLUENZA A, B, AND C

Disease Association: Upper and lower respiratory infections. Often responsible for serious acute respiratory tract illness and pneumonia.

Laboratory Diagnosis of Influenza A and B (influenza C is not routinely tested)

Virus isolation: Standard cell cultures of primary monkey kidney cells; cytopathogenic effect of degeneration and toxic appearance (often difficult to read) in 4 to 8 days.

Viral antigen detection: Immunofluorescence or enzyme immunoassay.

Serodiagnosis: Complement fixation useful for determining group antibodies in detecting seroconversion and in monitoring antibody levels. Hemagglutination inhibition required for determining antibody serotypes.

Specimens: Samples from upper and lower respiratory tract sites for virus isolation and for viral antigen detection. Submit clotted blood for serology.

The influenza viruses cause more life-threatening respiratory tract disease than do any of the other respiratory viruses. The viruses are transmitted through inhalation of respiratory droplets from infected individuals or by hand-to-hand transfer of secretions. Infections occur from December to March in the northern hemisphere. Symptoms of infection include rapid onset of high temperature, headache, and typical coldlike symptoms or "flu"; retro-orbital pain is common. Infections may progress to pneumonia. Both influenza A (Flu A) and influenza B (Flu B) present a greater threat to those who are immunocompromised or have underlying disease. Flu A and B infections are usually cyclic, on a 1- to 3-year cycle for Flu A and a 4- to 7-year cycle for Flu B. Pandemics of Flu A occur approximately every 10 years [1]. Influenza C has been described, but the related infections are usually subclinical or very minor, and this virus is not routinely tested for in most clinical virology laboratories.

Clinical samples should be collected from the respiratory tract and may include throat, nasal, and nasopharyngeal swabs as well as bronchial washings, aspirates, and lavages. The samples should be submitted to the laboratory for virus isolation and for viral antigen detection by immunofluorescence. For Flu A and B, enzyme immunoassay has been used for antigen detection [2]. Flu A and Flu B proliferate, usually in 5 to 7 days, in primary monkey kidney cells, although some subtypes of both viruses may not proliferate in standard cell cultures. Typical cytopathogenic effect (CPE) is degeneration and a toxic appearance to the cells; CPE may be very subtle and difficult to detect. Both Flu A and Flu B produce changes in the monolayer surface that allow erythrocytes to attach (hemadsorb). Hemadsorption testing (described in Chapter 3) is used to detect the presence of Flu A and B before CPE production.

Influenza cell culture isolates are usually tested by immunofluorescence to differentiate and identify them as Flu A or B. Subtyping of isolates, which is achieved through hemagglutination inhibition testing and is done more frequently with Flu A than with Flu B, depends on analysis of two glycoproteins found on the spikes or peplomers that protrude from the viral envelopes. One of these is a hemagglutinin (H), which is important in viral attachment and in initiation of infection, and the second is a neuraminidase (N), which functions in release of newly formed virus from infected cells [3]. After determination of the H and N types of the viruses, a common name is usually assigned; the names may reflect the geographical location in which the strain first produced epidemic disease or a location in which the infection was especially devastating. Names assigned for Flu A strains in the past include Asian flu and Hong Kong flu. Influenza isolates are usually typed only in situations in which the epidemiology of the infection is being investigated. Typing of influenza isolates is rarely helpful in diagnosis and management of infections and is usually offered by state health laboratories or in research facilities only.

Indirect immunofluorescence methods are often used for detection of Flu A and B antigens in clinical samples. Antigen tests for Flu A detect 67 to 84% of positive samples, and Flu B tests routinely detect approximately 87 to 90% of positive samples (see discussion of Respiratory Viral Antigen Profile data presented in Chapter 5). The immunofluorescence tests detect Flu A and B group antigens, so all of the serotypes should be detected. Enzyme immunoassay may be used for influenza antigen detection and such systems for detection of Flu A antigen are commercially available. Comparisons of the sensitivity and specificity of these methods with virus isolation are presented in Chapter 5.

Serological testing is routinely approached by the complement fixation method. A conversion from antibody negative to antibody positive or a fourfold increase in antibody level is evidence of current influenza infection. Presence of low levels of antibody may not be sufficient to determine immunity, so immune status determinations are not used routinely. Hemagglutination inhibition may be used in serodiagnosis, but this testing is subtype specific so that antibodies of only a single subtype will be detected.

Worldwide immunization programs have been effective in interrupting the pandemic cycle of Flu A. However, Flu A has the ability to change its H and N antigens; this involves complete changes resulting from genetic reassortment (antigenic shift) or periodic changes (antigenic drift). Such changes allow Flu A to be successful in infecting individuals who have been infected by or immunized against other Flu A strains. Immunity to the strains used in immunizations is transient; therefore, yearly immunizations are recommended for those who are elderly or immunocompromised. Flu B also demonstrates antigenic drift, but this is not as dramatic as the antigenic changes seen with Flu A. The antiviral agent amantadine can be used in treatment and prophylaxis of Flu A infections.

FAMILY: *PARAMYXOVIRIDAE* — VIRUS: MEASLES (OLD NAME: RUBEOLA)

Disease Association: Classic 7-day measles, characterized by rash and fever.

Laboratory Diagnosis

Virus isolation: Standard cell cultures of primary monkey kidney; CPE of syncytia and general deterioration (may be difficult to evaluate) in 7 to 10 days.

Viral antigen detection: May be performed by immunofluorescence but is not routinely available.

Serodiagnosis: Many methods (enzyme immunoassay, indirect immunofluorescence, complement fixation, hemagglutination inhibition) are used for determining immune status, detecting seroconversion, and monitoring changes in antibody level.

Specimens: Upper respiratory tract samples are most likely to yield virus in culture. Submit clotted blood for serology.

Classic 7-day measles caused by the measles (formerly called rubeola) virus was one of the common diseases of childhood in the United States before the implementation of a nationwide immunization program in 1968. Measles tends to occur in 1- to 3-year cycles during winter and spring. Measles is highly contagious, and transmission is by direct contact with or by inhalation of infected respiratory droplets. Seven-day measles is biphasic. The first phase is a 3- to 4-day prodromal phase that involves fever, cough, conjunctivitis, and an oral rash of bluish-white lesions of the buccal mucosa (Koplik's spots). The second phase is the rash phase characterized by a maculopapular rash that begins on the head and upper extremities and progresses to the lower extremities; the rash lasts about 6 days [4]. Although most cases are uncomplicated, 0.1 to 0.2% of infections involve complications such as encephalitis and secondary bacterial otitis media. A rare late-occurring fatal sequelae, subacute sclerosing panencephalitis which involves a progressive encephalitis that occurs 4 to 17 years after the initial infection, occurs in roughly one in each 1 million cases.

Since the implementation of vaccination programs, the incidence of measles has declined dramatically in children in the United States. The incidence of measles has decreased by 90%; only 2231 cases of measles in the United States were reported to the Centers for Disease Control in 1992 [5]. The immunization for measles is usually given in combination with rubella and mumps immunization to infants at age 15 months through the measles-mumps-rubella (MMR) vaccine. Sporadic outbreaks at present usually involve unimmunized children or previously immunized or nonimmunized older teenagers and young adults. The occurrence of measles in teenagers and young adults resulted in a recommendation for booster immunizations of all school-age individuals; this vaccination is in addition to the initial vaccination that is recommended for all children at age 15 months. Either infection or effective immunization is thought to result in lifelong immunity, and antibodies persist indefinitely at detectable levels in most individuals. Screening for measles antibodies is often included in pre-employment assessments for individuals involved in health care.

The occurrence of measles in partially immune individuals results in a milder infection that may not have typical symptoms and may be difficult for physicians to recognize. Partial immunity may result from presence of transplacental antibody, presence of measles antibodies caused by administration of immune serum globulin, immunizations with partially inactivated vaccines, or atypical response to immunizations [6].

For virus isolation, samples must be collected early in the disease. Upper respiratory tract secretions and blood should be submitted. The virus proliferates slowly in primary monkey kidney or may grow in continuous monkey kidney cells (Vero), usually requiring 7 to 10 days to produce CPE. The CPE consists of syncytia formation and generalized deterioration of the cell monolayer. CPE may be difficult to detect, and viral proliferation may be detected more quickly through hemadsorption testing (see discussion of hemadsorption in Chapter 3). Measles-infected cells hemadsorb rhesus erythrocytes but not guinea pig erythrocytes. The identity of isolated measles virus may be confirmed by immunofluorescence testing.

Clinical samples from the respiratory tract can be tested directly by immunofluorescence for measles antigens. However, because the disease is so rare at this time in the United States, most clinical laboratories do not offer this service routinely, and its sensitivity is not established relative to virus isolation techniques.

Serological testing is routinely approached at present by immunofluorescence or by enzyme immunoassay, although hemagglutination inhibition and complement fixation were used extensively in the past. A conversion from antibody negative to antibody positive or a fourfold increase in antibody level is evidence of current infection. Because antibodies are expected to persist lifelong after immunization or infection, immune status determinations are often performed. The complement fixation assay should not be used for immune status determinations because the measles antibody measured in this system disappears within a year after active disease.

FAMILY: *PARAMYXOVIRIDAE*   VIRUS: MUMPS

Disease Association: Classic mumps, characterized by inflamed pharynx and swollen parotid glands.

Laboratory Diagnosis
Virus isolation: Standard cell cultures of primary monkey kidney cells or human embryonic kidney cells; CPE of syncytia formation and cellular degeneration (may be difficult to read) in 6 to 8 days.

Box continued on following page

FAMILY: *PARAMYXOVIRIDAE Continued*   VIRUS: MUMPS

Viral antigen detection: May be performed by immunofluorescence but is not routinely available.

Serodiagnosis: Many methods (enzyme immunoassay, indirect immunofluorescence, hemagglutination inhibition) are used for determining immune status, detecting seroconversion, and monitoring changes in antibody level.

Specimens: Saliva and urine are most likely to yield virus in culture. Submit clotted blood for serology.

Classic mumps, caused by the mumps virus, was one of the "usual childhood illnesses" in children younger than 15 years in the United States before the implementation of a nationwide immunization program in 1977. The virus is spread from human to human through respiratory droplets and is highly contagious. The virus replicates initially in epithelial cells in the upper respiratory tract and in regional lymph nodes; initial replication is followed by viremia, which results in infection of the salivary glands and other sites [7]. Mumps infection may be subclinical in 20 to 40% of infections but when symptomatic is characterized by low fever, inflamed pharynx, and swollen parotid glands, with swelling lasting 7 to 10 days. Most mumps cases are uncomplicated, but 10 to 20% of the infections in postpubertal males involve the testicles, although sterility is rare. Although mumps infection involves the central nervous system in about half of all cases, only 1 to 10% show clinical symptoms [8].

Since the implementation of immunization programs, the incidence of mumps has declined dramatically in the United States. A total of 185,691 mumps cases were reported in 1967. This declined to 2982 cases by 1985 [9], and only 2485 cases were reported in the United States in 1992 [5]. A monovalent mumps vaccine is available, but a polyvalent vaccine that includes rubella and measles (MMR) is recommended for all children at 15 months of age. A second immunization is recommended for school-age children. Sporadic outbreaks at present usually involve unimmunized individuals.

Because the clinical features of classic mumps infection are usually so characteristic and the resulting illness is so mild, laboratory confirmation of infection has not been required. However, with the decreased incidence of mumps, the symptoms may be less familiar and not readily recognized, and the ever-increasing number of immunocompromised individuals may experience more severe illness. In such circumstances, laboratory confirmation may be more important.

For virus isolation, saliva, urine, and blood should be submitted. The virus proliferates slowly in primary monkey kidney cells and in human embryonic kidney cells, usually requiring 6 to 8 days to produce CPE. The typical CPE involves syncytia formation and cellular degeneration, but CPE may be difficult to detect. Hemadsorption testing may yield positive results before CPE is obvious or in strains that do not produce CPE. The identity of isolated mumps virus may be confirmed by immunofluorescence testing.

Clinical samples from the respiratory tract can be tested directly by immunofluorescence for mumps antigens. However, because the disease is so rare at this time in the United States, most clinical laboratories do not offer this service routinely, and its sensitivity is not established relative to virus isolation techniques.

Serological testing is routinely approached by complement fixation, hemagglutination inhibition, immunofluorescence, or enzyme immunoassay. A conversion from antibody negative to antibody positive or a fourfold increase in antibody level in paired sera collected 2 weeks apart is evidence of current infection. Because antibodies are expected to persist lifelong after immunization or infection, immune status determinations are often performed. Even very low levels of antibody indicate immunity. Complement fixation testing is not recommended for immune status determinations.

There are serological methods available for detection of mumps IgM. Mumps IgM is usually detectable within 2 days of the appearance of symptoms, and IgM detection is important in confirming acute infections.

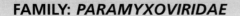

FAMILY: *PARAMYXOVIRIDAE*	VIRUS: PARAINFLUENZA 1, 2, 3, AND 4

Disease Association: Upper and lower respiratory infections.
Laboratory Diagnosis
  Virus isolation: Standard cell cultures of primary monkey kidney cells; CPE of syncytia (very subtle, difficult to read) in 4 to 8 days.
  Viral antigen detection: Immunofluorescence.
  Serodiagnosis: Complement fixation for determining type-specific antibodies in detecting seroconversion and monitoring changes in antibody levels. Hemagglutination inhibition is required for determining strain-specific antibodies.
Specimens: Samples from upper and lower respiratory tract sites for virus isolation and viral antigen detection. Submit clotted blood for serology.

Parainfluenza (Para) virus infections are transmitted by direct contact and by inhalation of aerosols. Para 1, 2, and 3 usually cause upper respiratory tract symptoms, including rhinitis and pharyngitis. Although Para viruses infect individuals of all ages, they are second only to respiratory syncytial virus in frequency of severe illness in children. Infections, especially those involving Para 1 and less frequently Para 2, may result in croup (laryngotracheitis). Para 3 may produce bronchiolitis and pneumonia and is a major cause of severe lower respiratory tract disease in infants and young children. Para 4 has been described but is less common and produces mild upper respiratory tract symptoms. Para 1 is most common in the fall (alternate years), Para 2 occurs in late autumn or early winter or sporadically year-round, and Para 3 occurs endemically throughout the year in some areas [1]. There are no accepted antiviral therapies available at present for treatment of Para infections.

For virus isolation, upper respiratory tract samples, including nose, throat, and nasopharyngeal swabs, should be submitted. Para proliferates slowly in primary monkey kidney cells, producing subtle, if any, CPE. The CPE usually consists of syncytia. Hemadsorption testing (described in Chapter 3) should be used to detect the virus. Para 4 hemadsorbs more strongly at 25 to 37°C. The identity of the isolated virus may be confirmed by immunofluorescence testing. Although most laboratories routinely differentiate only Para 1, 2, and 3, monoclonal antibodies are marketed for use in immunofluorescence testing for Para 4.

Indirect immunofluorescence methods are often used to detect Para 1, 2, and 3 antigens in clinical samples from the respiratory tract. The sensitivity of antigen detection varies among the para types, with 70 to 72% of Para 1, 65 to 67% of Para 2, and 70 to 74% of Para 3 detected (see discussion of Respiratory Viral Antigen Profile data in Chapter 5). Enzyme immunoassay can be used for antigen detection, but this is not widely available.

Several methods may be used for serological testing, including complement fixation and hemagglutination inhibition. Seroconversion or a fourfold or greater change in titer indicates a current infection. There is extensive cross-reactivity among Para types, so antibody titers may not effectively indicate which Para type is involved in the infection. Hemagglutination inhibition is used for determining strain-specific antibodies.

FAMILY: *PARAMYXOVIRIDAE*   VIRUS: RESPIRATORY SYNCYTIAL VIRUS

Disease Association: Most common cause of severe respiratory problems in infants and young children.

Laboratory Diagnosis

Virus isolation: Standard cell cultures of continuous human epithelial lines such as HEp-2 or HeLa, also infects primary monkey kidney cells; CPE of large refractile syncytia progressing to involve the entire monolayer in 4 to 10 days.

Viral antigen detection: Immunofluorescence or enzyme immunoassay.

Serodiagnosis: Many methods (complement fixation, indirect immunofluorescence) are used for detecting seroconversion and monitoring changes in antibody level.

Specimens: Samples from upper and lower respiratory tract sites for virus isolation and viral antigen detection. Submit clotted blood for serology.

Respiratory syncytial virus (RSV) is found worldwide and is the single most important cause of severe respiratory infections in infants and young children. It has been reported that all children are infected with RSV before they reach 4 years of age [10]. The infection, which is spread through respiratory droplets, tends to be very seasonal in temperate climates, usually occurring December through March. The virus replicates in the ciliated epithelial cells of the respiratory tract. Replication disrupts protein and nucleic acid synthesis resulting in death of the cells and release of enzymes, which trigger the complement cascade and initiate local inflammation. Mucus and fibrin, along with necrotic cells, clog the airways [11].

Although infants younger than 6 weeks are sometimes infected, they usually have mild disease, probably because of protection from maternal antibodies. Infants ages 6 weeks to 6 months acquire the most serious infections characterized by cough, fever, wheezing, and, in 25 to 40% of cases, bronchitis and pneumonia [1]; otitis media is a common complication of RSV infection. The illness usually lasts 7 to 12 days, and recovery is uneventful except in those with underlying heart or lung disease or with immunodeficiency syndromes. Supportive therapy of intubation and ventilation is required for severe cases as well as treatment with the RSV antiviral ribavirin. Older children and adults infected with RSV usually experience mild upper respiratory tract illness. This mild presentation may be related to the larger, less easily obstructed airways in older individuals and to protective antibodies produced in early infections. The elderly may experience severe RSV infections.

Clinical samples for RSV isolation and antigen detection should be collected from the upper respiratory tract. Nasal and nasopharyngeal swabs and washings are preferred. Samples should not be frozen before cell culture inoculation. RSV produces syncytia in 4 to 10 days in continuous human epithelial lines such as HEp-2 or HeLa cells and may show CPE in primary monkey kidney cells. Typical CPE is large refractile syncytia that progress to extensive syncytia involving the entire monolayer. The virus was named in keeping with its capacity to produce syncytia in cultured cells. RSV-infected cells do not hemadsorb. The identity of RSV isolates from cell cultures should be confirmed by immunofluorescence or by enzyme immunoassay.

Viral antigen detection by immunofluorescence or enzyme immunoassay often yields results that are comparable in sensitivity and specificity to virus isolation. See Chapter 5 for a comparison of RSV isolation and antigen detection by immunofluorescence and by enzyme immunoassay. The immunofluorescence assay for RSV antigen may detect 90 to 93% of all RSV-positive samples.

RSV infection can be confirmed serologically by complement fixation and indirect immunofluorescence. Seroconversion or a fourfold or greater change in antibody level is seen in current infection. RSV antibodies do not protect against infection, and reinfection is common. However, lower respiratory tract infection and severe disease are less common in those with antibodies.

FAMILY: *PICORNAVIRIDAE*   VIRUSES: COXSACKIEVIRUS, ECHOVIRUS, POLIOVIRUS, AND OTHERS

Disease Association: Various enteric, neuromuscular, and central nervous system infections have been reported.

Laboratory Diagnosis

Virus isolation: Most strains proliferate in standard cell cultures of primary monkey kidney cells in 2 to 5 days.

Viral antigen detection: Not used.

Serodiagnosis: Seroconversion and changes in antibody level can be detected reliably by viral neutralization. Immune status testing is helpful for poliovirus antibodies.

Specimens: For virus isolation, submit throat and rectal swabs and cerebrospinal fluid. Submit clotted blood for serology.

Three groups of viruses, the coxsackieviruses (A and B), echoviruses, and polioviruses, belong to the enterovirus genus in the *Picornaviridae* family. There are 24 serotypes of coxsackie A virus, 6 of coxsackie B virus, 33 of echovirus, and 3 of poliovirus; several additional serotypes have not been characterized fully but are named and numbered as enteroviruses. Enterovirus 72 is the numerical designation for hepatitis A virus. A discussion of hepatitis A follows this section. Coxsackie, echo, and polio viruses have been isolated from stools of infected individuals, most of whom have symptoms involving the gastrointestinal tract as well as the central nervous system or other organ systems. The viruses are transmitted via the fecal-oral route, especially during the summer months in temperate climates. The highest rates of infection are in infants of poor socioeconomic status. Many enteroviral infections are asymptomatic.

POLIOVIRUS. Poliovirus is the most well known of the enteroviruses. It produces classic paralytic polio. The virus enters through the mouth and replicates in the pharynx, tonsils, and gut. The virus then is transported via the lymphatic vessels to the blood and on to the target cells of the central nervous system. The virus replicates in the neurons of the gray matter of the anterior horn of the spinal cord and the motor nuclei of the pons and medulla. Symptoms include fever, sore throat, headache, and vomiting [12]. Poliomyelitis with paralysis occurs in only 0.1 to 1.0% of cases with central nervous system involvement and usually leaves extensive permanent paralysis. Poliovirus type 1 causes most paralytic disease.

Extensive vaccination programs in the United States since 1952 have dramatically reduced the incidence of polio infection. Initially, immunization involved inactivated polio virus (the Salk vaccine), which is administered subcutaneously. Subsequently, a live, attenuated polio virus (OPV, the Sabin vaccine), which is administered orally, was used. Only four confirmed cases of poliomyelitis in the United States were reported to the Centers for Disease Control in 1992, and all four of these cases were vaccine related [13]. On August 20, 1994, the Pan American Health

Organization reported that 3 years had passed since the occurrence of the last case of poliomyelitis associated with wild poliovirus isolation in the Americas [14].

The World Health Organization has adopted a resolution for global eradication of poliomyelitis by the year 2000 through emphasizing administration of OPV in young children, administering supplemental doses of oral vaccine to children in areas where wild poliovirus persists, and maintaining careful surveillance of the incidence of polio worldwide [13]. The number of polio cases reported worldwide decreased from 32,286 in 1988 to 9714 in 1993; most cases were reported in India, Southeast Asia, and Africa.

COXSACKIEVIRUSES. There are two groups of coxsackie viruses, group A and group B, but members of both groups produce similar infections and may be involved with a wide variety of clinical manifestations. These viruses produce most of the enteroviral disease in the United States. The viruses multiply initially in the throat and gut, and certain strains travel via the blood to other target organs, including the central nervous system, the heart, various striated muscles, the skin, and the respiratory tract. Coxsackieviruses are not as likely as the polioviruses to produce central nervous system complications but usually produce more serious infections than the echoviruses. Coxsackie A viruses have been associated with vesicular pharyngitis (herpangina), hand-foot-and-mouth disease, infantile diarrhea, aseptic meningitis, and paralysis. Coxsackie B viruses have been implicated more frequently in pericarditis and myocarditis as well as in infections similar to those of coxsackie A.

ECHOVIRUSES. The echoviruses (*e*nteric, *c*ytopathogenic, *h*uman, *o*rphan) have been isolated in various types of infections, but, as the "orphan" part of their acronym-based name suggests, their role in disease production is not well defined. Like the polioviruses and the coxsackieviruses, echoviruses enter through the mouth and multiply in the pharynx and small intestine; they are shed in the feces for approximately 1 month and in respiratory secretions for several days [15]. Echoviruses have been isolated in cases of aseptic meningitis, exanthem, diarrhea, and other types of infections but have also been found in apparently healthy individuals.

Specimens for isolation of coxsackie, echo, and polio viruses include stools, rectal swabs, throat swabs, and cerebrospinal fluid. Swabs from skin lesions may be productive in herpangina. Blood is seldom productive. Except for some strains of group A coxsackievirus that proliferate only in newborn mice, most enteroviruses will proliferate within 2 to 5 days in standard cell cultures of primary monkey kidney cells or in human fetal diploid cells. The identification of the isolated viruses is often reported as "enterolike" or "enterovirus—not specified" on the basis of typical CPE involving shrunken cells with "tails" or bridges of cytoplasm. Large empty areas in the monolayer where cells have lost their adherence and detached from the vessel wall are often seen with enteroviruses. Specific identification relies on neutralization of the enteroviral isolates by typing using the Lim Benyesh-Melnick pools. Neutralization testing is described in Chapter 2 and a procedure for typing of enterovirus isolates is included in the Appendix. This procedure is lengthy, expensive, and time consuming and is seldom offered except at larger laboratories for identification of isolates from cerebrospinal fluid or other critical sites. Monoclonal antibodies against some of the enteroviruses are now under development for use in immunofluorescence testing for enterovirus identification. These have not yet been thoroughly evaluated, and their sensitivity and specificity compared with neutralization testing have not been determined. The differentiation of the enteroviruses has little impact on patient management. At this writing, there is no antiviral agent that is effective against the enteroviruses.

Viral antigen detection tests are not used routinely, so the only alternative for laboratory confirmation other than virus isolation is serological confirmation. Neutralization testing remains the most important serological assay and is most effective when acute and convalescent sera are tested to evaluate changes in antibody level. Because some individuals have low levels of antibodies against some enteroviruses and because enterovirus antibodies tend to cross-react, a single antibody assay is not usually helpful. Complement fixation testing and other serological assays have been used to identify enteroviral group antibodies. These assays are not very helpful, and their use for enteroviral antibody detection is not encouraged.

FAMILY: *PICORNAVIRIDAE*   VIRUS: HEPATITIS A VIRUS

Disease Association: Classic "infectious" hepatitis.
Laboratory Diagnosis
  Virus isolation: Cannot be isolated in standard cell cultures.
  Viral antigen detection: Not available routinely.
  Serodiagnosis: Enzyme immunoassay for detecting seroconversion and monitoring changes in antibody levels.
Specimens: Submit clotted blood for serology.

Because of similarities in viral structure and routes of transmission, hepatitis A virus (HAV) has been classified, along with coxsackievirus, echovirus, and poliovirus, as an enterovirus, specifically enterovirus type 72 [16]. HAV may soon be reclassified because it differs from the other enteroviruses in its molecular structure and function.

Transmission of HAV (infectious hepatitis) is by the fecal-oral route, with most infections resulting from fecal contamination of food. Person-to-person spread is less common and is usually associated with crowded conditions and poor sanitary habits. HAV is endemic in many emerging countries, but the incidence in the United States is low; food-related outbreaks and custodial care institutions account for the majority of cases [17]. The incubation period lasts 2 to 6 weeks (average, 4 weeks). Up to two thirds of HAV infections may be asymptomatic, especially in children. Symptoms may include jaundice, fever, anorexia, vomiting, and fatigue. Dark urine and pale stools are associated with the beginning of jaundice. Acute disease usually lasts about 1 week and is generally mild. Recovery usually takes 2 to 4 weeks, and the infection is rarely life threatening [17]; the mortality rate is approximately 0.1% [18]. Chronic carriers are not found.

Because HAV does not proliferate in standard cell cultures and HAV antigen is usually not detectable in the serum or stool when symptoms of HAV infection first appear, diagnosis relies on antibody detection. At the onset of symptoms, IgM antibodies are detectable; these reach a maximum titer in 1 to 3 weeks. IgM falls to undetectable levels in 3 to 6 months and is replaced by IgG that persists for years, probably for life. In the clinical laboratory, testing for HAV includes determinations for IgM anti-HAV and for total (IgG and IgM) anti-HAV antibodies. The finding of IgM anti-HAV is highly diagnostic of current or very recent HAV infection in symptomatic patients. A positive result in the total anti-HAV test may signal current or past infection. By age 50 years, approximately 40% of the U.S. population have IgG anti-HAV [19]. More than 90% of the population in other parts of the world have IgG anti-HAV. Although increasing titers of total anti-HAV in sequential patient specimens may indicate an ongoing HAV infection, testing for total anti-HAV is primarily used to determine previous exposure to HAV.

FAMILY: *PICORNAVIRIDAE*   VIRUS: RHINOVIRUS

Disease Association: Upper respiratory infections, "common cold."
Laboratory Diagnosis
  Virus isolation: Some strains proliferate in standard cell cultures of primary monkey kidney cells incubated at 33°C; CPE of shrunken, rounded cells in 2 to 7 days.
  Viral antigen detection: Not available.
  Serodiagnosis: Not available in most clinical virology facilities.
Specimens: Submit throat, nose, and nasopharyngeal swabs for virus isolation.

The rhinoviruses are members of the *Picornaviridae* family but are not included in the designation "enterovirus" used to describe most of the other members of the family (i.e., coxsackie, echo, polio, hepatitis A). Rhinoviruses produce respiratory rather than enteric infections.

There are 102 serotypes of rhinovirus, which together are believed to cause one quarter to one half of all mild upper respiratory tract infections [1], better known as the "common cold." In temperate climates, rhinovirus infections are most common in the spring and fall but are also seen during the summer. They are not the major cause of colds during the winter [20]. Rhinoviruses replicate in the cells of the mucous membranes of the nose, causing sneezing, sore throat, and cough. Infected cells release bradykinin and histamine, which cause swelling and hyperemia and result in a watery discharge. Rhinoviruses may also be isolated in cases of otitis media. Serious acute lower respiratory tract disease or involvement of other organ systems is rare in rhinovirus infections, but such infections cause significant absenteeism from school and work. Person-to-person spread and aerosols are the major means of spreading rhinovirus infections.

The best culture specimens for rhinovirus isolation are nasal and nasopharyngeal swabs and washes. Culture tubes should be incubated at 33°C rather than at 35°C. Some strains of rhinoviruses will proliferate in 5 to 10 days in primary monkey kidney cells, producing a CPE of shrunken, rounded cells; some will produce rounding in 2 to 7 days in human diploid fibroblasts. Isolates are usually identified based on typical CPE alone. However, testing for acid stability, described in detail elsewhere [20,21], will differentiate the acid-labile rhinoviruses from the acid-stable enteroviruses.

Direct antigen detection methods are not available. Serodiagnosis is also not used routinely for confirming infection. In general, the diagnosis of rhinovirus infection in otherwise healthy individuals is made on a clinical basis, and laboratory testing is not usually undertaken. Laboratory confirmation of rhinovirus infection may be helpful in those with acute respiratory tract infection or other underlying disease.

FAMILY: *REOVIRIDAE*   VIRUS: ROTAVIRUS, OTHERS

Disease Association: Rotavirus produces diarrheal disease, especially in infants, young children, and the elderly. Other *Reoviridae* have no confirmed disease association.
Laboratory Diagnosis of Rotavirus
　Virus isolation: Cannot be isolated in standard cell cultures.
　Viral antigen detection: Enzyme immunoassay and latex agglutination.
　Serodiagnosis: Not available routinely.
Specimens: Submit stool samples and rectal swabs for viral antigen detection.

The *Reoviridae* family viruses were assigned their name based on an acronym: *r*espiratory, *e*nteric, *o*rphan. The name indicates that these viruses have been found in respiratory and stool specimens but that no characteristic disease was identified. The one known pathogen in the *Reoviridae* family is the virus rotavirus.

Rotavirus, which is transmitted primarily by the fecal-oral route, is one of the many agents that produce diarrheal disease in humans. The virus enters through the mouth or nose and enters the stomach, where it can survive the acid only when the pH is buffered by food. The virus passes into the small intestine, where it replicates in the enterocytes of the villi and impairs glucose and sodium transport [15]. Onset of symptoms is usually sudden, beginning with low fever and vomiting, which are followed by watery diarrhea. Although the infection is found in humans of all ages, the young (6 months to 3 years) and the elderly experience the most severe symptoms. In temperate climates, the infection occurs during the winter months and is the most common cause of diarrhea in children younger than 2 years. The infection often produces severe symptoms in young infants, and supportive therapy of fluid and electrolyte replacement is used when needed. There are, at present, no antiviral agents for treatment of rotavirus infections. Rotavirus gastroenteritis can cause death if the necessary supportive therapy is not provided and is thus a significant cause of mortality in many emerging nations.

The virus does not proliferate reliably in standard cell cultures, although isolation in shell vial cultures after an extraction-activation processing of the stool sample has been described for use in special circumstances [22]. The modified culture is more sensitive than antigen detection methods. The antibody response that may result from infection is not usually evaluated in the diagnostic laboratory because antibody production has been demonstrated in patients with asymptomatic infections. Laboratory confirmation of the infection relies on detection of the antigen in the feces of the infected individual. Although visualization of the viral particles by electron microscopy was for many years the only diagnostic method available, the newer antigen detection tests are now widely available and are reported to produce accurate results that are comparable or superior to electron microscopy. Enzyme immunoassay and latex agglutination are used for rotavirus antigen detection. Stool samples are the sample of choice for these assays, and both types of assays, of which many are available commercially, have been shown to yield acceptable results. These assays are not difficult to perform, and they require few if any specialized laboratory instruments or pieces of equipment.

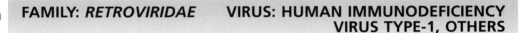

FAMILY: *RETROVIRIDAE*   VIRUS: HUMAN IMMUNODEFICIENCY VIRUS TYPE-1, OTHERS

Disease Association: AIDS
Laboratory Diagnosis
  Virus isolation: Cannot be isolated in standard cell cultures.
  Viral antigen detection: Enzyme immunoassay.
  Serodiagnosis: Enzyme immunoassay used extensively for confirmation of seroconversion; immunoblotting used to determine specificity of antibodies detected.
Specimens: Submit clotted blood for antigen and antibody detection.

HIV type 1 (HIV-1) is one of the several retroviruses that have been identified as significant in infections in humans. HIV-1 was identified in 1983 as one of the viruses associated with AIDS. After the initial HIV-1 infection, the patient may experience a mononucleosis-like syndrome, which includes fever, lymphadenopathy, headache, and sore throat. The symptoms last only a few weeks and are followed by a lengthy (estimated to average 8 years) asymptomatic period. As the infection progresses to AIDS, the immune system is depressed, specifically through inactivation or destruction of T lymphocytes of the CD4 subset. The ratio of the CD4 lymphocytes (helper T cells) to CD8 lymphocytes (suppressor T cells) is altered to allow predominance of suppressor cells rather than the normally predominant helper cells. This particular manifestation of immunodeficiency, along with other immune defects that are not as well defined, produce dramatic alterations in the individual's ability to respond to infection. Infecting agents that would be of little significance in otherwise healthy individuals often produce significant infection in HIV-1–infected patients, and these patients often suffer recurrent infections that are seldom experienced by immunocompetent individuals. Although HIV-1 infection can be confirmed through laboratory tests, the diagnosis of AIDS is not made until the evidence of an immunocompromised state manifests itself through susceptibility to infections. A list of the infections and other disease syndromes frequently seen in AIDS patients is provided in Table 9–1.

TABLE 9–1 LIST OF AIDS INDICATOR INFECTIONS

AIDS INDICATOR INFECTIONS AND CLINICAL SYNDROMES	
Infections	**Clinical Syndromes and Laboratory Findings**
Candidiasis (especially esophageal)	Cervical cancer (invasive)
Coccidioidomycosis	CD4 T lymphocytes: count of less than 200 per
Cryptococcosis	μl or percentage of total lymphocytes of
Cryptosporidiosis	less than 14%
Cytomegalovirus (especially retinitis)	Encephalopathy, HIV related
Herpes simplex	Kaposi's sarcoma
Histoplasmosis	Lymphoma (Burkitt's, immunoblastic, or
Isosporiasis	primary of brain)
Mycobacterium avium-intracellulare	Progressive multifocal leukoencephalopathy
complex or *kansasii*	Wasting syndrome of HIV
Mycobacterium tuberculosis	
Pneumocystis carinii pneumonia	
Pneumonia, recurrent	
Salmonella septicemia	
Toxoplasmosis (especially of brain)	

Data compiled from Centers for Disease Control. Revision of the CDC surveillance case definition for acquired immunodeficiency syndrome. MMWR 1987: 3S–15S; 1993 revised classification system for HIV infection and expanded surveillance case definition for AIDS among adolescents and adults. MMWR 1993: 1–19.

Pneumocystis carinii pneumonia is one infection that has become nearly synonymous with AIDS, and other infecting agents such as atypical mycobacteria and cryptosporidiosis are also more frequent in AIDS patients than in any other group.

Transmission of HIV-1 is through contaminated blood, blood products, and body fluids. This may involve body fluids exchanged through sexual contact, blood in needles shared by intravenous drug abusers, transfused blood, and transplanted organs. A second AIDS virus, HIV-2, also causes AIDS. This virus, along with several other related retroviruses, have been implicated in human infections, although HIV-1 and HIV-2 are the only ones that produce the syndrome defined as AIDS. Several of these retroviruses were identified at nearly the same time interval during the early 1980s, and all were initially named human T-lymphotrophic viruses (HTLV) and given numbers to differentiate them. Table 9–2 lists five of the original HTLV types and shows how these viruses have been reclassified according to the diseases they produce. HIV-1 is by far the most important of these viruses in the United States, although HIV-2 and HTLV-1 produce significant problems in other parts of the world. In the United States, the American Association of Blood Banks mandates that all transfused blood and blood products be tested for antibodies against HIV-1, HIV-2, and HTLV-1, although both HIV-2 and HTLV-1 are very rare in the United States.

TABLE 9–2 NAMING AND NUMBERING OF HUMAN T-CELL LYMPHOTROPHIC VIRUSES (HTLV)

ORIGINAL HTLV CLASSIFICATION	CURRENT NAMING AND DISEASE ASSOCIATION
HTLV-1	HTLV-1, tropical spastic paraparesis or HTLV-1–associated myelopathy and adult T-cell leukemia-lymphoma
HTLV-2	HTLV-2, disease association unknown
HTLV-3	HIV-1, AIDS
HTLV-4	HIV-2, AIDS
HTLV-5	HTLV-5, disease association unknown

None of the retroviruses will proliferate in standard cell cultures, although HIV-1 can be propagated in suspension cultures of phytohemagglutinin-stimulated human lymphocytes. Most individuals with detectable HIV antibody also have culturable virus in their peripheral blood mononuclear cells [23]. HIV-1 isolation is offered at some of the larger virology laboratories and at reference laboratories, and the culture protocol has been described in detail [24]. HIV-1 has been isolated from a variety of body fluids, but anticoagulated peripheral blood is the specimen of choice.

The viral antigen can be detected in the serum of infected individuals early in infection, often before the appearance of detectable antibody. The period between infection and antibody production is often called the "window" period. The length of the window interval for HIV-1 has not been definitively established but is believed to average about 6 to 12 weeks from infection. The antigen detection assay, which may detect HIV-1 antigen during the window period, may effectively "close the window" to allow early detection of HIV-1 infection. HIV-1 antigen presence in serum is transient, and when antibodies become detectable, the antigen usually becomes undetectable. The antigen remains routinely undetectable in serum until the patient's disease becomes severe, and the presence of detectable antigen typically signals increased viral replication and poor prognosis. Antigen detection assays rely on the enzyme immunoassay method in which HIV-1 antibodies are used to capture antigen in the sample. Then enzyme-labeled–HIV-1 antibodies are used to detect the bound antigen and produce a color change of the substrate. Enzyme immunoassay for antigen detection is described in Chapter 2. A positive HIV-1 antigen assay is usually confirmed by a blocking assay in which the reactivity of the antigen-positive serum is blocked by the addition of HIV-1–specific antibodies before performing the enzyme immunoassay.

Although both virus isolation and viral antigen detection for HIV-1 are available, the primary means of confirming HIV-1 infection is through demonstration of the presence of HIV-1 antibodies. Antibodies are reliably detectable usually 6 to 12 weeks after infection and throughout the course of AIDS. Most antibody assay protocols begin with an enzyme immunoassay that detects HIV-1 antibodies or HIV-1 and HIV-2 antibodies in combination. Each manufacturer of HIV antibody detection systems has a carefully defined protocol for performing the specific assay; these protocols must be followed without modification or alteration if the assay is expected to yield accurate results. All initially reactive samples are tested in duplicate by the same assay in another run of testing. This requirement guards against technical problems that might result in false-positive results in the enzyme immunoassays. Although a repeatedly positive HIV-1 antibody enzyme immunoassay result may be presumptive evidence of HIV-1 infection, these results alone are not sufficient to confirm HIV-1 infection. False-positive HIV-1 enzyme immunoassay results may occur in systems that use culture lysate antigen preparations. These preparations may contain human lymphocyte antigens from the human lymphocytes used in cultivation of the HIV-1 for use as the antigen in the HIV-1 test. Reactive results may be related to autoimmune or histocompatibility-related antibodies in some human sera that react with the lymphocyte-related antigens. Newer HIV antibody testing systems use cloned HIV antigens, but the potential for false positives as a result of antibodies directed against vector-related antigens (usually *Escherichia coli* or *Bacillus* species) exists. Confirmatory testing is required after repeated reactivity in the enzyme immunoassay system. Confirmatory testing may be approached in many ways, but immunoblotting (Western blotting) or immunofluorescence are used in most clinical laboratories.

The immunoblotting protocol is the most well accepted and widely used at this time. The concepts of immunoblotting are explained in Chapter 2. HIV-1 antibody–positive sera will yield bands of reactivity on the immunoblot test strips. Although all of the organizations involved with HIV-1 confirmatory testing do not agree completely on the criteria required to definitively identify HIV-1 antibodies, the Centers for Disease Control require the presence of any two of the following three bands: gp120/160, gp41, or p24. Most of the other agencies use criteria that are closely related to these.

An immunofluorescence assay using HIV-1–infected human lymphocytes as the substrate was approved in 1992 by the Food and Drug Administration in the United States for use in confirming HIV-1 antibody identity. This is an indirect immunofluorescence procedure that yields a simple positive or negative answer rather than relying on the presence of particular bands as with immunoblotting. This assay has been reported to correlate effectively with clinical HIV-1 infection and AIDS [25]. This newer immunofluorescence assay has not been used extensively at this point, and data are not widely available concerning its effectiveness.

Enzyme immunoassays for detection of HIV-2 and HTLV-1 antibodies are available commercially and are used in the United States for screening of blood and blood products. HIV-2 infection, which is associated with AIDS, is most common in western Africa, and HTLV-1 infection, associated with adult T-cell leukemia-lymphoma and HTLV-1-associated myelopathy (HAM) (also known as tropical spastic paraparesis or TSP and currently designated HAM-TSP), is most common in Japan and the Caribbean. When antibody assays for either of the two retroviral antibodies yields positive results, sera are usually referred to reference laboratories or to research laboratories for confirmatory testing.

FAMILY: *RHABDOVIRIDAE*   VIRUS: RABIES

Disease Association: Classic rabies
Laboratory Diagnosis
  Virus isolation: Cannot be isolated in standard cell cultures.
  Viral antigen detection: Not available in most laboratories.
  Serodiagnosis: Not available in most laboratories.
  Other: Diagnosis relies on detection of Negri bodies in brains of infected animals.
Specimens: Submit infected animal tissue to reference laboratory for exam for Negri bodies.

The rabies virus is associated with classic *rabies*. The infection has also been called *hydrophobia* because the infected individual has difficulty swallowing; swallowing may be very painful and produce throat contractions. The infected individual may experience periods of excitement and anxiety that alternate with quiet periods. Paralysis develops in the face and extremities, and death follows. The virus is transmitted to humans through contact with the saliva of infected animals, usually as the result of a bite. The rabies-infected animal demonstrates a unique type of insanity in which it attacks and bites any other animal or human. The incidence of rabies in the United States has decreased dramatically since 1960, when rabies immunizations became a requirement for all dogs. Nonbite aerosol transmission of rabies has been reported [26]. Since 1980 in the United States, eight rabies cases associated with bats have been reported. Only one of these had a history of bat bite; two had exposure to bats but no bites, and five had no known exposure to bats [27].

Rabies-related diagnostic services are not provided in most clinical diagnostic virology laboratories, and requests for such testing should be referred to state health laboratories or reference laboratories specializing in rabies diagnosis. For potentially infected humans, virus isolation in laboratory animals (usually mice) may be attempted, and throat and saliva samples may be stained with rabies antibodies to detect rabies antigen. For suspect animal infections, histological techniques may be used to detect rabies-specific cytoplasmic inclusion bodies known as Negri bodies in infected brain. Rabies antibodies may be measured using one of several sophisticated techniques.

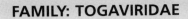

FAMILY: TOGAVIRIDAE · VIRUS: EASTERN AND WESTERN EQUINE ENCEPHALITIS

Disease Association: Encephalitis.
Laboratory Diagnosis
Virus isolation: Cannot be isolated in standard cell cultures.
Viral antigen detection: Not available.
Serodiagnosis: Hemagglutination inhibition and complement fixation used to determine seroconversion and monitor changes in antibody level.
Specimens: Submit clotted blood for serology.

Eastern equine encephalitis (EEE) virus and western equine encephalitis (WEE) virus are in the *Togaviridae* family as part of a group called the Alphaviruses, which includes other encephalitis viruses as well. All of these are arthropod-borne, with both EEE and WEE being transmitted by the bite of infected mosquitos. Infections are most common during the summer months when mosquitos are present. EEE is more common in the eastern United States, whereas WEE is found in the western United States. Both EEE and WEE may produce severe disease, but permanent impairment and death are not common for either. Neither EEE nor WEE will proliferate in standard cell cultures, and tests for detection of viral antigens are not available. The diagnosis relies on serological testing of paired sera. Such serological testing is usually available at state health laboratories and reference centers and is not offered at most clinical facilities.

FAMILY: TOGAVIRIDAE · VIRUS: RUBELLA

Disease Association: "German" or "three-day" measles; a mild febrile disease characterized by an erythematous rash.
Laboratory Diagnosis
Virus isolation: Proliferates slowly in standard cell cultures; produces no CPE; use challenge interference to detect viral presence.
Viral antigen detection: Not available.
Serodiagnosis: Many methods (hemagglutination inhibition, agglutination, enzyme immunoassay, immunofluorescence) used to determine seroconversion, monitor changes in antibody level, and determine immune status.
Specimens: Throat and nasal samples and urine for virus isolation and clotted blood for serology.

Rubella virus is the agent of German measles or three-day measles. The virus is transmitted from person to person through aerosols and is highly infectious. Rubella infection was common in children and young adults in the United States in years before the implementation of rubella immunizations for all children. Rubella typically produces mild symptoms for 3 days, including low-grade fever, headache, mild conjunctivitis, lymphadenopathy, and rash [28]. Complications of rubella infection in children are rare.

The most serious aspect of rubella infection involves pregnant women, particularly those in the first trimester of pregnancy, who become infected by the virus. The infection in the mother is not remarkable, but, during maternal viremia, the virus crosses the placenta and replicates within the fetus, leading to disseminated infection of fetal organs. Anomalies produced in the fetus by rubella virus infection include heart lesions, ocular complications, ear malfunctions, hepatosplenomegaly, meningoencephalitis, and lesions of the long bones [28]. The risk of fetal malformation after maternal rubella varies according to the time of the infection. In infections occurring during the first month of gestation, 30 to 50% of the fetuses will suffer malformations. Infection during the second month damages 22 to 25% of the fetuses, and infection occurring during the third month damages 6 to 8% [28]. Infections after the third month produce less frequent and less severe anomalies. Rubella is included in the TORCH group of infectious agents, which is responsible for most congenital infections.

A live, attenuated rubella vaccine has been available in the United States since 1969, and the current recommendation is that all children be vaccinated at age 15 months. The rubella is usually given in a polyvalent vaccine (MMR) that includes both measles and mumps vaccine as well. The number of rubella cases in the United States has declined dramatically, with only 157 United States cases reported to the Centers for Disease Control in 1992 [5]. No cases of congenital rubella were reported in the United States during 1992.

In the laboratory, the virus may be isolated from throat and nasal secretions and occasionally from urine or cerebrospinal fluid. Rubella virus will proliferate in primary African green monkey kidney cells, primary rabbit kidney,and BSC-1 cells, although an interference challenge test may be necessary to detect viral presence because CPE will be produced slowly and weakly, if at all. Interference challenge testing is described in Chapter 3. Virus isolation may be helpful in the diagnosis of congenital rubella but is not useful in other rubella infections. Viral antigen detection tests are not available.

In general, the serological approach is relied on to confirm a diagnosis of acquired rubella infection, to evaluate immune status, or to confirm congenital infection. Each of these circumstances and the appropriate serological protocols are described in Chapter 6. Many serological methods are used for detection of rubella antibodies. Hemagglutination inhibition has been a reference method for many years, although this method is not used extensively at present because of its cumbersome nature. Latex agglutination, enzyme immunoassay, and immunofluorescence are all used in rubella serology. IgM-specific serology testing is available at reference centers.

FAMILY: UNCLASSIFIED (?*FLAVIVIRIDAE*)   VIRUS: HEPATITIS C VIRUS

Disease Association: Hepatitis.
Laboratory Diagnosis
   Virus isolation: Cannot be isolated in standard cell cultures.
   Viral antigen detection: Not available routinely.
   Serodiagnosis: Enzyme immunoassay for detecting seroconversion and monitoring changes in antibody levels.
Specimens: Submit clotted blood for serology.

Hepatitis C virus (HCV) infections occur worldwide. Routes of transmission are not definitively identified at this time. Parenteral transmission through transfusions of blood and blood products, organ transplantation, and intravenous drug abuse is the most well-defined route, although other routes of transmission have not been ruled out. Approximately 20 to 40% of all hepatitis cases in the United States are thought to be due to HCV [17] as well as 95% of transfusion-related non-A, non-B hepatitis cases. The incubation period for HCV is 2 to 52 weeks, and most infected persons are asymptomatic. In symptomatic individuals, mild gastrointestinal symptoms and jaundice may be seen, but a small percentage can progress to severe disease. Greater than 75% of HCV patients experience chronic disease.

Little is known about the virus itself. This infection has been described for many years as non-A, non-B hepatitis because the diagnosis relied on ruling out infection by hepatitis A or hepatitis B virus. Recently, HCV was described and is reported to be similar to the viruses of the *Flaviviradae* or *Pestiviridae* families. It appears to be one of several non-A, non-B hepatitis viruses.

HCV will not proliferate in standard cell cultures, and tests for HCV antigen in serum are not available. Laboratory diagnosis of HCV involves testing for total anti-HCV antibodies. This is usually an enzyme immunoassay that uses beads coated with the recombinant HCV antigens c100-3, HC-31, and HC-34. Reactivity of patients' sera with these cloned antigens usually indicates that the patient has anti-HCV antibodies. Occasionally, a positive result may be due to antibodies directed against the vector or fusion proteins associated with the HCV recombinant antigens. Additional testing, usually by immunoblotting, may be used to confirm the specificity of HCV reactivity in samples that are repeatedly reactive in the enzyme immunoassay procedure.

OTHER RNA VIRUSES

The following viruses are described only briefly. They are either exceedingly uncommon in the United States or they cannot be diagnosed by routine clinical virology laboratory methods.

ASTROVIRUSES. These viruses are associated with gastrointestinal diseases. Little is known about them at this time. They are thought to cause disease in infants and young children and are possibly transmitted by the fecal-oral route. They have been observed by electron microscopy.

CALICIVIRIDAE: NORWALK. These viruses are the agent of sporadic gastroenteritis in older children and adults, usually associated with contaminated food. The infection is characterized by abrupt onset of vomiting and diarrhea, very similar to rotavirus. Diagnostic assays are not widely available and diagnosis usually depends on visualization of the viral particles in feces by electron microscopy.

CORONAVIRIDAE. These viruses, along with the rhinoviruses, are the major cause of the common cold, causing 5 to 10% of colds in adults and children [29]. Their infections are self-limiting and confined to the upper respiratory tract. Coronaviruses do not proliferate in standard cell cultures, and coronavirus antigen and antibody detection assays are not available in most laboratories. Diagnosis is made on clinical grounds alone.

FILOVIRIDAE: MARBURG AND EBOLA. These long, filamentous viruses are agents of severe, often fatal hemorrhagic fevers. They are found in Africa. Although they can be isolated in cell cultures of Vero cells, isolation should not be attempted except at reference facilities that meet the highest containment regulations.

HEPATITIS D VIRUS. Hepatitis D virus (HDV) can cause infection only in the presence of active hepatitis B (HBV) infection, and the symptoms of HDV are similar to those of HBV. Chronic HDV-HBV infection often results in progressive liver disease and fulminant hepatitis. HDV may be diagnosed by detecting anti-HDV antibodies [18].

HEPATITIS E VIRUS. Hepatitis E virus (HEV) is transmitted via the fecal-oral route and is associated with poor personal hygiene. The infection is not severe except in pregnant women. Infection occurs in epidemics or sporadically in Asia, North and West Africa, and Mexico. It rarely occurs in the United States. HEV may be a member of the *Caliciviridae* family but also resembles the *Picornaviridae*. No reagents are available commercially in the United States for detection of HEV antibodies [18].

REFERENCES

1. Akerlind-Stopner B, Mufson MA. Respiratory viruses. In Specter S, Lancz G (eds), Clinical Virology Manual, 2nd ed. New York: Elsevier, 1992, pp 321–340
2. Döller G, Schuy W, Tjhen KY, et al. Direct detection of influenza virus antigen in nasopharyngeal specimens by direct enzyme immunoassay in comparison with quantitating virus shedding. J Clin Microbiol 1992; 30:866–869
3. Wilson IA, Cox NJ. Structural basis of immune recognition of influenza virus hemagglutinin. Annu Rev Immunol 1990; 8:737–771
4. Fuccillo DA, Sever JL. Measles, mumps, and rubella. In Specter S, Lancz G (eds), Clinical Virology Manual, 2nd ed. New York: Elsevier, 1992, pp 571–584

5. Centers for Disease Control. Reported vaccine-preventable diseases—United States, 1993, and the childhood immunization initiative. MMWR 1994; 43:57–60

6. Schiff GM. Measles (rubeola). In Lennette EH (ed), Laboratory Diagnosis of Viral Infections, 2nd ed. New York: Marcel Dekker, Inc., 1992, pp 535–547

7. Kleiman MB, Leland DS. Mumps virus and Newcastle disease virus. In Lennette EH (ed), Laboratory Diagnosis of Viral, Rickettsial, and Chlamydial Infections. Washington, DC: American Public Health Association, 1995, pp 455–463

8. Ellner PD, Neu HC. Mumps and bacterial parotitis. In Understanding Infectious Disease. St. Louis: Mosby-Year Book, 1992, pp 233–235

9. Centers for Disease Control. Mumps prevention. MMWR 1989; 38:338–400

10. Chanock RM, Finberg L. Recovery from infants with respiratory illness of a virus related to chimpanzee coryza agent (CCA): II. Epidemiological aspects of infection in infants and young children. Am J Hyg 1957; 66:291–300

11. Ellner PD, Neu HC. Respiratory viruses. In Understanding Infectious Disease. St. Louis: Mosby-Year Book, 1992, pp 31–34

12. Zeichhardt H. Enteroviruses including hepatitis A virus. In Spector S, Lancz G (eds), Clinical Virology Manual, 2nd ed. New York: Elsevier, 1992, pp 341–360

13. Centers for Disease Control. Progress toward global eradication of poliomyelitis, 1988–1993. MMWR 1994; 43:499–503

14. Centers for Disease Control. Certification of poliomyelitis eradication—the Americas, 1994. MMWR 1994; 43:720–721

15. Ellner PD, Neu HC. Viral agents of gastroenteritis. In Understanding Infectious Disease. St. Louis: Mosby-Year Book, 1992, pp 183–186

16. Hollinger FB, Dreesman GR. Hepatitis viruses. In Rose NR, de Macario EC, Fahey JL, et al. (eds), Manual of Clinical Laboratory Immunology, 4th ed. Washington, DC: American Society for Microbiology, 1992, pp 634–650

17. Abbott Diagnostics Educational Services. Hepatitis Learning Guide, 2nd ed. Abbott Park, Il: Abbott Diagnostics, 1994.

18. Fody EP, Johnson DF. The serologic diagnosis of viral hepatitis. J Med Technol 1987;4:54–59.

19. Escobar MR. Viral heptatits. In Spector S, Lancz G (eds), Clinical Virology Manual, 2nd ed. New York: Elsevier, 1992, pp 397–423.

20. Couch RB. Rhinoviruses. In Lennette EH (ed), Laboratory Diagnosis of Viral Infections, 2nd ed. New York: Marcel Dekker, Inc., 1992, pp 709–729

21. Aarnaes S. Differentiation of rhinoviruses from enteroviruses: acid lability test. In Isenberg HD (ed), Clinical Microbiology Procedures Handbook. Washington, DC: American Society for Microbiology, 1992, pp 8.13.1–8.13.3.

22. Lipson SM. Cultivation of human rotaviruses. In Isenberg HD (ed), Clinical Microbiology Procedures Handbook. Washington, DC: American Society for Microbiology, 1992, pp 8.16.1–8.16.5

23. Wilber JC. Human immunodeficiency viruses: HIV-2 and HIV-2. In Lennette EH (ed), Laboratory Diagnosis of Viral Infections, 2nd ed. New York: Marcel Dekker, Inc., 1992, pp 477–494

24. Warfield DT, Feorino PM. Isolation and identification of human immunodeficiency virus type 1. In Isenberg HD (ed), Clinical Microbiology Procedures Handbook. Washington, DC: American Society for Microbiology, 1992, pp 8.15.1–8.15.11

25. Sullivan MT, Mucke H, Kadey SD, et al. Evaluation of an indirect immunofluorescence assay for confirmation of human immunodeficiency virus type 1 antibody in U.S. blood donor sera. J Clin Microbiol 1992; 30:2509–2510

26. Winkler WB, Baker EF, Hopkins CC. An outbreak of non-bite transmitted rabies in a laboratory colony. Am J Epidemiol 1972; 95:267–277

27. Centers for Disease Control. Human rabies—California, 1994. MMWR 1994; 43:455–457

28. Evans AS. Viral Infections of Humans, Epidemiology and Control. New York: Plenum, 1976

29. Ray G. Influenza, respiratory syncytial virus, adenovirus, and other respiratory viruses. In Ryan KJ (ed), Sherris Medical Microbiology, 3rd ed. Norwalk, CT: Appleton & Lange, 1994, pp 451–466

REVIEW QUESTIONS

1. Colds and upper respiratory infections are the most common disease association of which of the following RNA viruses?
   a. Rhinovirus
   b. Rotavirus
   c. Rubella
   d. Hepatitis A virus

2. Which of the pairs of viruses below are members of the same family?
   a. Coxsackie A virus and hepatitis C virus
   b. Rabies and rubella
   c. Measles and mumps
   d. Influenza and parainfluenza

3. Which of the following statements describes isolation of influenza viruses in standard cell cultures?
   a. Viruses grow rapidly (48 to 72 hours) in fibroblast cell lines.
   b. Cytopathogenic effect is distinctive, consisting of grapelike clusters.
   c. Hemadsorption testing may be helpful in detecting viral proliferation in cell cultures.
   d. Virus neutralization is the only method available for differentiating influenza A from influenza B.

4. Virus in a cerebrospinal fluid sample produced cytopathogenic effect within 48 hours after inoculation in a culture of primary monkey kidney cells. The cells were shrunken, had cytoplasmic "tails," and fell off the glass. Which virus is most likely?
   a. Enterovirus
   b. Encephalitis virus (eastern equine, western equine, or California encephalitis)
   c. Coronavirus
   d. Rotavirus

5. A physician suspects that his patient has eastern equine encephalitis (EEE). How should he proceed to obtain laboratory confirmation of this diagnosis?
   a. Collect a cerebrospinal fluid sample and submit it for routine viral culture.
   b. Submit acute and convalescent sera for antibody testing for EEE.
   c. Submit a fecal sample for enzyme immunoassay testing for EEE antigen.
   d. Collect a throat swab and request shell vial culture for EEE.

6. Which of the following statements accurately describes rabies and the rabies virus?
   a. The infection is characterized by vesicular lesions at the site of infection.
   b. The virus is transmitted by the bite of an arthropod vector.
   c. The virus proliferates rapidly in fibroblast cells.
   d. The virus is a member of the *Rhabdoviridae* family.

7. A rash or skin lesions typically accompany infections with each of the viruses listed below **except**
   a. Rubella
   b. Measles
   c. Variola
   d. Parainfluenza

8. Three hepatitis viruses have been named hepatitis A (HAV), hepatitis B (HBV), and hepatitis C (HCV). Which of the following statements describes these viruses?
   a. They are all members of the family *Picornaviridae*.
   b. They are all RNA viruses.
   c. None of them proliferate in standard cell cultures so they are usually diagnosed serologically.
   d. They are all transmitted via the fecal-oral route, especially in contaminated food.

9. The echoviruses are accurately described as follows:
   a. Named as they are because their mechanism of pathogenesis "echos" or mimics that of many other viruses
   b. Are members of the *Retroviridae* family
   c. Proliferate rapidly in primary monkey kidney cells, producing shrunken cells with cytoplasmic bridges
   d. Are conveniently identified by enzyme immunoassay

10. Which of the following statements describes laboratory diagnosis of human immunodeficiency virus type 1 (HIV-1) infection?
    a. A serum sample can be tested for HIV-1 antigen or antibody or both.
    b. The virus proliferates in 5 to 8 days in A 549 cells.
    c. Viral antigen can be detected in samples collected from genital lesions.
    d. There are no known culture systems for *in vitro* cultivation of HIV.

11. A fecal sample submitted to the virology laboratory was processed and inoculated into standard cell cultures. Which of the following viruses may be isolated by this approach?
    a. Rotavirus
    b. Coxsackie B virus
    c. Norwalk agent
    d. Astrovirus

12. A virus was isolated from a nasopharyngeal sample from a 5-month old child in January. The virus produced cytopathogenic effect of large, refractile syncytia in HEp-2 cells in 5 to 7 days and failed to hemadsorb guinea pig erythrocytes. Which virus is most likely?
    a. Measles
    b. Influenza
    c. Respiratory syncytial virus
    d. Parainfluenza

13. Hepatitis A virus (HAV) infection is characterized as follows:
    a. The virus is transmitted by the bite of an infected arthropod vector.
    b. Presence of IgG or total anti-HAV confirms active infection.
    c. The infection is seldom life threatening and chronic carriers are not found.
    d. Ninety-nine percent of infected individuals are jaundiced, have fever, and vomit for extended periods of time.

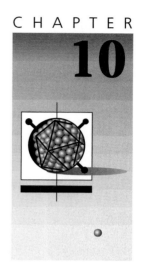

On the Horizon

INTRODUCTION

Chapters 1 to 9 of this text have focused on clinical diagnostic virology laboratory concepts and techniques that are well accepted and widely used in laboratories throughout the United States and on well-known viruses and their related infectious syndromes. In contrast, Chapter 10 highlights newer, less thoroughly explored diagnostic virology technology as well as several viruses that have become the focus of attention of both the medical community and the public in general. These viruses and contemporary technologies will undoubtedly impact the diagnostic virology laboratory. Included in this chapter are a discussion of antiviral agents and antiviral susceptibility testing; an introduction to two "newer" viruses, human herpesvirus type 6 and hantavirus; and a description of two contemporary technologies now being explored for viral disease diagnosis: the polymerase chain reaction (PCR) and engineered cell lines described as "enzyme-linked virus-inducible systems."

ANTIVIRALS AND ANTIVIRAL SUSCEPTIBILITY TESTING

Throughout this text, antiviral agents useful in treatment of certain viral infections have been named. The development of antivirals has been slow because the process of viral infection and replication involves intracellular viral reproduction that depends on host cell metabolic processes; it has been difficult to find compounds that can selectively and specifically inhibit viral replication while leaving host cell functions intact [1]. Progress in identifying effective, nontoxic antivirals has relied on the discovery that most human pathogenic viruses possess enzymes coded by the viruses themselves. These enzymes are not present in uninfected cells, and they are involved in viral nucleic acid synthesis. These enzymes have been the focus of most of the newer antivirals.

Because antivirals are now available, there is increased emphasis on rapid viral diagnosis. A definitive identification of the infecting virus ensures selection of the correct antiviral. Although antivirals are not used extensively except in serious viral infections, their use is becoming more frequent and important. However, resistance to antivirals, like resistance to antibiotics, is being experienced. Laboratory confirmation of resistance to antivirals is now being requested by physicians, and testing of the isolated virus against alternative antivirals is sought. Few diagnostic laboratories are offering antiviral susceptibility testing at this writing, although such services are available at reference facilities. There are many approaches for antiviral susceptibility testing,

TABLE 10–1   ANTIVIRALS AND THEIR CLINICAL APPLICATIONS

VIRUS	ANTIVIRAL	CLINICAL APPLICATIONS
CMV	Ganciclovir	Administered intravenously in CMV infections in immunocompromised patients and in prophylaxis in transplant recipients
	Foscarnet	Treatment of ganciclovir-resistant CMV
Hepatitis B and C	Interferon-α	Administered subcutaneously in hepatitis B chronic active liver disease and in hepatitis C chronic liver disease
HSV	Acyclovir	Administered orally, intravenously, or topically in localized and systemic herpes simplex infections and for prophylaxis in transplant recipients
	Foscarnet	Treatment of acyclovir-resistant herpes simplex
	Idoxuridine	Used to treat herpes keratitis
	Trifluridine	Used to treat herpes keratitis
	Vidarabine	Used to treat herpes encephalitis and neonatal infections; not used extensively at present
HIV-1	Didanosine	Treatment of HIV-1 in patients not responsive to zidovudine
	Zidovudine	Used to treat HIV infection
Influenza A	Amantadine	Prophylaxis and treatment of influenza A
	Rimantadine	Prophylaxis and treatment of influenza A
RSV	Ribavirin	Administered as an aerosol to treat severe respiratory syncytial virus infection; administered intravenously in hantavirus infections and Lassa fever
Varicella	Acyclovir	Used to treat localized and systemic varicella infections
	Foscarnet	Treatment of acyclovir-resistant varicella
	Vidarabine	Used for treatment of zoster in immunocompromised patients

CMV = cytomegalovirus; HSV = herpes simplex virus; RSV = respiratory syncytial virus.

several of which are presented here. As the list of available antivirals grows and the appearance of resistant viral strains accelerates, clinical diagnostic virology laboratories will be forced to decide whether to offer antiviral susceptibility testing, and, if such testing is to be offered, which method should be used for this testing.

A list of antivirals available at present is shown in Table 10–1 along with the names of viruses each is designed to treat and the clinical situations for use. The mechanism of action of each antiviral is described. Most antiviral agents are nucleoside analogues, which means that they are configured to "look like" the nucleoside bases needed for viral replication. When the antiviral reacts with virus-specific enzymes involved with replication in virus-infected cells, synthesis of viral DNA is blocked. Acyclovir, which is the drug of choice for serious herpes simplex virus (HSV) infections, is a guanosine analogue, which is phosphorylated by a virus-specific enzyme, thymidine kinase, to produce acyclovir monophosphate. Cellular kinases convert the acyclovir monophosphate to a triphosphate, which is then incorporated into newly synthesized viral DNA. The triphosphate can serve as a substrate for viral DNA polymerase during further viral DNA synthesis, but DNA synthesis is then blocked because the triphosphate does not have the chemical determinants required in linking to incoming nucleotides.

Almost all acyclovir resistance is associated with thymidine kinase gene mutation, although resistance may also result from changes or mutations in DNA polymerase. Widespread use of acyclovir, especially in bone marrow transplant recipients and others who are immunocompromised, gives rise to acyclovir-resistant herpes simplex and acyclovir-resistant varicella. It is important to have laboratory confirmation of acyclovir resistance in viruses that do not respond to therapy because alternative antiviral therapy is sometimes available. In the case of acyclovir-resistant HSV, foscarnet can often be used.

Ganciclovir, which is used in the treatment of severe cytomegalovirus (CMV) infections and is effective against herpes simplex, is a guanosine analogue. Virus-specific thymidine kinase in herpes-infected cells and an unidentified enzyme in CMV-infected cells convert ganciclovir to its monophosphate form; cellular kinases subsequently convert this to a triphosphate with activity similar to that of the triphosphate produced with acyclovir, which reacts with viral DNA polymerase and reduces viral replication. Ganciclovir-resistant CMV strains have been isolated from AIDS patients and other immunocompromised individuals. These isolates have either lost their ability to phosphorylate the ganciclovir or have mutations in their DNA polymerase genes.

Ribavirin is used in treatment of severe respiratory syncytial virus infection and also with hantavirus infections and Lassa fever. Ribavirin is a guanosine analogue. It is phosphorylated into monophosphate and triphosphate forms, both of which are active in inhibiting several steps in viral replication.

Vidarabine (adenine arabinoside, Ara-A) was used in the treatment of severe HSV infection. This was one of the first antivirals but is not used widely now because it has been replaced by the less toxic antiviral acyclovir. Vidarabine is a purine nucleoside. It is phosphorylated by cellular kinases to its triphosphate form, which acts as an inhibitor of viral DNA polymerase. Vidarabine-resistant viruses have not been reported to cause problems clinically.

Zidovudine (AZT) is a thymidine analogue used in treatment of HIV-1 infection. Cellular kinases convert AZT in HIV-infected cells into a triphosphate form, which competitively inhibits HIV reverse transcriptase, leading to chain termination. Another form of AZT, a monophosphate, competes with cellular thymidylate kinase, resulting in reduced production of thymidine triphosphate. HIV becomes resistant to AZT through mutations in the reverse transcriptase gene.

Two other antivirals do not act as nucleoside analogues. Amantadine, used in influenza A prophylaxis and treatment, prevents viral uncoating and release of viral RNA into the cytoplasm. Foscarnet, a pyrophosphate analogue used for treatment of acyclovir- and ganciclovir-resistant CMV and HSV, is a noncompetitive inhibitor of viral DNA polymerases.

In contrast to the antivirals just described, interferons are natural products. They are small proteins elaborated by eukaryotic cells in response to viral infection. These proteins signal to other noninfected cells to change their biochemical processes to make these cells resistant to subsequent viral infection. Interferons are described further in Chapter 1. At present, alpha interferons are available commercially for use in treatment of chronic hepatitis B or chronic hepatitis C infections. It is believed that a lack of natural interferon may be one of the reasons that some individuals are not able to naturally clear the hepatitis viruses and therefore experience chronic disease.

The clinical situations described next may warrant antiviral susceptibility testing [2]. When patients who are receiving acyclovir have persistent or worsening HSV or varicella infections, resistance should be evaluated. Alternative therapy with foscarnet can be initiated. For patients with persistent or worsening CMV retinitis, pneumonitis, or colitis that is not responding to ganciclovir, resistance should be evaluated; foscarnet can be used for treatment of resistant strains. For the purpose of evaluating clinical response with *in vitro* drug activity, it may be wise to test HIV isolates both before and after AZT therapy. In situations in which there is continuous shedding or transmission of influenza A despite amantadine prophylaxis in a population, the influenza isolates should be tested for resistance to amantadine.

Antiviral susceptibility testing is not used routinely at this writing, and susceptibility methods are not well standardized. Several of the methods used in antiviral susceptibility testing are described next.

Plaque Reduction Assay

Susceptible cells are inoculated with a measured dose of the viral isolate. The virus-infected cells are incubated with various concentrations of the antiviral. The assay is evaluated by counting the number of viral foci or plaques produced at each concentration. A decrease in numbers of viral plaques indicates effectiveness of the drug. Plaque reduction assays are cumbersome and reproducibility is low. The method has been criticized because it depends on the ability of the virus to grow *in vitro*. This may select for viral strains that are capable of replicating well *in vitro;* these strains may not necessarily represent the population that is causing problems in the patient [1].

SYNCYTIUM INHIBITION AND FOCI INHIBITION ASSAYS

These two assays are performed in similar fashion to the plaque reduction assay described previously and are criticized for the same reasons. The end point is determined by counting syncytia formed by the virus in the syncytium inhibition assay or through counting foci of infection after immunochemical staining in the foci inhibition assays.

ENZYME IMMUNOASSAY

Enzyme immunoassays are applied most frequently in antiviral susceptibility testing to measure the hemagglutinin of influenza virus or the p24 antigen of HIV-1 in the presence of their respective antiviral agents [2]. The end point is determined by comparing amounts of viral proteins formed in the presence of various concentrations of the drug.

Dye Uptake Assay

After virus-infected cells are incubated with various concentrations of antivirals, the amount of vital dye taken up by viable cells is measured; virus-damaged cells will not take up dye. The dye taken up by viable cells is eluted into a phosphate-alcohol buffer and measured colorimetrically. This assay has been found to be reproducible and reliable [3].

DNA Hybridization Assays

After incubation with the antiviral agent, the amount of inhibition of DNA synthesis of the virus is measured. A modification of the DNA hybridization assay has been developed and is available commercially. In this assay, a lysing agent is added to infected cell monolayers that have been incubated with antivirals. The lysing agent lyses the cells and denatures the DNA to single-stranded form. A filter membrane is then placed into the lysate, which allows the lysate to wick by capillary action onto the membrane. The wicked material is then hybridized with a radioiodinated DNA probe (Hybriwix probe systems, Diagnostic Hybrids, Inc., Athens, OH).

"NEW" OR EMERGING VIRUSES AND VIRUS-ASSOCIATED SYNDROMES

More viruses are being identified each day in association with disease in humans. Many factors can contribute to this disease emergence: changes in existing organisms; occurrence of known diseases in different geographical locations or in different human populations; appearance of previously unrecognized infections in populations undergoing ecological change; development of resistant strains; and breakdowns in public health measures for previously controlled infections [4].

Most of these emerging agents cannot be conveniently detected or identified by the standard diagnostic virology laboratory methods presented in this text. However, virologists need to be aware of these viruses and of their disease associations to discuss and recommend the virology reference laboratory services needed by physicians. Two of these newer or emerging viruses are discussed next.

Human Herpesvirus Type 6

One recently discovered virus has been named human herpesvirus, type 6 (HHV-6). Although this virus was identified in 1986 [5], its role in disease is constantly being defined and redefined as more and more information is gathered about the agent. HHV-6 was originally discovered in patients with lymphoproliferative disorders, including AIDS. The virus was isolated in B lymphocytes and was initially named human B-lymphotrophic virus (HBLV). On further characterization of the HBLV virus structure and genome, it was found that the structure was like that of the herpesviruses, with double-stranded DNA, an icosahedral capsid, and an envelope. The genome is closely related to that of the *Herpesviridae* family virus CMV.

It is now known that most HHV-6 infections occur in children younger than 3 years and that up to 95% of the adult population has antibody to the virus [6]. The mode of transmission is not clearly defined at this time but is suspected to be through respiratory droplets and exchange of body fluids. Regardless of the type of infection produced initially, the virus appears to establish latency. The virus is considered to be a lymphotrophic virus that can infect mononuclear cells, including T and B lymphocytes, megacaryocytes, and other types of cells. The name was changed from HBLV to HHV-6 after it was determined that the virus could infect cells other than B lymphocytes and that the virus closely resembled the *Herpesviridae* family viruses.

HHV-6 has been confirmed as the causative agent of roseola infantum, which is usually called *roseola* and is considered one of the common infections of childhood. Roseola is characterized by high fever, which lasts for 3 to 5 days and is followed by a maculopapular rash; the rash may recur repeatedly for weeks. Roseola does not require therapy and complications are rare.

HHV-6 has also been implicated in an infectious mononucleosis-like syndrome in children and young adults. Clinically, this syndrome closely resembles the mononucleosis of CMV and that of classic infectious mononucleosis associated with Epstein-Barr virus (EBV). The patient has fever, mild pharyngitis, cervical lymphadenopathy, and splenomegaly.

The association of HHV-6 with other immunodeficiencies is of great interest. Because HHV-6 infects peripheral blood mononuclear cells, it is sometimes isolated in lymphocyte cultures intended for HIV-1 isolation. Although laboratory studies have shown that coinfection of lymphocytes with HIV-1 and HHV-6 causes accelerated HIV-1 activity [7], AIDS patients have been shown to have lower titers of HHV-6 antibodies than control populations [8]. HHV-6 viremia and increased titers of antibodies have been reported in EBV-positive Burkitt's lymphoma, B-cell lymphomas, and other lymphoproliferative diseases. HHV-6 has also been linked to chronic fatigue syndrome [9]. The spectrum of clinical disease associated with HHV-6 has been expanded to include nonspecific febrile illness in young infants, recurrent febrile seizures, hepatitis, lymphadenopathy, and fever and pneumonitis in bone marrow transplant recipients.

Confirmation of HHV-6 infection at present may be approached by serological assessment. The service is available at reference laboratories and usually includes immunoglobulin (Ig) G and IgM detection. Detection of HHV-6 DNA by the molecular diagnostic technique of PCR is becoming popular. Isolation of HHV-6 in cell cultures of human lymphocytes is usually performed in research laboratories only. At present, laboratory confirmation of most of the HHV-6 associated syndromes is not sought by physicians. However, in complicated cases, especially in immunocompromised patients, the importance of HHV-6 infection requires further assessment, of which laboratory confirmation of infection is an essential part.

Hantavirus

In the southwestern United States (New Mexico, Colorado, Utah, Arizona) in May 1993, several otherwise healthy people died from a mysterious illness. They initially experienced a flulike illness with fever and muscle aches. Eventually their lungs filled with fluid, and they died. Although plague was suspected, laboratory assays did not confirm this cause. Blood and tissue sent to the Centers for Disease Control were analyzed and a viral cause, hantavirus, was identified. The mystery disease was called hantavirus pulmonary syndrome. A total of 83 cases of hantavirus pulmonary syndrome had been confirmed in the United States by July 1994; 45 have died [10].

Hantaviruses are RNA viruses in the family *Bunyaviridae*. Hantaviruses have been identified in other parts of the world in the past in association with hemorrhagic fever and renal syndrome in association with Korean hemorrhagic fever. No human infections resulting from hantavirus were reported in the United States until the 1993 outbreak of hantavirus pulmonary syndrome. Since this outbreak in the southwestern United States, hantavirus pulmonary syndrome has been identified in more than 12 states, from California to Florida and Rhode Island [4]. The mortality rate was initially 60 to 80%, but now the infection is being recognized earlier and appropriate supportive therapy is provided. The antiviral ribavirin is now used for treatment.

The hantaviruses have rodent hosts. Several strains of hantavirus have been identified in association with hantavirus pulmonary syndrome, each with its own reservoir. Hantavirus in the southwest, called the Muerto Canyon strain, is carried by deer mice. Hantavirus in Florida and throughout the southeast is carried by the cotton rat. Infected rodents, which show no illness from the infection, shed virus in their saliva, urine, and feces, and humans become infected when rodent saliva or excreta is inhaled as aerosols. Infection may also result from rodent bites. Person-to-person transmission has not been documented [11].

Laboratory confirmation of hantavirus infection initially relied on demonstration of viral antigen in tissue. The hantavirus antigen can be identified in human tissue samples via immunohistochemical staining. Enzyme-labeled hantavirus antibodies are applied to paraffin-embedded tissues and bind to hantavirus antigens characteristically located in endothelial cells. Serological testing is also available. Human hantavirus antibodies are identified by enzyme immunoassay or by immunoblotting using recombinant hantavirus antigen in the test system. Virus isolation in cell culture is not used at present for hantavirus detection.

CONTEMPORARY APPROACHES FOR VIRAL DISEASE DIAGNOSIS

Although the traditional technologies of virus isolation, viral antigen detection, and viral serodiagnosis are the mainstay of viral disease diagnosis, the applications of new technologies are constantly being expanded. Only through careful attention to these new technologies and assessment of their usefulness in the clinical diagnostic virology laboratory will the laboratory keep pace and continue to offer the most up-to-date and clinically useful services. Two new technologies are described next. One is the molecular technique called PCR, which is used to multiply *in vitro* target nucleic acid sequences of infecting viruses so that the sequences may be detected and identified. The second technology is a new approach to virus isolation in which the cell culture host is genetically altered to allow it to produce a specific enzyme only when it is stimulated by a specific virus. Both of these technologies hold enormous potential for enhancing diagnostic virology in the future.

Polymerase Chain Reaction

PCR reaction technology has been in use for more than 10 years, although applications to viral disease diagnosis are still under assessment. PCR is described in Chapter 2. PCR is simply an amplification method that allows many copies of a nucleic acid sequence, usually a DNA sequence, to be produced *in vitro* in a very short time period. This has been applied in infectious disease diagnosis as an adjunct to molecular diagnostic techniques that rely on detection of nucleic acids of the infecting agent to define the cause of the infection.

The PCR technique has many possible advantages. Although certain viruses can be isolated in standard or modified cell culture systems within 24 to 48 hours of culture inoculation, a physician's decision may be aided dramatically if results could be made available more quickly. Such quick and sensitive detection may be available soon through the use of PCR, which may yield results within 5 to 10 hours after the sample is received in the laboratory. PCR may also be applied for detecting viruses that are nonculturable in the standard cell culture systems available in most clinical diagnostic virology laboratories. PCR may be the ideal (and only!) approach for direct demonstration of the presence of nonculturable viruses.

PCR technology may also be very helpful in analyzing clinical samples that are typically small in size (i.e., a biopsy sample) or of small volume (i.e., a cerebrospinal fluid sample). Often many laboratory analyses are desired on these tiny samples, and a technique such as PCR, which has the capacity to replicate the nucleic acid within the sample, could be very helpful. Likewise, the fact that a sample may contain only dead or inactivated virus, which is, therefore, incapable of infecting cell cultures, is not a problem for PCR. The technique does not rely on viability of the virus or even on the presence of intact genome. PCR can also be used for analysis of samples that have been previously paraffin embedded. Because PCR multiplies the amount of nucleic acid present in the sample, it is better than direct antigen detection techniques that yield positive results only if a sufficient amount of viral antigen is present. Another advantage of PCR is that only the target nucleic acid is multiplied; this target is noninfectious and is not capable of future independent biological activity. This is in contrast to replication of infective virus in cell cultures that results in high titers of infective and sometimes dangerous viruses in the laboratory.

There are currently some disadvantages of PCR. The technology is sophisticated, requiring special patented DNA polymerase and a thermocycler to facilitate the reaction. At this writing, the reagents and equipment are expensive, and the procedures require considerable expertise in their performance. Although the sensitivity of the technique, owing to the amplification of the target sequences, is excellent, the extreme sensitivity may also be the most significant obstacle in the inclusion of the technique into routine clinical laboratories [12]. This is true because it is possible for laboratory surfaces, reagents, and equipment to become contaminated with amplified target sequences (amplicons). These amplicons may inadvertently be introduced into patients' samples before the amplification process, allowing further amplification of the sequence and resulting in a false-positive result for the samples. Improved systems for PCR are under development, and protocols for minimizing or eliminating amplicon contamination are under development and should enhance the usefulness of PCR in the clinical laboratory.

PCR is applied to detect a specific target nucleic acid sequence. This limits each assay to detection of only one agent. This is in contrast to viral cultures that involves inoculation of several types of susceptible hosts and provides for isolation of a range of viruses. However, some of the newer PCR protocols are designed as multiplex systems that allow for simultaneous amplification of several targets at the same time. Simultaneous detection of CMV, EBV, HHV-6, HSV, and varicella virus in a single PCR reaction requiring only 100 μl of patient's sample has been reported [13]. Such modified protocols may provide for broader applications of PCR technology.

Many viruses and types of clinical samples have been tested by PCR. This technology has been applied for detection of nonculturable or difficult-to-culture viruses such as parvovirus B19, hepatitis B and hepatitis C virus, EBV, and human papilloma virus. It has also been used with culturable viruses such as CMV and HSV. The results of some of these PCR studies are described next.

CYTOMEGALOVIRUS. Although CMV can be isolated in standard cell cultures and often the culture results using centrifugation-enhanced inoculation of shell viral cultures (described in Chapter 4) are available within 24 to 48 hours of culture inoculation, physicians may rely on PCR to provide results more quickly. Because CMV, like all of the herpesviruses, may establish latency and reactivate on stress of the host, a positive CMV PCR result may not definitively identify CMV as the source of the clinical symptoms. PCR, performed in quantitative fashion, may be able to contribute to differentiating actual CMV-related syndromes from insignificant CMV reactivation disease that is secondary to another infection or complication. When the CMV nucleic acid is present in high titer, there is enhanced likelihood that the infection is actually due to CMV.

CMV has been associated with retinitis, especially in those who are immunocompromised. This retinitis clinically resembles herpes simplex keratitis, but the differentiation is important because the treatments (acyclovir for herpes simplex or ganciclovir or foscarnet for CMV) are not the same [14]. PCR can be used to test small samples of aqueous fluid to make this differentiation rapidly.

ENTEROVIRUSES. Most serotypes of enteroviruses proliferate well in standard cell cultures. However, PCR for enterovirus detection has been reported to be more sensitive than cell culture. When magnetic beads were used to extract enteroviral RNA from various clinical samples (cerebrospinal fluid, stool, saliva, blood, pericardial fluid, urine, and formalin-fixed solid tissue) and reverse transcription was used to prepare DNA from the RNA, PCR amplification of the DNA was more sensitive for enteroviral detection that standard cell cultures [15].

HEPATITIS VIRUSES. The hepatitis viruses do not proliferate in standard cell cultures so the serological approach has been the major avenue for disease diagnosis. In hepatitis B infection, antibody detection may not differentiate past from present infection; presence of viral nucleic acid detected by PCR in serum is evidence of current infection. In hepatitis C, antibodies may not be produced in response to infection, especially in immunocompromised individuals. PCR detection of hepatitis C may be the only laboratory method available to reliably confirm hepatitis C infection.

HERPES SIMPLEX VIRUS. Although herpes simplex virus grows quickly and produces dramatic cytopathogenic effect (CPE) in many types of standard cell cultures, there are several situations in which PCR has been applied with advantage. One of these is with patients suffering from HSV infections of the eye involving intraocular manifestations. HSV is usually present at low concentrations in ocular fluid, and only 50 to 100 µl of fluid can be safely removed for testing. This small volume of fluid is sufficient for the highly sensitive PCR method [13]. Cerebrospinal fluid from 257 patients with suspected HSV encephalitis were analyzed by PCR for HSV. PCR was positive in all nine cases confirmed by serological assessment and in an additional 14 cases that could not be confirmed by serology but were clinically indicated [16].

HUMAN IMMUNODEFICIENCY VIRUS. Although HIV can be isolated in suspensions of phytohemagglutinin-stimulated lymphocytes, this culturing is not offered in most clinical virology facilities often because isolation of the virus in high titer is dangerous for laboratory employees and requires specialized isolation facilities. With PCR, HIV sequences can be detected in neonates, and the presence of these sequences correlates with the presence of development of clinical HIV disease. PCR for HIV can also be used to monitor the viral load in those receiving antiviral therapy.

HUMAN PAPILLOMA VIRUS. Human papilloma virus cannot be isolated in cell cultures, and serological assessment of infection is not helpful. Through PCR, the virus can be detected and serotyped.

PARVOVIRUS B19. This virus cannot be isolated in traditional cell cultures, and reagents for serological assessment are not widely available. Through PCR, parvovirus B19 DNA can be detected in fetal and placental tissues from cases of intrauterine death.

ENZYME-LINKED VIRUS-INDUCIBLE SYSTEM

Molecular cloning technology has been used to prepare a cell line that will express an enzyme only after infection with a specific virus [17]. In this case the specific virus is HSV type 1 or type 2, and the cell line is a line of baby hamster kidney cells into which an *Escherichia coli LacZ* gene has been inserted behind an inducible promoter from HSV-1 UL 39. The promoter encodes ICP6, an important part of ribonucleotide reductase. This promotor has no expression in uninfected cells, is activated specifically by HSV types 1 and 2, and expresses within hours after infection with HSV-1 or -2. When HSV-1 or -2 containing the protein VP16 enters the cell and triggers the HSV promoter, the *LacZ* gene is stimulated by ICP6 to express B-galactosidase. The *LacZ* gene is described as a "reporter" gene because it "reports" the stimulation by HSV-1 or HSV-2 by producing the enzyme β-galactosidase. The β-galactosidase is detected by adding a solution of β-D-galactopyranoside, which turns blue in the presence of β-galactosidase. This system has been named enzyme-linked virus inducible system (ELVIS).

In the ELVIS system (ELVIS, Diagnostic Hybrids, Inc., Athens, OH), cell monolayers are supplied in either 24-well microplates or in shell vials. Processed clinical samples are placed directly on the monolayer, and the plates or vials are spun in the centrifuge at 700 *g* for 10 to 30 minutes. Cell culture medium is added, and the cultures are incubated at 35°C for 16 to 24 hours. After incubation, the medium is decanted, and the cell monolayer is dried and then fixed in formalin. A staining solution of galactopyranoside is added, and the cells are incubated at 35°C and observed within 1 to 5 hours for the presence of blue color. Many positive results can be detected macroscopically. HSV types 1 and 2 are not differentiated by this test.

The ELVIS system was compared with traditional cell cultures (primary rabbit kidney and MRC-5) for isolation of herpes simplex virus. Ninety-six specimens were tested, and 31 were positive by both ELVIS and cell culture. Although viral CPE was not observed for 2 or more days in 15 of the positive cultures, all were positive by ELVIS within 16 to 24 hours [18].

In a study of 435 samples conducted at a major reference laboratory, ELVIS was compared with isolation in shell vials for detection of HSV types 1 and 2. Two ELVIS vials were inoculated for each sample along with two shell vials. The shell vials were stained with fluorescein-labeled monoclonal antibodies, one with HSV type 1 antibodies and the other with HSV type 2. All 143 samples that were positive in shell vial were positive by ELVIS, and 13 samples were positive by ELVIS alone [19].

REFERENCES

1. Bean B. Antiviral therapy: current concepts and practices. Clin Microbiol Rev 1992;5:146–182
2. Swierkosz EM. Antiviral susceptibility testing: coming of age. ASM News 1992;58:83–87
3. Hill EL, Ellis MN. Antiviral drug susceptibility testing. In Specter S, Lancz G (eds), Clinical Virology Manual, 2nd ed. Elsevier, New York: 1992, pp 277–284
4. Centers for Disease Control. Addressing emerging infectious disease threats: a prevention strategy for the United States. MMWR 1994;43:1–18
5. Salahuddin SZ, Ablashi DV, Markham PD, et al. Isolation of a new virus, HBLV, in patients with lymphoproliferative disorders. Science 1986;234:596–601
6. Levy JS, Ferro F, Greenspan D, Lennette ET. Frequent isolation of HHV-6 from saliva and high seroprevalence of the virus in the population. Lancet 1990;1:1047–1050
7. Lusso P, Ensoli B, Markham PD, et al. Productive dual infection of human CD4+ T lymphocytes by HIV-1 and HHV-6. Nature 1989;337:370–373
8. Spira TJ, Bozeman LH, Sanderlin KC, et al. Lack of correlation between human herpesvirus-6 infection and the course of human immunodeficiency virus infection. J Infect Dis 1990;161:567–570
9. Holmes GP, Kaplan JE, Gantz NM, et al. Chronic fatigue syndrome: a working case definition. Ann Intern Med 1988;108:387–389
10. Yablonsky T. The mystery of the hantavirus. Lab Med 1994;25:557–565
11. Zon RT, Slama TG. Hantavirus pulmonary syndrome in Indiana. Indiana Med 1994;May/June:216–218
12. Persing DH. Polymerase chain reaction: trenches to benches. J Clin Microbiol 1991;29:1281–1285
13. Werner JC, Wiedbrauk DL. Polymerase chain reaction for diagnosis of herpetic eye disease. Lab Med 1994;25:664–667
14. Drew WL, Buhles W, Ehrlich KS. Herpesvirus infections (cytomegalovirus, herpes simplex virus, varicella zoster virus): how to use ganciclovir (DHPG) and acyclovir. Infect Dis Clin North Am 1988;2:495–509
15. Muir P, Nicholson F, Jhetam M, et al. Rapid diagnosis of enterovirus infection by magnetic bead extraction and polymerase chain reaction detection of enterovirus RNA in clinical specimens. J Clin Microbiol 1993;31:31–38
16. Puchhammer-Stockl E, Heinz FX, Kundi M, et al. Evaluation of the polymerase chain reaction for diagnosis of herpes simplex virus encephalitis. J Clin Microbiol 1993;31:146–148
17. Stabell EC, Olivo PD. Isolation of a cell line for rapid and sensitive histochemical assay for the detection of herpes simplex virus. J Virol Methods 1992;38:195–204
18. Stabell EC, O'Rourke SR, Storch GA, Olivo PD. Evaluation of a genetically engineered cell line and a histochemical B-galactosidase assay to detect herpes simplex virus in clinical specimens. J Clin Microbiol 1993;31:2796–2798
19. Owen JA, Minshew BH. Comparison of an enzyme linked inducible system and rapid centrifugation shell vial culture for herpes simplex virus detection. Presented at the annual meeting of the Pan American Group for Rapid Viral Diagnosis, Clearwater, FL, 1994

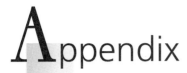

Appendix

PREPARING TRANSPORT AND CELL CULTURE MEDIA

Principle

Transport media are used for transport of viral culture samples. They contain proteins to stabilize viruses, buffers to control pH, antibiotics to keep contaminating bacteria and fungi from overgrowing the viruses, and a color indicator [1]. Many types of transport media are available commercially. However, suitable transport media can be prepared in house. The base of one transport medium is Hanks balanced salt solution (BSS), which can be purchased in liquid form. Fetal bovine serum and antibiotics are added. The medium is then dispensed into tubes to be used when viral culture specimens are collected. The same instructions for addition of fetal bovine serum (FBS) and antibiotics can be followed for enriching media for use as cell culture media in the virology laboratory. For cell culture media, Minimum Essential Medium Eagle with Earles BSS with L-glutamine (or other suitable medium) is used rather than Hanks BSS.

Materials

Equipment: sterile pipettes, individually wrapped (1, 10, and 25 ml), sterile 15-ml screw-capped tubes (conical centrifuge tubes work well for this), filters, labels

Reagents: Hanks BSS (500-ml bottle) or Minimum Essential Medium Eagle with Earles BSS with L-glutamine (500-ml bottle), sterile heat-inactivated FBS, gentamicin sulfate (50 mg/ml), amphotericin B (250 µg/ml)

Procedure for Preparing Transport Medium

1. Thaw and filter sterilize 10 ml of heat-inactivated FBS.

2. Open one 500-ml bottle of Hanks BSS.

3. Add 10 ml of filter sterilized FBS, 1 ml of gentamicin sulfate (50 mg/ml), and 1 ml of amphotericin B (250 µg/ml) to the Hanks BSS. The final concentrations of the antibiotics are 100 µg/ml for gentamicin and 0.5 µg/ml for amphotericin B. Mix by inverting the bottle.

4. Label the bottle with the date, additives, and expiration date as follows:
   2% FBS
   100 µg/ml gentamicin
   0.5 µg/ml amphotericin B (Fungizone)
   Date: [insert current date]
   Expires: 1 year from date prepared

5. Aliquot 3 ml of medium into each sterile screw-capped tube. Keep lids tightly closed after medium is dispensed.

6. Label each tube with the following information: VIRAL TRANSPORT MEDIUM for use with virology samples. Store at 4°C. DO NOT FREEZE. Expires [insert date 1 year from date prepared].

7. Store tubes and any medium remaining in the bottle at 2 to 8°C.

Procedure for Preparing Cell Culture Medium

To prepare cell culture medium: Substitute one 500 ml bottle of Minimum Essential Medium Eagle with Earles BSS with L-glutamine (or another suitable medium) for the Hanks BSS in step 2. Follow steps 1 to 3. On the label on the side of the bottle, mark the date and list the substances added. Store the medium at 2 to 8°C until needed.

R E F E R E N C E S

1. Leland DS. Concepts of clinical diagnostic virology. In Lennette EH (ed), Laboratory Diagnosis of Viral Infections, 2nd ed. New York: Marcel Dekker, Inc., 1992, pp 3–43.

PROCESSING OF ANTICOAGULATED BLOOD SPECIMENS FOR VIRAL CULTURE

. . . .

Specimens

Anticoagulated whole blood is required. A fresh (within 2 to 6 hours of collection) specimen is preferred. Heparin, EDTA, and acid citrate dextrose may be used as anti-coagulants. At least 3 ml of blood is needed. Hold blood at room temperature (18–22°C) after collection [1].

Principle

Density centrifugation is used to separate mononuclear cells from the other components of anticoagulated peripheral blood. Before centrifugation, the blood is mixed with commercially available PMN isolation medium, formerly Polymorphprep, which is a mixture of sodium metrizoate and dextran 500. The density of the PMN medium is 1.113 ± 0.001 g/ml, which allows differential migration during centrifugation of both mononuclear leukocytes and polymorphonuclear leukocytes. These cells are used as inoculum for viral cultures.

Materials

Equipment: sterile pipettes (Pasteur and 1 ml and 5 ml serologicals), sterile-screw-capped 15 ml conical centrifuge tubes, swinging-bucket centrifuge, vortex mixer

Reagents: PMN isolation medium (store unopened bottles at room temperature and opened bottles at 4–6°C), balanced salt solution (BSS) (500-ml Hanks BSS with 100 μg/ml gentamicin sulfate and 0.5 μg/ml amphotericin B), Minimum Essential Medium Eagle with Earles salts (MEM-E), and lysing buffer (ammonium chloride, pH 7.4). Ammonium chloride lysing buffer: Use 1.00 g potassium bicarbonate, 0.3729 disodium EDTA, and 8.29 g ammonium chloride. Add distilled water to reach a total volume of 1000 ml. Adjust pH to 7.4. Filter to sterilize.

Procedure for Use with PMN Isolation Medium (Robbins Scientific Corp., Mountain View, CA).

1. Bring blood to room temperature if it has been refrigerated. Place 3.5 ml of well-mixed room temperature PMN medium (invert bottle two to three times) in a sterile 15-ml screw-capped conical centrifuge tube.

2. Draw the room temperature anticoagulated blood sample into a 5-ml pipette. Holding the centrifuge tube at a 45-degree angle to the work surface, place the pipette tip against the side of the centrifuge tube slightly above the level of the PMN medium (Fig. A–1). Slowly allow 3 to 5 ml of anticoagulated blood to flow on top of the PMN medium solution without mixing PMN medium with the blood. Hold the centrifuge tube securely to avoid any unnecessary movement. Replace the lid on the tube.

3. Spin the centrifuge tube at room temperature (18–22°C) at 450 to 500g for 30 minutes in a swinging-bucket rotor centrifuge.

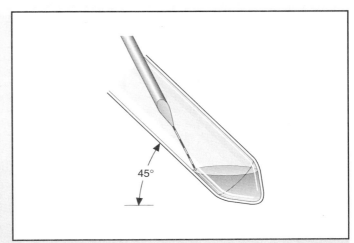

. . . .
FIGURE A–1 ADDITION OF BLOOD TO PMN ISOLA-TION MEDIUM. Anticoagu-lated blood is layered on the surface of the separation me-dium by tilting the centrifuge tube at a 45-degree angle.

4. When centrifugation is complete, carefully remove the tube from centrifuge and examine the layers that have formed. Six layers should be visible. Layers are as follows, starting at the top of the tube (Fig. A–2): (1) plasma, (2) mononuclear leukocyte (MN) band, (3) PMN medium, (4) polymorphonuclear leukocyte (PL) band, (5) PMN medium, (6) red blood cell (RBC) pellet.

5. Using a sterile pipette, draw off the plasma layer (layer 1) and discard it. Take care not to disturb layer 2 (the MN layer).

6. Using a clean sterile pipette, transfer the MN layer (layer 2) and the PL layer (layer 4) along with the small PMN medium layer 3 to a clean sterile 15-ml conical screw-capped centrifuge tube. Add 2 to 5 ml of BSS.

7. Spin the centrifuge tube at room temperature (18–22°C) at 400*g* for 10 minutes.

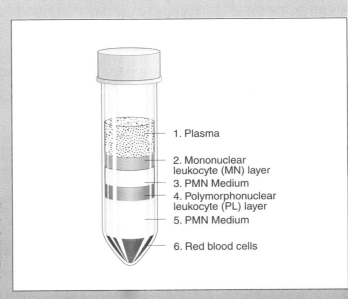

1. Plasma

2. Mononuclear leukocyte (MN) layer

3. PMN Medium

4. Polymorphonuclear leukocyte (PL) layer

5. PMN Medium

6. Red blood cells

. . . .
FIGURE A–2 LAYERS THAT APPEAR AFTER CENTRIFU-GATION OF PERIPHERAL BLOOD LAYERED OVER PMN ISOLATION MEDIUM. Leuko-cyte layers 2 and 4 are harvested and used for cell culture inocula-tion.

8. When centrifugation is complete, carefully remove the tube from the centrifuge. There will be a small pellet of packed cells in the bottom of the tube. Aspirate and discard the supernatant, add 5 ml BSS, mix using a vortex mixer, mark the number 2 on the tube to indicate that this is the second rinse, and spin as directed in step 7.

9. Using a clean, sterile Pasteur pipette, draw off the supernatant and discard it. Mix the tube contents with a vortex mixer to resuspend the cell pellet. Observe the mixture for presence of RBC contamination. If no RBC contamination is present, resuspend the pellet in 2.5 ml of MEM-E and continue with step 10. If RBC contamination is present:

    a. Add 10 ml of cold lysing buffer (ammonium chloride pH 7.4) to the resuspended pellet.

    b. Refrigerate (4°C) the tube for 30 minutes. Invert the tube several times during the incubation period to resuspend any RBCs that may have settled to the bottom of the tube.

    c. Centrifuge the tube for 15 min as directed in step 7.

    d. Aspirate and discard the supernatant and add 2 to 5 ml of sterile BSS. Invert to mix, and centrifuge the sample again as directed in step 7. Repeat this wash one additional time.

    e. Aspirate and discard the supernatant, and resuspend the pellet in 2.5 ml of MEM-E. Continue with step 10.

10. Use the cell mixture to inoculate cell cultures.

Expected Values

Two bands containing leukocytes should be seen. The top band contains mononuclear leukocytes (MN), and the lower layer contains polymorphonuclear leukocytes (PL). The bands may be harvested and used separately or together (as directed in this procedure).

DISCUSSION

Lower temperatures increase the chance of not resolving distinct bands. Maximal separation is accomplished when the blood is processed within 2 hours of collection; however, separation can be obtained for up to 6 hours of storage at room temperature. Severely anemic individuals and those with recurrent infections or chronic granulomatosis disease as well as those receiving aspirin, indomethacin, prednisone, aurothioglucose, intravenous cefamandole, trimethoprim-sulfamethoxazole, pseudoephedrine sulfate (Drixoral), and theophylline (Theo-Dur) may have blood that does not separate well using this procedure.

More than 95% of the harvested cells are viable. Only 2 to 6% of harvested cells are contaminating erythrocytes [1].

REFERENCES

1. Miller M. Isolation of leukocytes from anticoagulated peripheral blood. In Isenberg HD (ed), Clinical Microbiology Procedures Handbook. Washington, DC: American Society for Microbiology, 1992, pp 8.4.1–8.4.4.

HEMADSORPTION TESTING

Specimens

Cell cultures, usually primary monkey kidney, that have been inoculated with a suspension of virus or with clinical samples are used for hemadsorption testing. After the infected cultures have incubated for the desired time, usually 5 to 14 days, hemadsorption testing is performed.

Principle

Certain viruses have the capacity to alter the surface of cells they infect to make the cells have an affinity for erythrocytes; this affinity is demonstrated through the hemadsorption test. Viral hemagglutinating proteins, specified by the viral genome and expressed in the plasma membrane of virus-infected cells [1], are responsible for this affinity for erythrocytes. Hemadsorption is described in Chapter 3. Many of the viral respiratory pathogens, including the influenza and parainfluenza viruses, induce hemadsorption. In hemadsorption testing, the cell culture medium is replaced with a suspension of erythrocytes from the appropriate species (guinea pig erythrocytes are used routinely) and are examined microscopically to determine whether the erythrocytes have adhered to the cell monolayer. This procedure is used in various ways [2]. In many laboratories it is used as a screening test at the completion of the 14-day incubation period for cell culture tubes that have not shown cytopathogenic effect (CPE). Cell cultures, such as primary monkey kidney cells, that are known to support the growth of respiratory viruses are usually tested by hemadsorption. Often this procedure is performed after 3 to 5 days of cell culture incubation during seasons when respiratory viruses are common. Hemadsorption is independent of CPE, so hemadsorption may occur in CPE-negative cultures, either before the appearance of CPE or with viruses that do not produce CPE. Hemadsorption may also be used to test inoculated cell culture tubes that are producing CPE, suggestive of a hemadsorbing respiratory virus such as influenza or parainfluenza.

Materials

Equipment: 50-ml sterile screw-capped centrifuge tubes, sterile graduated cylinder, slanted stationary rack, sterile pipettes (10 ml), refrigerator, microscope, centrifuge

Reagents: guinea pig erythrocytes in Alsever's solution, sterile phosphate-buffered saline (PBS; pH 7.6), negative control tube (uninoculated cell culture tubes from the same lot as those being tested), and positive control tube (cell culture tube inoculated with a hemadsorbing virus such as influenza or parainfluenza).

Procedure for Preparation of Guinea Pig Erythrocyte Suspension

1. Transfer the bottled guinea pig erythrocytes to a 50-ml centrifuge tube.
2. Spin the erythrocyte suspension at 400g for 10 minutes and remove supernatant.
3. Resuspend cells in PBS, pH 7.6, and spin as just described.
4. Repeat steps 2 and 3 until supernatant is clear (usually three washes).

5. After the final wash, mix 2 ml of the packed erythrocytes and 50 ml PBS to prepare a stock concentration of 4%.

6. For use in hemadsorption testing, a 0.08% working dilution is prepared daily. This is done by diluting 1 ml of the 4% stock erythrocytes in 49 ml of cell culture medium.

Hemadsorption Test Proper (Combination Hemadsorption-Hemagglutination Method)

1. Prepare a 0.08% guinea pig erythrocyte suspension in a sterile graduated cylinder by making a 1:50 dilution of the 4% stock solution in tissue culture medium. Two milliliters of the 0.08% suspension is required for each culture tube that is to be tested.

2. Remove culture medium from monkey kidney cell culture tubes from 7-day-old and 14-day-old (testing date may vary from laboratory to laboratory) respiratory cultures. Also include one uninoculated cell culture tube from the same lot of cell cultures as those being tested (i.e., a negative control) and one cell culture tube inoculated with influenza or parainfluenza virus and incubated for 3 to 5 days (i.e., a positive control). Deliver 2 ml of the 0.08% erythrocyte suspension to each tube.

3. Refrigerate tubes for 30 minutes at 4°C in a slanted rack.

4. Examine tubes microscopically for hemadsorption and any agglutination. Specific hemadsorption is observed as rosettes of erythrocytes covering the cell surface. A diagram of a positive hemadsorption test result is shown in Chapter 3. Tap or rotate each tube gently to evaluate whether the erythrocytes have settled onto the monolayer or are truly hemadsorbed to the monolayer. Hemadsorbed erythrocytes will not float free when the tube is moved, whereas settled cells will be easily dislodged. Nonspecific "suspicious" hemadsorption is sometimes seen in monkey kidney cells. To identify nonspecific hemadsorption, compare the appearance of any suspicious reactions in the inoculated tubes with the reaction in the uninoculated negative control tube. If the suspicious reaction is seen in both the inoculated and uninoculated tubes, the reaction is nonspecific and can be ignored.

5. The positive control tube should show hemadsorption, and the negative control tube should not show hemadsorption. If control tubes have given the expected results, proceed with step 6. If the control tubes have not given the expected results, do not proceed. Consult with a supervisor and take appropriate remedial action.

6. Incubate any cell culture tubes that were negative for hemadsorption at 35°C for 30 minutes and re-examine to detect parainfluenza type 4 virus, which may hemadsorb at 35°C but not at 4°C [3].

7. For any culture tube that is showing hemadsorption, rinse the monolayer with sterile cell culture medium to remove erythrocytes and then harvest the infected cells for testing to identify the isolated virus definitively. Immunofluorescence can be used to identify many hemadsorbing viruses. See Appendix: Preparing Antigen Smears for Immunofluorescence Testing. If immunofluorescence will not be used for the definitive identification, prepare the infected cell culture material as needed for testing by the method that will be used.

8. For any culture tubes that do not show hemadsorption, allow the tubes to sit vertically at room temperature for 3 hours or until a compact cell button forms in the bottom of each tube. A button of unagglutinated cells confirms a negative test.

If the cell button is absent and agglutinated cells are spread over the bottom of the tube, the presence of a hemagglutinating virus is indicated. Viruses that are capable of hemagglutinating guinea pig erythrocytes include influenza, parainfluenza, and mumps. If hemagglutination is observed, rinse the culture to remove the erythrocytes, and perform follow-up testing as described in step 6. For tubes that are negative and are at the end of their 14-day incubation period, discard the tubes. For tubes that are to be returned to the incubator to complete their incubation, rinse the monolayers with sterile cell culture medium, and add 2 ml of cell culture medium to each tube. Return these tubes to the 35°C incubator.

Expected Values

A positive result should be observed with cell cultures infected with influenza A or B, parainfluenza 1, 2, 3, or 4, or mumps virus. A negative result should be observed with uninfected cultures or with cultures infected with viruses other than influenza, parainfluenza, and mumps.

Discussion

Strong hemadsorption is easy to read because rotating the tube gently usually dislodges nonspecifically absorbed cells and leaves only those that are strongly hemadsorbed. Weak hemadsorption may be more difficult to interpret, and nonspecific hemadsorption is common. Nonspecificity is easier to interpret if uninoculated control tubes are tested or if a large number of inoculated tubes from the same lot cell cultures are hemadsorbed at the same time. If all monolayers show the same pattern of hemadsorption, nonspecificity is likely. Bacterial contamination may also cause hemadsorption or hemagglutination [4].

R E F E R E N C E S

1. Fenner F, White DO. Medical Virology, 2nd ed. New York: Academic Press, 1976.
2. Swenson PD. Detection of viruses by hemadsorption. In Isenberg HD (ed), Clinical Microbiology Procedures Handbook. Washington, DC: American Society for Microbiology, 1992, pp 8.8.1–8.8.5.
3. Mufson MA. Parainfluenza viruses, mumps virus, and Newcastle disease virus. In Schmidt NJ, Emmons RW (ed), Diagnostic Procedures for Viral, Rickettsial, and Chlamydial Infections, 6th ed. Washington, DC: American Public Health Association, 1989, pp 669–691.
4. McIntosh K, Clark JC. Parainfluenza and respiratory syncytial viruses. In Lennette EH, Hausler WJ Jr, Herrmann KL et al (eds), Manual of Clinical Microbiology, 4th ed. Washington, DC: American Society for Microbiology, 1985, pp 763–768.

PREPARING ANTIGEN SMEARS FOR IMMUNOFLUORESCENCE TESTING

. . . .

Specimens and Principle

Immunofluorescence testing requires an antigen smear on a glass microscope slide. The smear may be prepared in the laboratory from virus-infected cells from a cell culture tube or from patients' clinical samples. Useful clinical samples include biopsy and autopsy samples, spinal fluid, and swabs from genital lesions, nose or throat, skin lesions, and eyes. Most "swab" samples will be received in the laboratory in transport medium. Smears from clinical samples received in transport medium are prepared in the virology laboratory; mucus is removed and cells are concentrated by centrifugation and placed on the microscope slide in small areas that allow for efficient staining and examination of results. Urine, anticoagulated blood, stools, and rectal swabs are not appropriate for immunofluorescence testing.

Smears for immunofluorescence testing may be prepared at bedside and sent to the laboratory. Large smears containing mucus, watery secretions, and blood are not acceptable. Smears must contain infected cells.

Most of the human viral pathogens that proliferate in standard cell cultures can be identified by immunofluorescence. This includes adenovirus (group only, not type); herpes simplex types 1 and 2; influenza A and B; measles; mumps; parainfluenza 1, 2, 3, and 4; respiratory syncytial virus; and varicella-zoster. In contrast, enteroviruses are usually identified by neutralization. Attempts to identify cytomegalovirus antigens in clinical samples and in cells from standard cell cultures demonstrating cytopathogenic effect are not usually successful, although cytomegalovirus immediate early antigens produced in shell vial cultures (see Chapter 4) are readily detectable by immunofluorescence.

Materials

Equipment: sterile screw-capped centrifuge tubes, sterile pipettes (1 ml, 2 ml), glass microscope slides (Teflon-coated slides with precut wells are preferred), centrifuge, vortex mixer, 25-μl fixed volume pipette, disposable pipette tips

Reagents: acetone

Procedure (For In-Laboratory Preparation of Antigen Smears) [1]

1. For **transport medium tubes containing clinical samples** on swabs, mix the tube contents with a vortex mixer while the swab is immersed in the transport medium to dislodge cells trapped within the swab fibers. For sputum or other mucus-filled respiratory specimen, add a small amount of liquid transport medium and pipette the mixture up and down to disperse mucus [1]. For **cell culture tubes,** use a sterile 1-ml disposable pipette, rubber policeman, or other type of scraper to remove the monolayer from the surface of the tube. For **tissue biopsies for impression smears,** transfer the tissue sample to a Petri dish and cut the tissue to expose a fresh surface [2]. Place the tissue on a flat surface and press a glass slide against the cut surface. Prepare several spots and proceed to step 7.

2. Using a sterile 2-ml pipette, transfer the fluid (either transport medium or cell culture medium containing infected cells) to a sterile 15-ml conical centrifuge tube.

3. Spin the tubes at 1500g for 10 minutes.

4. Using a sterile 2-ml pipette, remove supernatant and transfer it to a sterile centrifuge tube. (Supernatant may be used for inoculation of cell cultures if virus isolation has been requested on the specimen or for passage of infected cell cultures.)

5. Resuspend cell pellet in an equal volume of residual supernatant using a vortex mixer.

6. Using a 25-µl sampler (with a clean disposable tip), spot cells on Teflon-coated glass slides with the appropriate number of test wells. Label the slide with the specimen log number and names of the viral antigens to be tested.

7. Allow smears to air dry in a biological safety cabinet.

8. When smears are dry, fix in acetone for 10 minutes. Rinse in distilled water. If immunofluorescence testing will be performed immediately, proceed with immunofluorescence procedure. If immunofluorescence will not be performed within 8 hours, freeze the smear at −20°C.

Procedure (For Bedside Preparation of Antigen Smears)

1. Use two frosted-end glass slides. Place the specimen on the clear portion of the front side (same side as the frosted surface) of the slide. Record the patient's name and identification number on the frosted end (use pencil).

2. For lesions, remove the outer layer of crust and press a glass microscope slide against the lesion. Make several spots on each of two glass slides. For throat, nasal, or genital swabs, collect the swab specimen according to the usual protocol for collection of viral culture specimens (see Chapter 3 for specimen collection guidelines). Use the swab to smear the collected material in two 1- to 2-cm circular areas on each of two glass microscope slides.

3. Allow the slides to air dry.

4. Prepare test request forms indicating which viral antigens should be tested.

5. Place slides in a protective container and send them with the test request to the laboratory.

6. When prepared smears are received in the laboratory, follow step 8 (presented previously).

REFERENCES

1. Leland DS. Concepts of clinical diagnostic virology. In EH Lennette (ed), Laboratory Diagnosis of Viral Infections, 2nd ed. New York: Marcel Dekker, Inc., 1992, pp 3–43.
2. Keller EW. Preparation of cell spots for immunofluorescence. In Isenberg HD (ed), Clinical Microbiology Procedures Handbook, Washington, DC: American Society for Microbiology, 1992, pp 8.10.1–8.10.9.

PREPARING CONTROL SMEARS FOR IMMUNOFLUORESCENCE TESTING

Specimens

Uninfected cell cultures and cell cultures infected with known viruses are used to prepare control smears.

Materials

Equipment: glass microscope slides (teflon-coated slides with precut antigen wells are preferred), sterile pipettes (1 ml), centrifuge, 35°C incubator, cell scraper, 100-μl fixed volume pipette, disposable pipette tips

Reagents: cell cultures (in tubes), stock viruses, phosphate-buffered saline (PBS; pH 7.6) containing 2% fetal bovine serum

Procedure for Positive Control Smears

1. Retrieve an aliquot of the appropriate stock virus from freezer storage. Thaw at room temperature.

2. Identify a virus-susceptible cell type, and inoculate five cell culture tubes (more tubes may be used, if desired) of susceptible cells using 0.1 to 0.2 ml of thawed virus mixture per tube.

3. Incubate cell culture tubes at 35°C and observe until 50 to 75% of the cell monolayer demonstrates cytopathogenic effect.

4. Harvest the infected cultures and an equal number of fresh, uninfected cell cultures of the same cell type by scraping the cells from the vessel surface. Use a sterile pipette, a rubber policeman, or other scraper to remove monolayers from the cell culture tubes.

5. Combine all cells in a centrifuge tube, spin at 800g for 10 minutes, and decant the supernatant fluid.

6. Resuspend packed cell button in 0.1 ml of PBS (pH 7.6) containing 2% fetal bovine serum. Add more PBS if the cell suspension is too thick. Mix by aspiration to disperse cells.

7. Prepare smears using new teflon-coated slides with precut antigen wells. The arrangement and number of wells is determined by the testing protocol in which the smears will be used. Sample arrangements for control smears for herpes simplex types 1 and 2 antigen testing and for parainfluenza 1, 2, and 3 antigen testing are illustrated in their respective procedures included in this Appendix. Using a 100-μl sampler (with a clean disposable tip) as a dispenser, gently touch the pipette tip to the slide to deliver the desired number of small drops of cell mixture to the antigen wells of each slide.

8. Allow the smears to air dry.

9. Fix dry smears in acetone for 10 minutes. Air dry.

10. Label each slide with the date prepared, cell type, and virus type. Indicate contents of individual wells as needed.

11. Freeze slides at −20°C. Slides may be stored indefinitely.

Procedure for Negative Control Smears

Harvest the desired number of cell cultures of uninfected cells of the same type as those used to prepare positive control smears. Scrape the cells from the vessel surface. Follow steps 5 to 11 of the procedure for preparation of positive control smears.

Note: Perform the following for all types of control smears, if all antigens cannot be applied to the slides on the same day:

1. If the application of antigens will be completed within the next 24-hour period, fix smears in acetone, and store them at room temperature until all antigens are applied. Then fix (again) in acetone and store frozen.

2. If additional antigens will be added 24 hours or longer after the first antigen, acetone fix the smears after application of the first antigens, and store smears frozen. For applying the remaining antigens, thaw smears and apply antigens. Then fix (again) in acetone and store frozen.

R E F E R E N C E S

1. French MLV, Leland DS. Concepts of clinical diagnostic virology. In Lennette EH (ed), Laboratory Diagnosis of Viral Infections. New York: Marcel Dekker, Inc., 1985, pp 1–39.

HERPES SIMPLEX VIRUS TYPES 1 AND 2 ANTIGEN DIRECT IMMUNOFLUORESCENCE

. . . .

Specimens

Specimens should be collected according to guidelines for collection of specimens for viral culture (see Chapter 3) or smears may be prepared at bedside (see Appendix: Preparing Antigen Smears for Immunofluorescence Testing). Useful clinical samples include biopsy and autopsy samples, spinal fluid, and swabs from genital lesions, nose or throat, skin lesions, and eyes. Urine, anticoagulated blood, stools, and rectal swabs are not acceptable. This procedure is also appropriate for definitive identification of virus in infected cells from cell cultures.

Principle

This herpes simplex antigen immunofluorescence test is a direct method. Fluorescein-labeled mouse monoclonal antibodies, one against herpes simplex virus type 1 (HSV-1) and another against herpes simplex virus type 2 (HSV-2), are used. The labeled antibodies are added to smears of material fixed on glass microscope slides. If the antibodies recognize viral antigen within the sample, the antibodies will bind. After incubation and rinsing to remove unattached antibodies, the smear is viewed with a fluorescence microscope. If antibodies bound to antigen in the sample, fluorescence will be seen. If the antibodies did not bind to antigens in the sample, no fluorescence will be seen. Direct immunofluorescence is discussed in Chapter 2.

Materials

Equipment: glass microscope slides (Teflon-coated slides with precut antigen wells are preferred), Tri-Chem liquid waterproof marker (if plain microscope slides are used), no. 1 coverslips, humidity chamber, fluorescence microscope, 100-µl fixed volume pipette, disposable pipette tips

Reagents: acetone, fluorescein isothiocyanate–conjugated mouse monoclonal anti-HSV-1 and anti-HSV-2 antibody preparations in Evans Blue counterstain (Bartels Immunodiagnostic Supplies, Inc.), phosphate-buffered saline (PBS, pH 7.4 ± 0.2), buffered glycerol mounting medium, control smears of HSV-1–infected cells, HSV-2–infected cells, and uninoculated cells

Procedure for Use with HSV Types 1 and 2 Direct Antigen Detection System (Bartels Immunodiagnostic Supplies, Inc.)

1. Using a 2-well glass microscope slide, prepare two smears from each sample (see Appendix: Preparing Antigen Smears for Immunofluorescence Testing). Air dry smears.

2. Fix smears in acetone for 10 minutes and air dry. Store fixed smears at 2 to 8°C if the test will not be performed immediately. Freeze fixed smears at −20°C if the test will not be performed within 8 hours.

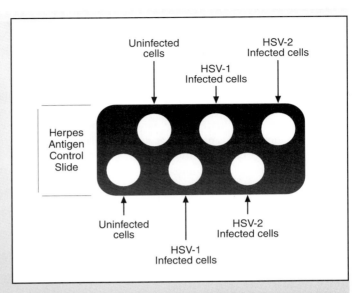

Uninfected cells

HSV-1 Infected cells

HSV-2 Infected cells

Herpes Antigen Control Slide

Uninfected cells

HSV-1 Infected cells

HSV-2 Infected cells

FIGURE A–3 CONTROL SMEAR FOR USE IN IMMU-NOFLUORESCENCE TESTING FOR HERPES SIMPLEX VIRUS (HSV) TYPES 1 AND 2 ANTI-GEN. Herpes type 1 monoclonal antibody is added to one "row" of test wells, including one smear of uninfected cells, one smear of herpes type 1–infected cells (HSV-1), and one smear of herpes type 2–infected cells (HSV-2). Herpes type 2 monoclonal antibodies are added to the other "row" of test wells, which includes the same types of smears as those used for the herpes 1 antibodies.

3. Thaw herpes antigen control slide (see Appendix: Preparing Control Smears for Immunofluorescence Testing). The control slide has acetone-fixed smears of uninfected cells as well as cells infected with HSV-1 or HSV-2.

4. If smears are prepared on a plain glass slide, encircle all smears with all-purpose liquid waterproof marker (Tri-Chem). This ink will serve to hold the staining compounds on the smear area. *Be sure ink is dry before starting the next step!*

5. Use Bartels Immunodiagnostic Supplies, Inc. HSV-1/HSV-2 monoclonal antibodies:

   a. *Use a 100-μl fixed-volume pipette with a clean tip. To one smear of each specimen and to one "row" of a control slide (includes one smear of HSV-1 infected cells, one smear of HSV-2 infected cells, and one smear of uninfected cells) (Fig. A–3), add sufficient fluorescein-labeled anti-HSV-1 antibody to completely cover the smear.*

   b. *Use a 100-μl fixed-volume pipette with a clean tip. To the second smear of each specimen and to the second "row" of the control slide (includes one smear of HSV-1 infected cells, one smear of HSV-2 infected cells, and one smear of uninfected cells) (see Fig. A–3), add sufficient fluorescein-labeled anti-HSV-2 antibody to completely cover the smear.*

6. Incubate slides in a moist, dark chamber at 35°C for 30 minutes.

7. Rinse slides individually in phosphate buffered saline using a squirt bottle to direct the flow of PBS gently over the slide. *Do not* aim flow of liquid directly at smear; direct force may wash away cells.

8. Place slides in a wash rack. Rinse in PBS (pH 7.6) with gentle agitation for 10 minutes.

9. Dip slides in a dish of distilled water several times. Air dry slides. (Slides may be dried by incubating them in the 35°C incubator, if desired.)

10. Add one drop of mounting fluid to each smear area, and carefully place a coverslip on the slide. Expel any air bubbles.

11. Scan the smears using the 25 × objective of the fluorescence microscope, and count the cells that are observed. Specimens that do not contain at least 20 cells

per smear have insufficient cells for a definitive reading and should be reported as "specimen unsatisfactory; insufficient cells." If adequate cells are present, evaluate yellow-green fluorescence. Reminder: Evans Blue counterstain, included in the antibody preparation, will stain uninfected cells a red color. Disregard stained cell debris, staining that is a flat, nonfluorescent green color, and staining of the cell periphery ("rimming") in the absence of characteristic cytoplasmic staining.

True HSV fluorescence may be in the nucleus and cytoplasm. HSV-1 generally produces strong perinuclear staining. HSV-2 produces homogeneous staining. Record results as follows [1]:

    0 = no visible fluorescence
    ± = very dim yellow-green fluorescence
    1+ = dim yellow-green fluorescence
    2+ = dull yellow-green fluorescence
    3+ = bright yellow-green fluorescence
    4+ = glaring yellow-green fluorescence

Smears with fluorescence of 1+ or greater are reported as positive. The manufacturer (Bartels Herpes Simplex Virus Type-Specific Fluorescent Monoclonal Antibody Test, Bartels Immunodiagnostic Supplies, Inc., Bellevue, WA) recommends that quantities of less than two positively stained cells per smear should be ignored, and the result should be considered negative. Consult the supervisor, if necessary, for this evaluation.

12. Check controls:

   a. The uninfected cells should be 0 for both the type 1 and the type 2 antibodies.
   b. The HSV-1 infected cells should be 3 to 4+ with the type 1 antibody and 0-± with the type 2 antibody.
   c. The HSV-2 infected cells should be 0-± with the type 1 antibody and 3 to 4+ with the type 2 antibody.

If the controls have given the expected results, read and report patients' results as described in step 13. If controls have not given the expected results, do not evaluate or report patients' results. Report control values to the supervisor, and take appropriate remedial action.

13. Report patient results:

   a. Specimens giving 0 fluorescence with type 1 and type 2 antibodies are reported as negative for HSV-1 and HSV-2.
   b. Specimens yielding 1 to 4+ fluorescence with the HSV-1 antibody are reported as positive for HSV-1. (No fluorescence should be observed with the HSV-2 antibody on these samples.)
   c. Specimens yielding 1 to 4+ fluorescence with the HSV-2 antibody are reported as positive for HSV-2. (No fluorescence should be observed with the HSV-1 antibody on these samples).
   d. If 2 to 4+ fluorescence is observed with both the HSV-1 and HSV-2 antibodies, consult the virology supervisor. Dual infections with both HSV-1 and HSV-2, although rare, may be diagnosed by identifying characteristic fluorescent staining in both reagent wells (Bartels Herpes Simplex Virus Type-Specific Fluorescent Monoclonal Antibody Test, Baxter Immunodiagnostic Supplies, Inc., Bellevue, WA).

Expected Values

Smears prepared from cells infected with herpes simplex virus should yield positive results. Uninfected cells should yield negative results. Comparisons of the sensitivity and specificity of direct immunofluorescence and virus isolation for detection of herpes simplex virus are presented in Chapter 5.

Discussion

The monoclonal antibodies used in this assay are type specific for HSV-1 or HSV-2. The antibodies clearly differentiate HSV-1 from HSV-2; a differentiation that was difficult to make with polyclonal HSV antibodies.

R E F E R E N C E S

1. U.S. Department of Health, Education, and Welfare, Centers for Disease Control. Manual—Immunofluorescence Methods in Virology. Atlanta, GA: U.S. Public Health Service, 1978.

PARAINFLUENZA VIRUS TYPES 1, 2, AND 3 ANTIGEN INDIRECT IMMUNOFLUORESCENCE

. . . .

Specimens

Specimens should be collected according to guidelines for collection of specimens for viral culture (see Chapter 3) or smears may be prepared at bedside (see Appendix: Preparing Antigen Smears for Immunofluorescence Testing). Useful clinical samples include respiratory biopsy and autopsy specimens and swabs or washes from nose or throat. Urine, anticoagulated blood, stools, and rectal swabs are not acceptable. This procedure is also appropriate for definitive identification of virus in infected cells from cell cultures.

Principle

This parainfluenza 1, 2, and 3 antigen immunofluorescence test is an indirect method. Mouse monoclonal antibodies against parainfluenza 1, parainfluenza 2, and parainfluenza 3 are added to smears of material fixed on glass microscope slides. If the antibodies recognize viral antigen within the sample, the antibodies will bind. After incubation and rinsing to remove unattached antibodies, fluorescein-labeled antimouse antibodies are added. These will bind to previously bound antibodies. After incubation and rinsing, fluorescence will be visible when the smear is viewed with a fluorescence microscope. If the monoclonal antibodies did not bind to antigen in the sample, the fluorescein-labeled antibodies will not bind, and no fluorescence will be seen. Indirect immunofluorescence is discussed in Chapter 2.

Materials

Equipment: glass microscope slide (Teflon-coated slides with precut antigen wells are preferred), Tri-Chem liquid waterproof marker (if plain microscope slides are used), no. 1 coverslips, humidity chamber, fluorescence microscope, 100-µl fixed-volume pipette, disposable pipette tips.

Reagents: acetone; liquid waterproof marker; parainfluenza 1, 2, and 3; mouse monoclonal antibodies; fluorescein isothiocyanate (FITC)-conjugated goat antimouse antibodies with Evans Blue counterstain; phosphate-buffered saline (PBS; pH 7.4 ± 0.2); buffered glycerol mounting medium; controls smears of uninfected cells and cells infected with parainfluenza 1, parainfluenza 2, or parainfluenza 3.

Procedure for Use with Baxter Bartels Viral Respiratory Screening and Identification Kit, Parainfluenza 1, 2, and 3 Antibodies and FITC-Conjugated Antimouse IgG (Fab′)$_2$*

1. Using a glass microscope slide, prepare three smears from each respiratory specimen or from infected cell culture material. Air dry. See Appendix: Preparing Antigen Smears for Immunofluorescence Testing.

---

*Bartels Viral Respiratory Screening and Identification Kit, Baxter Diagnostics Inc., Deerfield, IL (1).

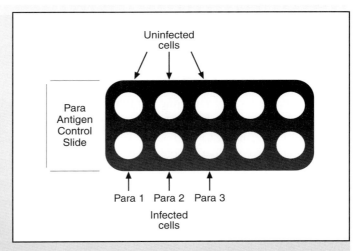

FIGURE A–4 CONTROL SLIDE FOR PARAINFLUENZA 1, 2, AND 3 ANTIGEN IMMUNOFLUORESCENCE TESTING. Parainfluenza 1 monoclonal antibodies are added to one smear of uninfected cells and to the smear of parainfluenza 1 (Para 1)–infected cells. The parainfluenza 2 and 3 monoclonals are added to corresponding smears of uninfected and infected cells.

2. Fix smears in acetone for 10 minutes and air dry. Store fixed smears at 2 to 8°C if test will not be performed immediately. Freeze fixed smears at −20°C if test will not be performed within 8 hours.

3. Thaw one parainfluenza control slide (see Appendix: Preparing Control Smears for Immunofluorescence Testing). The control slide has acetone-fixed smears of uninfected monkey kidney cells as well as cells infected with parainfluenza 1, 2, or 3.

4. If smears are prepared on a plain glass slide, encircle all smears with all-purpose liquid waterproof marker (Tri-Chem). This ink will serve to hold the staining compounds on the smear area. *Be sure that ink is dry before starting the next step!*

5. Add parainfluenza monoclonal antibodies to the patient's smears and to the control slide (Fig. A–4) as follows:
  a. *Use a 100-μl fixed-volume pipette with a clean tip. To one smear of each test specimen and to one smear of parainfluenza 1 (P1)–infected cells and one smear of uninfected cells on the control slides, add sufficient P1 monoclonal antibody to completely cover the smear.*
  b. *Use a 100-μl fixed-volume pipette with a clean tip. To one smear of each test specimen and to one smear of parainfluenza 2 (P2)–infected cells and one smear of uninfected cells on the control slides, add sufficient P2 monoclonal antibody to cover the smear completely.*
  c. *Use a 100-μl fixed-volume pipette with a clean tip. To one smear of each test specimen, one smear of parainfluenza 3 (P3)–infected cells, and one smear of uninfected cells on the control slides, add sufficient P3 monoclonal antibody to completely cover the smear.*

6. Incubate slides in a moist, dark chamber at 35°C for 30 minutes.

7. Rinse slides individually in PBS using a squirt bottle to direct the flow of PBS gently over the slide. *Do not* aim flow of liquid directly at smear; direct force may wash away cells.

8. Place slides in a wash rack, and place the rack in a staining dish containing PBS (pH 7.6). A staining dish with a magnetic stirrer is recommended. Allow slides to rinse for 10 minutes.

9. Dip slides in a dish of distilled water several times. Air dry slides. (Slides may be dried by incubating in the 35°C incubator, if desired.)

10. To each specimen and control smear, add sufficient FITC-labeled goat antimouse IgG (Fab')$_2$ antibody to completely cover the smear.

11. Repeat steps 6, 7, 8, and 9.

12. Add one drop of mounting fluid to each smear area and carefully place a coverslip on the slide. Expel any air bubbles.

13. Scan the smears using the 25 × objective of the fluorescence microscope, and count the cells that are observed. Specimens that do not contain at least one cell per field have insufficient cells for a definitive reading and should be classified as "specimen unsatisfactory; insufficient cells." If adequate cells are present, evaluate yellow-green fluorescence. Reminder: Evans Blue counterstain included in the antibody preparation will stain uninfected cells a red color. Disregard stained cell debris and mucus, staining that is a flat, nonfluorescent green color, and staining of the cell periphery ("rimming") in the absence of characteristic cytoplasmic staining.

Cells from infected cell cultures or clinical samples that are positive for parainfluenza virus types 1, 2, or 3 will exhibit cytoplasmic fluorescence that is punctate with irregular inclusions (Bartels Viral Respiratory Screening and Identification Kit product information, Baxter Diagnostics Inc., Deerfield, IL). Record results as follows:

> 0 = no visible fluorescence
> ± = very dim yellow-green fluorescence
> 1+ = dim yellow-green fluorescence
> 2+ = dull yellow-green fluorescence
> 3+ = bright yellow-green fluorescence
> 4+ = glaring yellow-green fluorescence

Smears with fluorescence of 1+ or greater in two or more cells are reported as positive. The manufacturer recommends that quantities of fewer than two positively stained cells in the entire smear should be ignored, and the result should be considered negative. Consult the supervisor, if necessary, for this evaluation.

For smears prepared from infected cell cultures: Both positive and negative cells should be observed. Smears from culture tubes with less than 25% cytopathogenic effect (CPE) may yield false-negative results because of an inadequate number of infected cells in smear. Culture tubes that have greater than 25% CPE and demonstrate no specific staining on stained smears should be reported as negative.

14. Check controls:

a. The uninfected control cells should be 0 with each of the three monoclonal antibodies.

b. The parainfluenza 1, 2, and 3 infected control cells should be 3 to 4+ when stained with their corresponding monoclonal antibody. If the controls have given the expected results, read and report patients' results as described in the next step. If controls have not given the expected results, do not evaluate or report patients' results. Report control values to the supervisor, and take appropriate remedial action.

15. Report patient results:

a. Specimens giving less than 1+ fluorescence or 1+ or greater fluorescence in fewer than two cells are reported as negative for parainfluenza 1, 2, and 3.

b. Specimens yielding 1 to 4+ fluorescence in two or more cells stained with parainfluenza 1 antibodies and less than 1+ fluorescence with parainfluenza 2 and 3 antibodies are reported as positive for parainfluenza 1.

c. *Specimens yielding 1 to 4+ fluorescence in two or more cells stained with parainfluenza 2 antibodies and less than 1+ fluorescence with parainfluenza 1 and 3 antibodies are reported as positive for parainfluenza 2.*

d. *Specimens yielding 1 to 4+ fluorescence in two or more cells stained with parainfluenza 3 antibodies and less than 1+ fluorescence with parainfluenza 1 and 2 antibodies are reported as positive for parainfluenza 3.*

e. *Results of specimens yielding 1 to 4+ fluorescence in two or more cells of more than one of the stained preparations should be interpreted with caution. Consult supervisor for this interpretation.*

Expected Values

Smears prepared from throat and nasal swab samples collected from parainfluenza-infected individuals and smears prepared from parainfluenza-infected cell cultures should yield positive results.

In clinical evaluations of fluorescent antibody staining of patients' direct respiratory specimens, the manufacturer obtained sensitivity and specificity values as shown for parainfluenza type 1 and type 3. No data were generated for parainfluenza type 2.

PARAINFLUENZA TYPE	SENSITIVITY	SPECIFICITY
1	52%	100%
3	85%	99%

Discussion

The monoclonal antibodies used in this assay are type specific for parainfluenza viruses. They cannot be used for differentiating parainfluenza strains within each type.

R E F E R E N C E S

1. Baxter Healthcare Corporation MicroScan Division. Product Information for Bartels Indirect Fluorescent Antibody Viral Respiratory Panel. Bartels Immunodiagnostic Supplies, Inc., 1989.

VIRAL TITRATION PROCEDURE

. . . .

Specimens

Viruses proliferating in cell cultures or stored in stock solutions are suitable for use in titration procedures.

Principle

Before their use in neutralization procedures, viruses must be titrated to determine their quantity (strength, "dose"). This is done to ensure that the virus and the other reactants in neutralization testing will be in optimal quantities relative to each other. The titration is performed by preparing serial 10-fold dilutions of the viruses. Each dilution is then inoculated into susceptible cell cultures, which are observed for evidence of viral proliferation. The end point of the titration is the highest dilution that produces viral proliferation in 50% of the cell cultures inoculated. [1] This end-point dilution is defined as one tissue culture infective dose—50% ($TCID_{50}$). The titration does not provide the exact "quantity" of the virus but rather indicates the dilution at which the virus still is present to proliferate. Viral titration is discussed in Chapter 3.

Materials

Equipment: sterile snap-top tubes (12×75 mm), sterile pipettes (1 ml), slanted rack, 35°C incubator, 100-µl fixed-volume pipette, sterile pipette tips, light microscope, vortex mixer

Reagents: cell cultures grown in tubes, stock virus or virus-infected cells from cell cultures, cell culture medium

Procedure

1. Label eight sterile tubes (12×75 mm) as follows: −1, −2, −3, −4, −5, −6, −7, and −8. (These are the logs of the dilutions.) Pipette 0.9 ml of cell culture medium into each tube.

2. Prepare the viral suspension. If the virus is an **adenovirus** or an **enterovirus** from an infected cell culture monolayer, freeze and thaw the monolayer as follows to prepare the viral suspension: Place the cell culture tube in the −70°C freezer with the medium covering the monolayer. When the medium is frozen, thaw tube contents by holding tube under running water. Repeat this cycle once. Then transfer the fluid into a centrifuge tube and spin at 1500*g* for 10 minutes. Use the supernatant fluid for the titration. **For all other viruses,** use the culture medium from an infected cell culture tube for the titration.

3. Use a 100-µl fixed-volume pipette with a sterile tip to add 0.1 ml of well-mixed virus suspension into the first dilution tube. Cap the tube securely and mix using a vortex mixer.

4. Using a fresh pipette or tip, transfer 0.1 ml of dilution from the −1 tube into the −2 tube and mix well. Continue this serial dilution through the −8 tube using a fresh pipette or tip for each transfer. In preparing viral dilutions, it is important to discard pipette tips or pipettes between each dilution to avoid carrying virus particles on the outside of the pipette or tip to the next dilution; failure to do so results in misleadingly high infectivity end points [2].

5. Label two tubes of a susceptible type of cell culture to correspond with the serial dilutions (−1 through −8).

6. Using a clean pipette or tip for each dilution, transfer 0.1 ml of each dilution into each of the two corresponding cell culture tubes.

7. Incubate cell cultures at 35°C in a slanted cell culture tube rack. Observe microscopically at intervals over a 7-day period (or longer for slower growing viruses).

8. The end point of the titration is the highest dilution showing cytopathogenic effect (CPE) in at least one of the two cell culture tubes inoculated. The end point of a titration is the dilution which contains one $TCID_{50}$. In viral identification procedures, a dilution containing 100 $TCID_{50}$ or 1000 $TCID_{50}$ of virus is used. To calculate the dilution containing 100 $TCID_{50}$, a factor of +2 (the log of 100) is added to the log of 1 $TCID_{50}$. To calculate the dilution containing 1000 $TCID_{50}$, a factor of +3 is added to the log of 1 $TCID_{50}$.

For example, if the end point of the viral titration is the 10^{-6} dilution, then 1 $TCID_{50}$ is contained in 0.1 ml of a 10^{-6} dilution of the inoculum.

$$-6.0 \text{ (log of 1 } TCID_{50})$$
$$\underline{+2.0 \text{ (log of 100)}}$$
$$-4.0 = \text{log of dilution of viral suspension}$$

containing 100 $TCID_{50}$ in a volume of 0.1 ml (10^{-4} is the working dilution)

Expected Values and Discussion

Ideally each viral titration dilution should be inoculated into six to eight hosts to make accurate determinations of $TCID_{50}$. Likewise, a calculation method such as Reed-Muench or Karber [3], which determine the 50% end point based on the total number of hosts, can be used to determine the 50% end point. Although the titration described here does not include either a large number of hosts or a calculation method for determining the 50% end point, this type of titration provides an acceptable approach for titering, provided that reactions occur predictably for the dilutions tested. If reactions do not occur in the expected pattern (e.g., if CPE is not observed at a low dilution but is observed at higher dilutions), the end point is probably inaccurate, and the test should be repeated [3].

R E F E R E N C E S

1. Schmidt NJ. Tissue culture technics for diagnostic virology. In Lennette EH, Schmidt NJ (eds), Diagnostic Procedures for Viral and Rickettsial Infections, 4th ed. New York: American Public Health Association, Inc., 1969, pp 78–179.
2. Ballew HC. Neutralization. In Spector S, Lancz GJ (eds), Clinical Virology Manual. New York: Elsevier, 1986, pp 187–200.
3. Hawkes RA. General principles underlying laboratory diagnosis of viral infections. In Lennette EH, Schmidt NJ (eds), Diagnostic Procedures for Viral, Rickettsial, and Chlamydial Infections, 5th ed. Washington, DC: American Public Health Association, Inc., 1979, pp 3–48.

NEUTRALIZATION IN IDENTIFICATION OF ENTEROVIRUSES USING THE LIM BENYESH-MELNICK ANTISERUM TYPING POOLS

. . . .

Specimens

Stock virus or unknown virus isolated in cell cultures are suitable for use in neutralization testing. Each virus must be titrated before use to determine the tissue culture infective dose ($TCID_{50}$). See Appendix: Viral Titration Procedure.

Principle

The Lim Benyesh-Melnick (LBM) antiserum pools named with letters A through H consist of 42 equine antisera combined into eight pools, each pool containing 10 to 11 antisera. The eight pools prepared in 1984 under World Health Organization sponsorship will correctly identify the 42 enteroviruses listed in the identification table (Table A–1). Seven additional pools named with letters J through P contain 19 coxsackievirus A sera.

In viral neutralization, viral antibodies are mixed with the virus. Then the mixtures are inoculated into susceptible cell cultures. If the antibodies bind to the viruses to inactivate or "neutralize" them, the viruses will be unable to proliferate in the susceptible cell cultures. If the antibodies do not bind to the viruses, the viruses are not neutralized and remain viable and able to infect susceptible cell cultures [1]. Viral neutralization is discussed in Chapter 2, and the applications of the technique are described in Chapter 3.

Materials

Equipment: sterile snap-top tubes (12×75 mm); 35°C incubator; light microscope; sterile disposable pipettes (1 ml, 5 ml, 10 ml); 56°C water bath; vortex mixer; fixed-volume pipette; sterile, disposable pipette tips

Reagents: LBM pools A-H; Hanks balanced salt solution (BSS) with 100 µg/ml of gentamicin and 0.5 µg/ml of amphotericin B; Minimum Essential Medium Eagle with Earles salts (MEM-E) with 2% fetal bovine serum (FBS), 100 µg/ml gentamicin, and 0.5 µg/ml amphotericin B; monkey kidney cell culture tubes

Procedure

LBM pools arrive in lyophilized form from the State Serum Institute in Copenhagen, Denmark. Each vial should be rehydrated with 10 ml of sterile cell culture medium, which contains antibiotics. Melnick's Medium B is suggested [2]. However, Hanks BSS with 100 µg/ml of gentamicin and 0.5 µg/ml of amphotericin B is used in this laboratory. Each 0.1 ml of the working dilution contains 50 antibody units of each antiserum contained in the pool. Refrigerate pools at 2 to 8°C when not in use or aliquot in small volumes and freeze at −20°C. Before performing the neutralization test, the unknown virus must be prepared and titrated as described in the viral titration procedure (see Appendix: Viral Titration).

TABLE A–1 IDENTIFICATION OF ENTEROVIRUSES USING LIM BENYESH-MELNICK POOLS

ACCORDING TO POOL

If Neutralized by Pool	Virus is	If Neutralized by Pool	Virus is
A	E15	CD	E6
B	E21	CE	CB5
C	E24	CF	P1
D	E25	CG	CB3
E	E11	CH	E12
F	E27	DE	E13
G	E31	DF	E14
H	CA16	DG	E16
AB	CA7	DH	P3
AC	CB1	EF	E18
AD	E33	EG	E17
AE	CB4	EH	E22
AF	E7		
AG	E4	FG	E20
AH	E1	FH	CB6
BC	E2	GH	E23
BD	CB2		
BE	P2	ACF	E29
BF	E19	AEG	E5
BG	CA9	BDF	E26
BH	E3	BFH	E9
		CEG	E30
		DEH	E32

ACCORDING TO VIRUS

Virus	Neutralizing Pool	Virus	Neutralizing Pool
CA1	J	CA13	M
CA2	KL*	CA14	JO
CA3	OP*	CA15	K†
CA4	JP	CA17	KO‡
CA5	JN	CA18	LM
CA6	L	CA19	MP
CA8	P*	CA20	JL
CA10	O	CA21	MN
CA11	KN†	CA22	LO
CA12	JMN		

*Tests with CA3 and CA8 monovalent sera are required for firm identification.
†Tests with CA11 and CA15 monovalent sera are required for firm identification.
‡CA17 virus may also be neutralized by heterologous pools J, L, M and N in mice. Final identity should be established using A17 monovalent serum.

1. Label eight sterile tubes (12 × 75 mm) with snap tops with letters A through H and the log number of the unknown virus to be tested. Mix each rehydrated LBM antiserum pool using a vortex mixer. Dispense 0.2 ml of each LBM antiserum pool into the corresponding tube. Heat inactivate the LBM serum by incubating the tubes in a 56°C water bath for 30 minutes.

2. Retrieve the isolate to be tested from the −70°C or liquid nitrogen freezer. Thaw in cold water in a covered container.

3. Prepare 3 ml of the working dilution by making serial 10-fold dilutions of the unknown virus. The working dilution is the dilution of the unknown virus that contains from 100 to 300 $TCID_{50}$ per 0.1 ml. The working dilution should have been determined previously by the viral titration procedure (see viral titration procedure in this Appendix). **The same virus stock must be used in the neutralization procedure as was used in the titration procedure.**

4. To each of the eight tubes (A–H), add 0.2 ml of the working dilution. Mix each tube using a vortex mixer.

5. Incubate the serum-virus mixtures at 35°C for 2 hours. Incubate the tube containing the remainder of the working dilution of virus; this will be used in the back titration to determine the actual strength or dose of the working dilution.

6. Return the remaining unknown virus to the freezer.

7. During this incubation period, label tubes to be used to prepare the back titration, which will consist of three 10-fold serial dilutions of the virus working dilution. Label three 12×75-mm sterile pop-top tubes as shown, and add 0.9 ml of Hanks BSS to each tube as follows (BT = back titration, WD = working dilution):
　　Tube 1: BT $10^{-(WD + 1)}$
　　Tube 2: BT $10^{-(WD + 2)}$
　　Tube 3: BT $10^{-(WD + 3)}$
Example: If WD = 10^{-5}, label tubes as follows:
　　Tube 1: BT 10^{-6}
　　Tube 2: BT 10^{-7}
　　Tube 3: BT 10^{-8}

8. During this incubation period, label monkey kidney cell culture tubes as follows:
　　a. Eight tubes: with one each of the LBM pool letters A to H
　　b. Eight tubes: two for the working dilution and two for each of the three dilutions prepared in step 7

9. Refeed all of the monkey kidney cell culture tubes with MEM-E with 2% FBS, 100 µg/ml gentamicin, and 0.5 µg/ml amphotericin B.

10. After the incubation period is over, inoculate 0.2 ml of each serum-virus mixture (A–H) into the corresponding monkey kidney cell culture tube labeled in step 8. Use a fresh pipette or tip for each serum-virus mixture.

11. Transfer 0.1 ml of the working dilution to the sterile back titration tube 1 (pop-top tubes prepared in step 7) and mix. With a fresh pipette or tip, transfer 0.1 ml from tube 1 to tube 2 and mix. With a fresh pipette or tip, transfer 0.1 ml from tube 2 to tube 3. Inoculate the two corresponding monkey kidney culture tubes with 0.1 ml from the working dilution and from each of the three serial dilutions tubes.

12. Incubate all monkey kidney cell culture tubes at 35°C and observe them daily for 5 to 7 days.

13. Read and record results as follows:
　　+ = evidence of viral replication
　　0 = no evidence of viral replication

14. Check back titration: Read and record back titration results. Evidence of viral replication should be seen in at least one of the two cell culture tubes of the back titration dilutions containing greater than or equal to 1 $TCID_{50}$ of virus. If the challenge virus was prepared to contain 100 $TCID_{50}$, then two 10-fold serial dilutions ($1:10$ and $1:100$) should contain 10 and 1 $TCID_{50}$, respectively. The third 10-fold serial dilution ($1:1000$) should not contain any virus. For example,

VIRUS DILUTIONS	CALCULATED TCID	EVIDENCE OF VIRAL REPLICATION*
Working dilution (WD) = 10^{-5}	100	+
$1:10$ dilution of WD = 10^{-6}	10	+
$1:100$ dilution of WD = 10^{-7}	1	+ or 0
$1:1000$ dilution of WD = 10^{-8}	0	0

*+ = Evidence of viral replication; 0 = no evidence of viral replication.

If the controls have given the expected results, evaluate results of the unknown virus. If the controls have not given the expected results, do not evaluate or identify the unknown virus. Report control results to the supervisor, and take appropriate remedial action.

Note: A known positive control virus is not routinely inoculated as part of this procedure. However, it may be wise to test each new lot of LBM pools with a known stock virus, preferably Coxsackie virus B or Echovirus type 11 to ensure the quality of the antisera.

15. The unknown virus should give a 0 reaction when mixed with its homologous antiserum. The results of neutralization are checked against the scheme for identity (see Table A–1). Often a tentative identification can be made on the third or fourth day if the dose of virus is high or if the virus has proliferated rapidly. Slower growing viruses may require a full 7 days of incubation. Complete neutralization on the seventh day with a dose of virus from 100 to 300 $TCID_{50}$ constitutes a firm identity. Complete neutralization through the fourth day and then evidence of a slow breakthrough is probably due to small aggregates of virus in the virus culture. In this situation, identification is considered adequate, although it may be deemed advisable to confirm the identification by the use of type-specific monovalent antiserum.

16. Echovirus 22-23 Complex: Echovirus 22 antiserum appears in pools E and H and Echovirus 23 antiserum in pools G and H. Unless large doses of virus are used, the two viruses are not clearly distinguished but may be neutralized by pools E, G, and H. Titration of the isolate against both Echovirus 22 and Echovirus 23 antisera is required for positive identification of the subtype. With some strains of echovirus 22, heterotopic neutralization may occur with pool B. However, none of the other enteroviruses can be identified by the combination of pools BEH.

Expected Values

Enteroviruses of the types included in antiserum pools A to H (Table A–1) should be neutralized, resulting in their identification. Other enteroviruses will not be identified; some of these may be identified by neutralization using the LBM pools J to F.

Discussion

The LBM pools combine antisera against the more common enteroviruses. Through neutralization testing with these pools, the viruses should be identified. Additional testing may be necessary for viruses that are not neutralized or for viruses that are neutralized but not clearly differentiated (see steps 16 and 17). Neutralization testing is the only method that has been demonstrated conclusively to provide accurate identification of the enteroviruses.

The LBM pools were prepared many years ago, and their availability is very limited at this time. The following recommendations have been made in hopes of conserving the pools [3]: (1) Use a microtiter assay; (2) use LBM pools to identify prevailing types, and identify subsequent isolates by using individual type-specific antiserum; and (3) limit use of LBM pools to isolates associated with severe or unusual illnesses.

REFERENCES

1. Schmidt NJ. Tissue culture techniques for diagnostic virology. In Lennette EH, Schmidt NJ (eds), Diagnostic Procedures for Viral and Rickettsial Infections, 4th ed. New York: American Public Health Association, Inc., 1969, pp 78–179.
2. World Health Organization. Procedure for Using the Lyophilized LBM Pools for Typing Enteroviruses. Geneva: World Health Organization; Houston, TX; Copenhagen, Denmark: Collaborating Center for Virus Reference and Research.
3. Melnick JL, Mordhorst CH, Bektimirov T. Policy statement: new LBM antiserum available for typing enteroviruses. Houston, TX: World Health Organization Center for Virus Research and Research, Baylor College of Medicine; Copenhagen, Denmark: State Serum Institute; Geneva: Virus Disease Laboratory, World Health Organization.

VIRAL BACK TITRATION PROCEDURE

. . . .

Specimens

Any prepared dilution of live virus can be tested in the back titration.

Principle

The back titration is performed as a part of procedures that require live viral antigens that have been diluted to contain an amount of virus that yields a specified level of activity. The optimal dilution is determined by performing a viral titration (see Appendix: Viral Titration). In the viral titration procedure, the tissue culture infective dose ($TCID_{50}$) of the virus is determined, and a working dilution of the virus is prepared that should contain the calculated number of $TCID_{50}$. This dilution is used in the given procedure; for example, the neutralization test. If the results of the neutralization are to be accepted as valid, there must be proof that the virus was actually used at the optimal strength or dilution. By using the back titration, the actual strength of the virus dilution can be confirmed [1, 2]. Most viral techniques that use calculated dilutions of live virus require either 100 or 1000 $TCID_{50}$ of virus. The procedure that follows includes instructions for back titrations for these amounts. However, the procedures should serve as examples, and the viral back titration should be suitable for modification for use with amounts other than those shown.

Materials

Equipment: sterile snap-top test tubes (12×75 mm), sterile pipettes (1 ml and 5 ml or sterile pipette tips), light microscope, 35°C incubator, stationary slant rack

Reagents: prepared dilution of live virus, cell culture medium, cell cultures growing in cell culture tubes

Procedure for Use with Virus Dilutions Expected to Contain 100 $TCID_{50}$ (A Procedure for Use with Virus Dilutions Containing 1000 $TCID_{50}$ Follows Step 7):

1. Label three sterile test tubes as follows:
    1 = 1 : 10
    2 = 1 : 100
    3 = 1 : 1000

2. Using a sterile pipette, add 0.9 ml of cell culture medium to each tube.

3. To tube 1, add 0.1 ml of virus dilution that has been prepared to contain 100 $TCID_{50}$. Mix with a vortex mixer. Discard the pipette or tip.

4. Using a new sterile pipette or tip, remove 0.1 ml of fluid from tube 1 and transfer it to tube 2. Mix with a vortex mixer. Discard the pipette or tip. Repeat this step using a new sterile pipette or tip to transfer fluid from tube 2 to tube 3.

5. Inoculate two cell culture tubes with 0.1 ml from each virus mixture (in tubes 1, 2, and 3) and from the original virus dilution used in the test. Incubate the cell cultures for 5 to 7 days at 35°C and observe cultures.

6. Predict expected results as follows:

VIRUS DILUTION	CALCULATED TCID$_{50}$	EVIDENCE OF VIRAL REPLICATION*
Original virus dilution	100	+
Tube 1 (1:10 dilution)	10	+
Tube 2 (1:100 dilution)	1	+ or 0
Tube 3 (1:1000 dilution)	0.1	0

*One or greater TCID$_{50}$ should produce evidence of viral replication; + = evidence of viral replication, 0 = no evidence of viral replication.

7. Read and record back titration results. Viral CPE in at least one of the two cell cultures inoculated for the dilution is evidence of viral proliferation at that dilution. The recorded results should approximate the calculated results if the appropriate amount of virus was contained in the original virus dilution. If all tubes give a + result, too much virus was used in the test. If all tubes give a 0 result, too little virus was used in the test system. When the results of the viral back titration are not acceptable, the entire assay in which the virus dilution was used should be repeated using a new and perhaps different dilution of virus. If deemed appropriate, the initial titration procedure should be repeated to identify any errors resulting from incorrect titration results.

Procedure for Use with Virus Dilutions Expected to Contain 1000 TCID$_{50}$:

1. Label four sterile test tubes as follows:
   1 = 1:10
   2 = 1:100
   3 = 1:1000
   4 = 1:10,000

2. Using a sterile pipette, add 0.9 ml of cell culture medium to each tube.

3. To tube 1, add 0.1 ml of virus dilution that has been prepared to contain 1000 TCID$_{50}$. Mix using a vortex mixer. Discard the pipette or tip.

4. Using a new sterile pipette or tip, remove 0.1 ml of fluid from tube 1 and transfer it to tube 2. Mix using a vortex mixer. Discard the pipette or tip. Repeat this step using new sterile pipettes or tips to transfer fluid from tube 2 to tube 3 and from tube 3 to tube 4.

5. Inoculate two cell culture tubes with 0.1 ml from each virus mixture (in tubes 1, 2, 3, and 4) and from the original virus dilution used in the test. Incubate the cell cultures for 5 to 7 days at 35°C and observe cultures.

6. Predict expected results as follows:

VIRUS DILUTION	CALCULATED $TCID_{50}$	EVIDENCE OF VIRAL REPLICATION*
Original virus dilution	1000	+
Tube 1 (1:10 dilution)	100	+
Tube 2 (1:100 dilution)	10	+
Tube 3 (1:1000 dilution)	1	+ or 0
Tube 4 (1:10,000 dilution)	0.1	0

*One or greater $TCID_{50}$ should produce evidence of viral replication; + = evidence of viral replication, 0 = no evidence of viral replication.

7. See step 7: procedure for use with virus dilutions containing 100 $TCID_{50}$.

Expected Values and Discussion

The actual viral dose and the expected (calculated) viral dose should be comparable if the initial viral titration provided accurate results and if the viral dilution was prepared and maintained appropriately. When the back titration results and the expected dose are not comparable, there is doubt concerning the accuracy of the procedure in which the virus dilution was used. Do not report results of any procedure in which the virus back titration signals that an incorrect dose of virus was used. Perform a new viral titration and prepare fresh dilutions of the virus before repeating the procedure in question.

R E F E R E N C E S

1. Ballew HC. Neutralization. In Specter S, Lancz GJ (eds), Clinical Virology Manual. New York: Elsevier, 1986, pp 187–200.
2. Grist NR, Ross CA, Bell EJ. Diagnostic Methods in Clinical Virology, 2nd ed. Oxford, England: Blackwell Scientific Publications, 1974.

INOCULATION OF SHELL VIAL CULTURES

. . . .

Specimens

Suspensions of stock virus or clinical samples processed for inoculation into viral cultures as described in Chapter 3 (Table 3–4) are appropriate for inoculation into shell vial cultures.

Principle

Cultured cells grown on coverslips contained in 1-dram shell vials can be inoculated with processed clinical material. The inoculum is placed directly on the coverslip monolayer, and the entire shell vial assembly is centrifuged at low speed. Excess inoculum is drawn off and discarded, cell culture medium is added to the vial, and the culture is incubated for a designated time period. At the conclusion of the incubation period, the cells on the coverslip are tested to detect or identify virus proliferating within the cells [1]. The detection test is usually a fluorescent antibody staining method. Staining is performed while the coverslip is contained in the vial. The stained coverslip is then withdrawn from the vial, mounted on a microscope slide, and viewed with a fluorescence microscope.

This system, although originally used for isolation of chlamydia, is now widely used in viral isolation and provides a rapid method for viral detection. Cytomegalovirus (CMV), which usually requires 18 to 21 days to produce cytopathogenic effect in traditional cell cultures, can be identified in shell vials in 24 to 48 hours after inoculation in 85 to 95% or more of CMV-positive urine samples [2]. The shell vial system has also been used for other viruses [3].

Materials

Equipment: aspiration system with sterile Pasteur pipettes, sterile disposable serologic pipettes (1 ml, 2 ml), centrifuge, 35°C incubator

Reagents: cell monolayers growing on coverslips contained in shell vials, culture medium with 2% fetal bovine serum (FBS) and antibiotics, and sterile phosphate-buffered saline (PBS).

Procedure

1. Label two shell vials (of appropriate cell lines for virus to be isolated) for each sample. Use three shell vials of fibroblast cells for peripheral blood samples for CMV detection.

2. Decant cell culture medium from each shell vial, and place 0.2 ml of processed clinical sample (see Chapter 3) on the cell monolayer growing on the coverslip in the bottom of the vial.

3. Position vials in a centrifuge and spin them at 700*g* for 40 to 60 minutes at 33 to 35°C.

4. Remove vials from the centrifuge and draw off residual sample using a sterile disposable Pasteur pipette with vacuum suction. Use a different sterile pipette for each patient's vials.

5. To each vial, add 2 ml of sterile PBS. Using a sterile disposable Pasteur pipette with vacuum suction (use a different sterile pipette for each patient's vials), draw off and discard the PBS.

6. To each vial, add 2 ml of culture medium containing 2% FBS and antibiotics. Close vial lids tightly and incubate vials at 35°C in an upright position. Vials will be evaluated and tested according to established protocols for the virus in question. For CMV detection by immunofluorescence, see this Appendix: Cytomegalovirus Early Antigen Detection in Shell Vials by Direct Immunofluorescence.

REFERENCES

1. Leland DS. Concepts of clinical diagnostic virology. In Lennette EH (ed), Laboratory Diagnosis of Viral Infections, 2nd ed. New York: Marcel Dekker, Inc., 1992, pp 3–43.
2. Leland DS, Hansing RL, French MLV. Clinical experience with cytomegalovirus isolation using both conventional cell cultures and rapid shell vial techniques. J Clin Microbiol 1989;27:1159–1162.
3. Wold AD. Shell vial assay for rapid detection of viral infections. In Isenberg HD (ed), Clinical Microbiology Procedures Handbook. Washington, DC: American Society for Microbiology, 1992, pp 8.6.1–8.6.10.

CYTOMEGALOVIRUS EARLY ANTIGEN DETECTION IN SHELL VIALS BY DIRECT IMMUNOFLUORESCENCE

. . . .

Specimens

This procedure is intended for use with cell culture monolayers grown on coverslips in shell vials. After centrifugation-enhanced inoculation of these monolayers with clinical samples (see Appendix: Inoculation of Shell Vial Cultures) and appropriate incubation, the cells on the coverslip are stained to determine whether cytomegalovirus (CMV) early antigen is present in the cells.

Principle

After shell vials inoculated with clinical samples are incubated for the appropriate time, fluorescent antibody staining is performed on the cells growing on the coverslip in the bottom of each vial. Staining is performed while the coverslip is still in the vial. Fluorescein-labeled monoclonal antibodies are available for detection of early antigen of CMV. The staining procedure is a direct fluorescent antibody staining method. The monolayer is covered with fluorescein-labeled monoclonal antibody against CMV early antigen. Unattached antibody is rinsed away. The coverslip is mounted on a slide and viewed using a fluorescence microscope. Fluorescence in the area of the cell nucleus is a positive result. Absence of fluorescence is a negative result.

Materials

Equipment: Pasteur pipettes (nonsterile 5¾ in.), vacuum assembly for aspiration and discard of liquids, 1-ml tuberculin syringe with 1½-in. needle with bent tip, 4½-in. sharp point forceps, frosted-ended microscope slides, fluorescence microscope assembly

Reagents: methanol, 1-dram shell vials with coverslip monolayers of MRC-5 or human foreskin cells (Bartels Immunodiagnostics, Bellevue, WA), Merifluor Cytomegalovirus Identification Reagent—mouse monoclonal antibodies against CMV early antigens—in Evans Blue counterstain (Meridian Diagnostics Inc., Cincinnati, OH), phosphate-buffered saline (PBS)—pH 7.6—distilled water, mounting fluid (phosphate-buffered glycerol FA mounting medium), shell vial with fixed CMV-infected cells (positive control)

Procedure for Use with CMV Early Antigen Antibodies from Meridian Diagnostics

1. Perform staining for CMV early antigen detection on two vials for each clinical sample; stain one after 16 to 24 hours of incubation and one after 40 to 48 hours of incubation (other time intervals may be used and numbers of vials per sample may vary).

2. Prepare a laboratory work sheet with a list of the culture or log numbers of the shell vials that will be evaluated. Label frosted-end glass slides with the culture or log numbers of the shell vials that will be evaluated; two or three coverslips may be mounted on each slide.

3. Remove and discard the cap from each shell vial, and aspirate the cell culture medium using a nonsterile 5¾-in. disposable Pasteur pipette with vacuum apparatus.

4. Rinse the coverslip twice by adding and then withdrawing 2 ml of PBS.

5. Use a pump dispenser to add 3 ml of methanol to each vial. Aspirate and discard the methanol.

6. Use the pump dispenser to fill each vial with methanol. Leave the methanol on the cells for 20 minutes. Withdraw and discard as much of the methanol as possible. Allow any residual methanol to evaporate before continuing with the procedure. If the staining procedure cannot be continued at this time, recap the vials and store them at 4°C for up to 5 days or at −70°C for longer periods [1].

7. Include a positive control vial in testing. Control vials with methanol-fixed coverslips containing MRC-5 or human foreskin cells infected with CMV may be prepared ahead and stored in a −20°C freezer. (See note after Discussion.) Remove and discard the cap of the positive control vial.

8. Examine all vials carefully to ensure that the cell monolayer is facing upward in the vial. To evaluate this, look for a cloudy appearance of the surface of the coverslip, indicating that cells are growing on that surface. If the surface is shiny, the coverslip has likely turned over during the fixation process, and the monolayer is facing downward. If the cell monolayer is not facing up, use a Pasteur pipette with vacuum to carefully lift coverslip and invert it.

9. Rinse coverslips once by adding and then withdrawing 2 ml of PBS.

10. Add 0.1 ml of monoclonal CMV antibody to each vial. Tilt the vial, as needed, to ensure that the antibody covers the entire coverslip. Incubate vials at room temperature (18–25°C) for 15 minutes.

11. Add 2 ml of PBS to each vial. Draw off and discard the PBS. Repeat this step once.

12. Add 2 ml of distilled water to each vial. Draw off and discard the water.

13. For each coverslip, place one drop of mounting fluid on the labeled slides. Using a tuberculin syringe with a 1½-in. needle bent near the point, insert the needle point under the edge of the coverslip in the vial. Circle the needle point around the coverslip and pull upward gently. The coverslip should come out of the bottom of the vial. Grasp the coverslip with pointed forceps and place it, cell monolayer down, in the drop of mounting medium on a slide.

14. Examine the coverslips to ensure that all are mounted with the cell monolayer facing downward toward the surface of the slide. If any of the coverslips are inverted, use forceps to carefully slide the coverslip off the edge of the microscope slide. Grasp the coverslip, and replace it in the mounting fluid on the slide with the cell monolayer facing down.

15. Examine the coverslips using the 25 × dry objective of the fluorescence microscope. Switch to the 40 × dry objective to examine any questionable cells that are found. A positive result will appear as bright yellow-green fluorescence localized in the nucleus of the monolayer cells. The staining pattern can vary from small, bright nuclear inclusions in early infections to a uniform staining of the entire nucleus of the infected cell (Cytomegalovirus Identification Reagent package insert, Meridian Diagnostics, Inc., Cincinnati, OH). Grade fluorescence as follows:

  0 = no visible fluorescence
  ± = very dim yellow-green fluorescence
  1+ = dim yellow-green fluorescence
  2+ = dull yellow-green fluorescence
  3+ = bright yellow-green fluorescence
  4+ = glaring yellow-green fluorescence

Fluorescence of ± or greater in one or more cells per coverslip is reported as a positive result for CMV early antigen. A negative result appears as an absence of nuclear fluorescence and indicates an absence of CMV early antigen. Negative cell nuclei and the cytoplasm of all nonfluorescing cells will appear red because of the Evans Blue counterstain.

Uneven or overlapping monolayers or large clumps of cells or debris from the specimen may cause nonspecific trapping of reagent. Restrict microscopic observations to uniform areas of the monolayer that have the thickness of a single cell layer. The presence of *Staphylococcus aureus* on the cell monolayer may result in some faint yellow fluorescent staining of these organisms (Cytomegalovirus Identification Reagent package insert, Meridian Diagnostics, Cincinnati, OH).

16. Check the result of the coverslip from the positive control vial. The coverslip must have more than one cell per low-power field showing fluorescence greater than or equal to 2+. If the positive control has given the expected result, read and report patients' results as described in step 17. If the control has not given the expected result, do not evaluate or report patients' results. Report the control value to the supervisor, and take appropriate remedial action.

17. Evaluate patients' results as described in step 15. Report positive for patients with one or more cells showing ± or brighter fluorescence. Report negative for patients with no fluorescing cells.

18. If all cells are missing from coverslips from both vials of any specimen as a result of specimen toxicity, retrieve the processed original sample stored in freezer storage; make a 1:10 dilution of the stored processed material, and inoculate fresh vials.

Expected Values

A positive result should be observed with specimens that contain infectious CMV. A negative result should be observed with specimens that do not contain infectious CMV. Not all CMV will be detected. See Chapter 4 for comparisons of CMV isolation in shell vials and in traditional cell cultures.

Discussion

Detection of CMV early antigen in shell vial depends on the presence of infectious virus. Improper specimen collection or handling may result in inactivation of CMV, which will cause a false-negative result. The sensitivity of shell vial versus traditional cell culture varies according to specimen source [2].

Note: Shell vials for use as positive controls in this procedure can be prepared in advance and stored frozen until needed. When excess fibroblast shell vials are available, the vials can be inoculated with CMV instead of discarding them. After a suitable incubation period, one vial is fixed in methanol and stained with CMV monoclonal antibodies. If this vial does not show positive results, continue incubating vials and test again at a later time interval. If this vial yields satisfactory results, all of the inoculated vials can be fixed in methanol and then allowed to dry completely. On completion of drying, the vials can be recapped and stored at $-20°C$. One of these vials can be used with each run of shell vial staining to serve as a positive control.

R E F E R E N C E S

1. Wold AD. Shell vial assay for the rapid detection of viral infections. In Isenberg HD (ed), Clinical Microbiology Procedures Handbook, Washington, DC: American Society for Microbiology, 1992, pp 8.6.1–8.6.10.
2. Leland DS, Hansing RL, French MLV. Clinical experience with cytomegalovirus isolation using both conventional cell cultures and rapid shell vial techniques. J Clin Microbiol 1989;27:1159–1162.

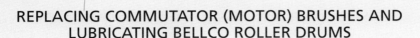

REPLACING COMMUTATOR (MOTOR) BRUSHES AND LUBRICATING BELLCO ROLLER DRUMS

Principle

As routine maintenance for roller drums, commutator brushes should be changed according to a regular schedule. Series 2RD and 3RD motor brushes are replaced every 3 months; series 3RDB and 3RDBB motor brushes are replaced every 6 months. This schedule should be planned ahead and each replacement recorded in a maintenance log.

Equipment

Bellco roller drum, screw drivers, lubricant WD40, replacement commutator brushes

Procedure (For Use with Bellco Roller Drums [1], Series 2RD and 3RD and Series 3RDB and 3RDBB) (if roller drums are not from Bellco or are not of the series identified, do not use this procedure; consult manufacturer for instructions for changing commutator brushes):

1. Remove the roller drum test tube rack from the drive unit and unplug the unit.

2. Position the drive unit on a bench top. (A laboratory coat and gloves should be worn during this procedure because the drive units often have dust and oil residue inside. These may stain clothing and be difficult to remove from hands.)

3. For 3RDB and 3RDBB series drive units, remove the six screws securing the rear belt guard to the drive unit and remove the guard (Fig. A–5). For 2RD and 3RD series drive units, there is no rear belt guard.

4. For all models loosen and remove the two screws on each side of the cover of the drive unit. Lift the cover from unit exposing the interior of the chassis and the motor.

5. Remove the brush screw caps on either side of the motor of the 3RDB and 3RDBB models. For the 2RD and 3RD models the brush screw caps are on the top and bottom of the motor. The motor must be removed to access these screw caps. To remove the motor, loosen the four hex head screws that secure the motor to the rear of the chassis. If the motor will not rotate, loosen the hex head set screw on the lower-most drive pulley and remove pulley.

6. When the brush screw caps are removed, the motor brushes, which are spring loaded, may pop out. If not, pull out the worn brushes, and install new brushes that correspond with the series being replaced. For the 2RD and 3RD series, the brush curvature must follow the curvature of the motor. For the 3RDB and 3RDBB series, the brush and spring must be joined before placing brush into motor.

7. Replace the brush screw caps.

8. To reassemble, reverse the above disassembly procedure.

9. Clean the drum shaft and grease it lightly with WD40.

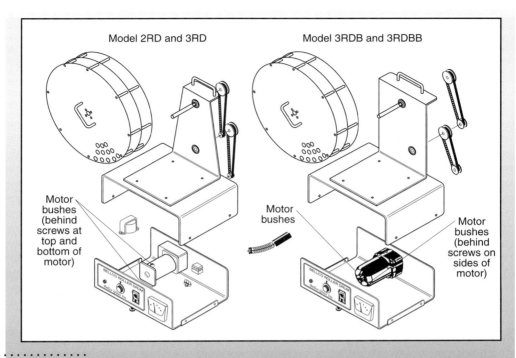

Model 2RD and 3RD

Model 3RDB and 3RDBB

Motor bushes (behind screws at top and bottom of motor)

Motor bushes

Motor bushes (behind screws on sides of motor)

FIGURE A–5 SCHEMATIC OF DRIVE OF BELLCO ROLLER DRUMS. The commutator (motor) brushes of roller drums must be replaced periodically. These are located on the motor. Diagrams show the location of the motor brushes for two models of roller drums for the Bellco Glassware Company.

10. Clean the exterior of drive unit with suitable cleaning solvent (i.e., Alconox).

11. Record the information, including maintenance activities completed and the date on the maintenance record card for each roller drum serviced.

R E F E R E N C E S

1. Bellco Glass, Inc. Maintenance instructions for Bellco roller drums. Vineland, NJ: Bellco Glass, Inc., 1973 and 1992.

ANSWERS TO REVIEW QUESTIONS

Chapter 1
1. 4, 3, 2, 1
2. elec, light, light, elec
3. b
4. c
5. c, e, a, d, b
6. DNA, *herpesviridae*
   DNA, *hepadnaviridae*
   DNA, *herpesviridae*
   RNA, *retroviridae*
7. d
8. c
9. c
10. b
11. b
12. d

Chapter 2
1. c
2. c
3. c
4. a
5. b
6. d
7. a, h, e, b, b, g, h, c, f, d, i
8. d
9. c

10. b
11. a
12. d
13. b

Chapter 3
1. b, e, c, a
2. d
3. a
4. c
5. d
6. b
7. Primary (b, e, i)
   Diploid (d, f, h)
   Established (a, c, g, j)
8. b
9. b
10. b
11. T
12. F
13. F
14. T
15. F
16. T

Chapter 4
1. d
2. c
3. d
4. a
5. c
6. a

7. b

Chapter 5
1. d
2. d
3. b
4. a
5. c
6. b
7. c

Chapter 6
1. c
2. a
3. b
4. c
5. d
6. c
7. a
8. a
9. a
10. a
11. b
12. F
13. F
14. T

Chapter 7
1. b
2. d
3. a
4. d
5. c
6. d

7. b
8. c
9. a
10. T
11. F

Chapter 8
1. a
2. c
3. d
4. c
5. b
6. a
7. d
8. b
9. a
10. c
11. c

Chapter 9
1. a
2. c
3. c
4. a
5. b
6. d
7. d
8. c
9. c
10. a
11. b
12. c
13. c